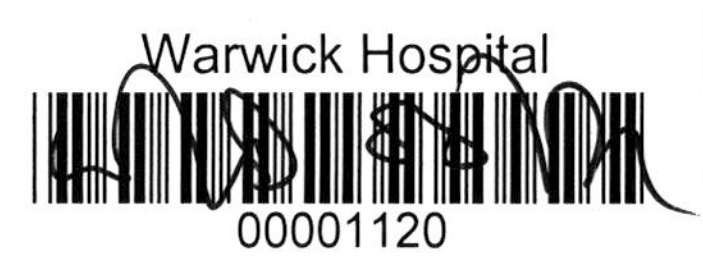
Warwick Hospital
00001120

D0302738

Atlas of Contact Dermatitis

Atlas of Contact Dermatitis

Robert L Rietschel MD
Department of Dermatology
Ochsner Clinic
New Orleans, USA

Luis Conde-Salazar MD
National Institute of Occupational Medicine
Madrid, Spain

An Goossens RPharm, PhD
Department of Dermatology (Contact Allergy Unit)
University Hospital
Leuven, Belgium

Niels K Veien MD
The Dermatology Clinic
Aalborg, Denmark

MARTIN DUNITZ

First published in the United Kingdom in 1999 by
Martin Dunitz Ltd
The Livery House
7–9 Pratt Street
London NW1 0AE

A CIP catalogue record for this book is available from the British Library

ISBN 1-85317-554-4

Distributed in the United States by:
Blackwell Science Inc.
Commerce Place, 350 Main Street
Malden, MA 02148, USA
Tel: 1–800–215–1000

Distributed in Canada by:
Login Brothers Book Company
324 Salteaux Crescent
Winnipeg, Manitoba, R3J 3T2
Canada
Tel: 204–224–4068

Distributed in Brazil by:
Ernesto Reichmann Distribuidora de Livros, Ltda
Rua Coronel Marques 335, Tatuape 03440–000
Sao Paulo
Brazil

A 35-mm slide set, based on this Atlas,
is available from the publishers:
ISBN 1-85317-847-0

Composition by Scribe Design, Gillingham, Kent
Printed and bound in Spain by Grafos, S.A. Arte Sobre papel

Contents

	Preface	vii
1	**Introduction and Background**	1
2	**Patch Test and Prick Test Techniques**	21
	Patch test technique 21	
	Prick test technique 35	
3	**Management of Contact Dermatitis**	39
4	**Contact Dermatitis by Specific Body Region**	47
	Face and scalp 49	
	Ears 58	
	Trunk and axillae 60	
	Extremities and genitalia 72	
	Hands 78	
	Nails 103	
	Feet 107	
5	**Patterns of Contact Dermatitis**	115
	Systemic contact dermatitis 115	
	Non-eczematous contact dermatitis 125	
	Phototoxic and photoallergic reactions 134	
	Airborne contact dermatitis 143	
	Contact urticaria and protein contact dermatitis 150	
6	**Specific Categories of Contact Allergens**	157
	Medications 157	
	Medical devices 177	
	Cosmetics 185	
	Metals 192	

Plants and woods 196
Textiles, clothing and shoes 207

7 Occupational Contact Dermatitis 215
Agriculture 217
Construction industry 223
Health care 230
Acrylates, epoxy and other resins 242
Rubber 252
Metals and metal lubricants 262
Hair care 271
Floristry, horticulture and woodwork 277
Photography and graphic arts 285

8 Unique cases 299

Apppendix: European and US Standard Patch Test Series 307

Index 311

Preface

Contact dermatitis is among the most common dermatoses encountered by dermatologists, and recognizing patterns of dermatitis is very helpful in making a specific diagnosis. The authors of this Atlas have collected many typical and also some unusual cases of contact dermatitis in an effort to illustrate the wide spectrum of this area of dermatology.

This Atlas is intended as a supplement to existing contact dermatitis textbooks, rather than as a textbook in itself. Therefore, the main body of information is contained in the legends to the many figures. The accompanying pages of text provide a summary of fundamental aspects of contact dermatitis.

Following a general introduction, the Atlas presents sections on regional contact dermatitis, patterns of contact dermatitis, specific categories of causative substances, occupational contact dermatitis, and, finally, unusual cases. This organization is intended to assist the reader in finding the cause of contact dermatitis based on the information available, i.e. the area of involvement, clinical symptoms, suspected causative substance, or suspected occupational cause.

RLR
LCS
AG
NKV

1

Introduction and Background

Contact dermatitis is a pruritic, epidermal and dermal inflammatory reaction caused or aggravated by items in contact with the skin. Eczematous dermatoses can be classified as shown in the box.

Dermatitis caused by external factors (contact dermatitis)
- Irritant contact dermatitis
- Allergic contact dermatitis
- Phototoxic contact dermatitis
- Photoallergic contact dermatitis
- Non-immunological contact urticaria, including protein contact dermatitis
- Immunological contact urticaria, including protein contact dermatitis

Dermatitis caused by constitutional factors
- Atopic dermatitis
- Seborrhoeic dermatitis
- Nummular dermatitis
- Pompholyx (recurrent, vesicular hand dermatitis)
- Hyperkeratotic palmar dermatitis
- Eczematous psoriasis

Other types
- Stasis dermatitis
- Lichen simplex chronicus
- Microbial dermatitis

Common examples of contact dermatitis include irritant contact dermatitis caused by soaps, detergents, oils and plants, while allergic contact dermatitis is commonly caused by metals, perfumes, rubber, preservatives and drugs. These two types of contact dermatitis are often interwoven. Primary irritant contact dermatitis damages the barrier function of the epidermis, thus giving access to sensitizing chemicals that cause secondary allergic contact dermatitis. Primary allergic contact dermatitis makes the skin more susceptible to irritants. Therefore, irritant contact dermatitis is frequently superimposed on, for example, allergic contact dermatitis of the hands. Clinically, contact dermatitis is often described as acute, subacute or chronic (Lever and Schaumburg-Lever, 1990).

Contact dermatitis is most commonly located on the hands, forearms, face and legs. The diagnosis is made by combining information about the history of the patient, the clinical findings, diagnostic tests and, possibly, exposure tests.

IRRITANT AND ALLERGIC CONTACT DERMATITIS

Numerous studies have shown that it is difficult to distinguish between irritant and allergic reactions, both experimentally and in clinical practice (Hoefakker et al, 1995). Extreme examples of the two major types of reactions do show distinct differences, but as both reactions become milder and more chronic, the distinctions blur.

Although mechanisms for irritant contact dermatitis are thought to be non-immunological and allergic contact dermatitis is generally considered a delayed hypersensitivity disease, recent studies of the immunology of irritant contact dermatitis show almost no difference between the two (Rietschel, 1997).

Traditional concepts of irritant contact dermatitis

Irritant contact dermatitis is a condition that can be induced in anyone by a sufficiently corrosive material. The onset of symptoms is generally rapid (minutes to hours) after skin contact with an irritant; these symptoms may include stinging, burning and itching. The morphology is likely to consist of erythema and oedema at onset, with vesicles or bullae forming only in very strong irritant reactions. Epidermal necrosis may occur and appear initially as a glazed or parched-looking surface. The reaction seldom extends beyond the area of direct physical contact. If no further exposure occurs, the dermatitis usually begins to fade within a few days, and resolves fully within about two weeks. Patch testing is generally negative in irritant contact dermatitis, and testing with known irritants is not recommended. The diagnostic criteria for irritant contact dermatitis are listed in Table 1.1.

Traditional concepts of allergic contact dermatitis

Allergic contact dermatitis will only occur in those individuals with the genetic potential to recognize and process a hapten, and therefore some individuals will be incapable of developing this reaction regardless of the nature of the exposure. A period of exposure is required to induce the sensitized state; this is usually from 10 to 14 days with strong allergens, but the induction period may be much longer. Once the induction period is past, a period of time will elapse between the contact of skin with an allergen and the actual onset of dermatitis. This is the elicitation phase of allergic contact dermatitis, and most commonly the period of time is between two and seven days. The primary symptom is itching and the classic morphological change is the development of vesicles and/or bullae. The

Table 1.1 Diagnostic criteria for irritant contact dermatitis

- **Subjective major criteria**

1. Onset of symptoms within minutes to hours of exposure.
2. Pain, burning, stinging, or discomfort exceeding itching, especially early in the clinical course.

- **Subjective minor criteria**

1. Onset of dermatitis within two weeks of environmental exposure. (This is often difficult history to elicit except in special settings where the irritant is a relatively novel rather than ubiquitous substance.)
2. Many people in the environment similarly affected. (If this information is based solely on history provided by the patient, its validity is suspect unless verified by an examining physician.)

- **Objective major criteria**

1. Macular erythema, hyperkeratosis, or fissuring predominating over vesicular change. (Vesicles and bullae may be present in irritant reactions, especially on the palms, with *strong* irritants. When vesicles predominate, the likelihood of allergy increases.)
2. Glazed, parched or scalded appearance of the surface of the skin.
3. The healing process proceeds without plateau upon withdrawal of exposure to the substance in question. (If not, then endogenous disease, such as atopic dermatitis or psoriasis should be strongly considered.)
4. Patch testing with known environmentally relevant allergens is negative.

- **Objective minor criteria**

1. Sharp circumspection of the dermatitis.
2. Evidence of gravitational influences, such as a dripping effect.
3. Lack of tendency for spread of dermatitis. (This can be properly evaluated only on sequential examinations.)
4. Vesicles juxtaposed closely to patches of erythema, erosions, bullae or other morphological changes that suggest that small differences in concentration or contact time produce large differences in skin damage.

intensity of the immune response can lead to extension of the dermatitis beyond the area of physical contact. If no further exposure occurs, the dermatitis may continue for several weeks and actually intensify for several days after the first day of dermatitis. Patch testing is generally done to confirm a diagnosis of allergic contact dermatitis. The immunological mechanisms that underpin allergic contact dermatitis have recently been reviewed (Belsito, 1997).

ACUTE CONTACT DERMATITIS – MILD TO MODERATE

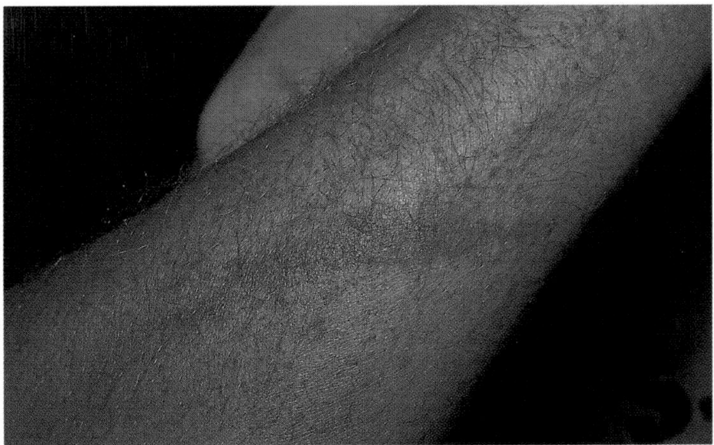

Figure 1.1 *Irritant:* Brisk erythema and a stinging sensation occurred on the forearm of this young man within 20 minutes of his leaning against a post freshly painted with creosote at a riding stable. The reaction was sharply demarcated and did not spread. This was a mild, acute, irritant reaction.

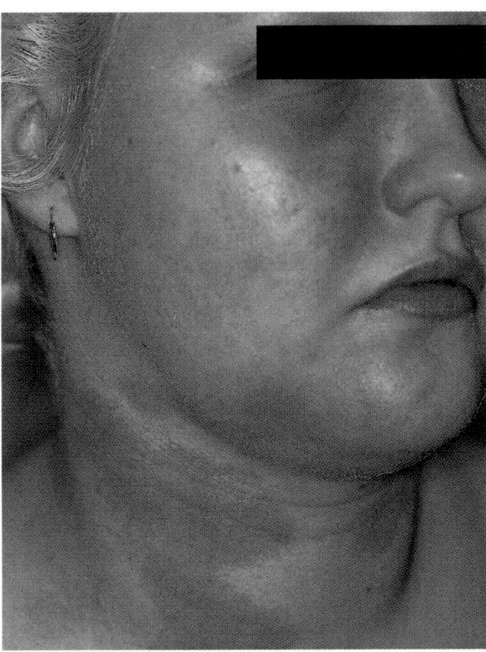

Figure 1.2 *Irritant:* This 19-year-old woman had acute dermatitis on her face and neck after using a new, scented shampoo. Patch testing with standard screening allergens was negative, and testing with the shampoo showed an irritant reaction to a 1:10 dilution, while there was no reaction to a 1:100 dilution. The sharply demarcated erythema is characteristic of an acute, irritant reaction.

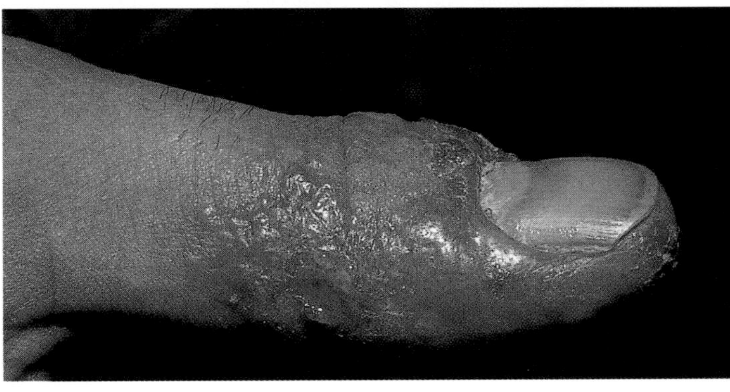

Figure 1.3 *Allergic:* This is a classic example of allergic contact dermatitis, showing typical clinical lesions, with vesicles, blisters and exudation.

ACUTE CONTACT DERMATITIS – MODERATE TO SEVERE

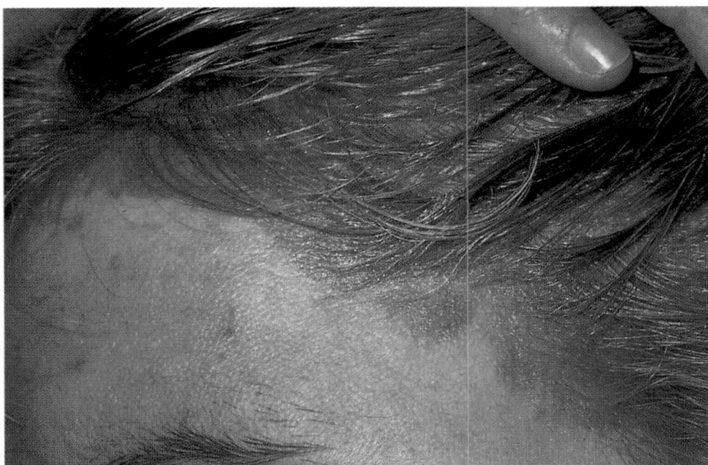

Figure 1.4 *Irritant:* This acute, irritant reaction on the scalp was due to hair bleach. Such reactions can vary widely in intensity – this is a moderate reaction.

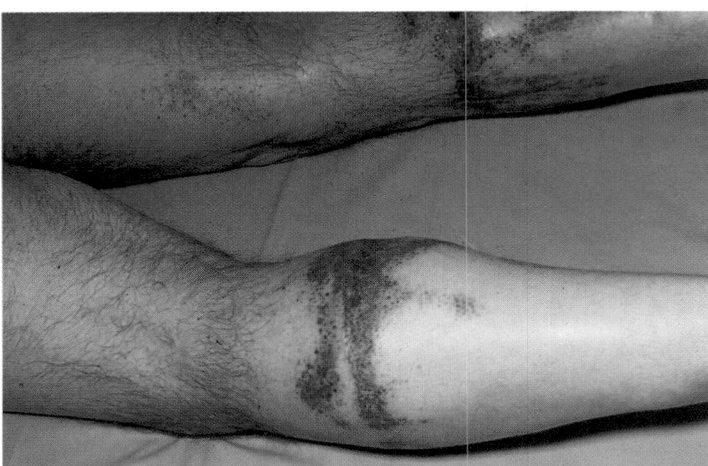

Figure 1.5 *Irritant:* Cement is very alkaline and very caustic. Irritant reactions known as cement burns can occur as seen here. The localization is explained by boots that protected the worker up to the middle of the calf. This is moderate to severe irritant contact dermatitis.

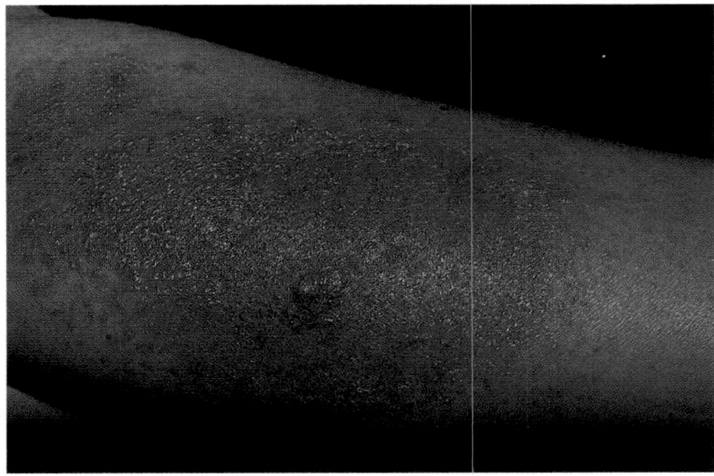

Figure 1.6 *Allergic:* Spreading vesicular dermatitis is seen on the forearm of this man. The dermatitis occurred three days after he cleaned out vines in his garden. This is the typical appearance of poison ivy dermatitis, a classic cause of acute allergic contact dermatitis of moderate to severe intensity.

ACUTE SEVERE IRRITANT CONTACT DERMATITIS

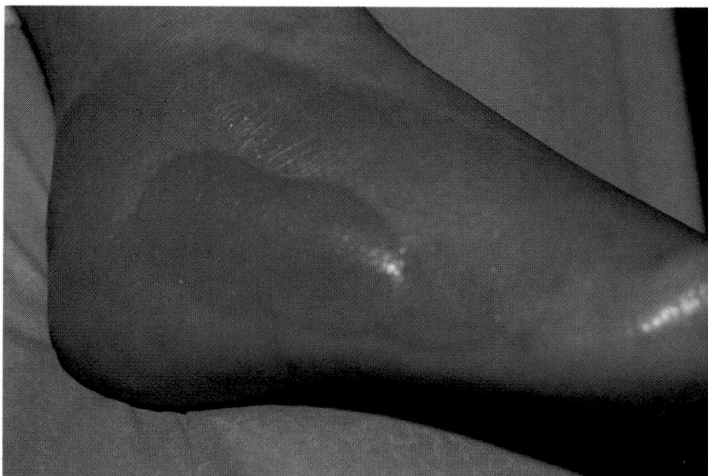

Figure 1.7 Severe irritant reactions can be accompanied by bulla formation, as noted in this patient who, owing to a mistake made by a pharmacist, used phenol instead of formaldehyde to treat hyperhidrosis of the feet.

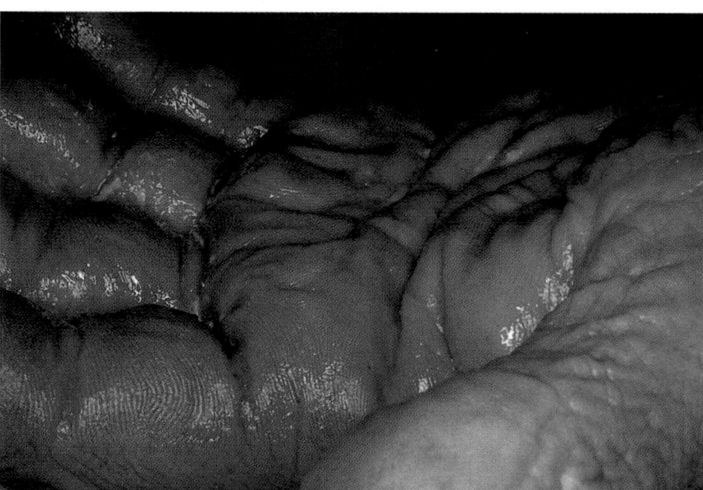

Figure 1.8 This case of irritant contact dermatitis was caused by handling dimethylformamide.

SUBACUTE CONTACT DERMATITIS

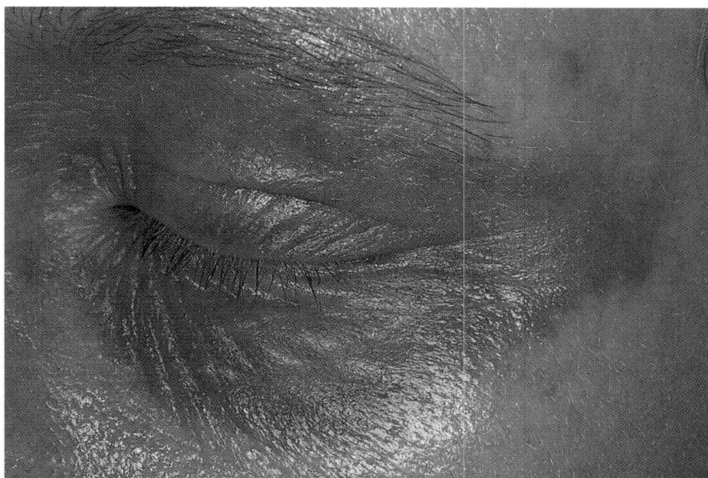

Figure 1.9 *Irritant:* Erythema and a change in the surface texture of the skin are seen in this subacute, irritant reaction due to eye cosmetics in a 45-year-old woman.

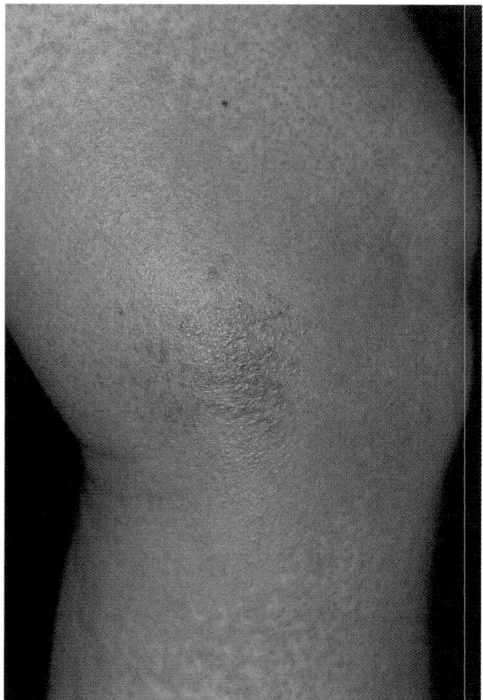

Figure 1.10 *Allergic:* This acute to subacute allergic contact dermatitis occurred in a fragrance-sensitive woman.

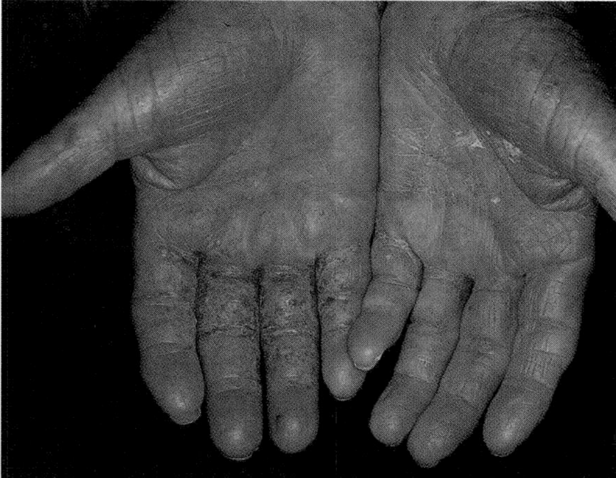

Figure 1.11 *Allergic:* Vesicles have given way to superficial erosions on the palm of this patient who was found to be allergic to colophony. This is a subacute form of allergic contact dermatitis.

CHRONIC CONTACT DERMATITIS

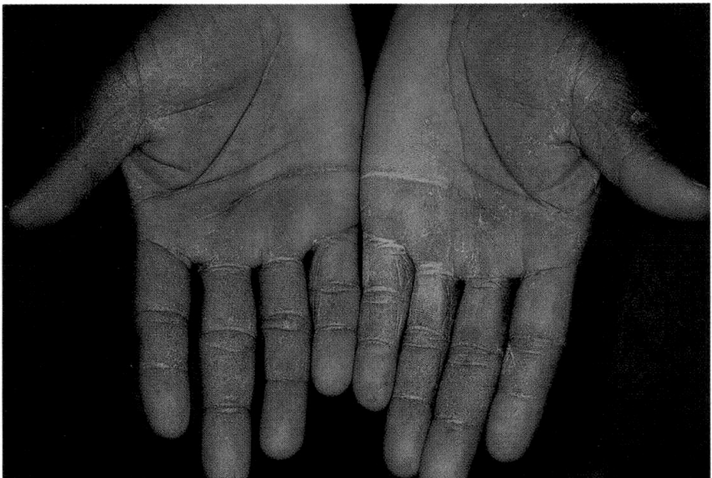

(a)

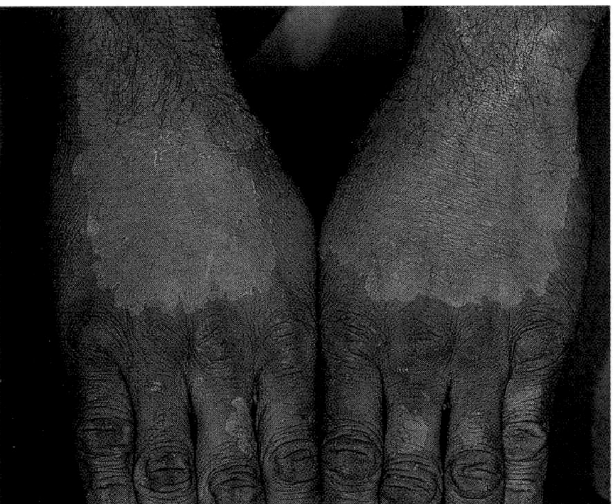

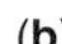

(b)

Figure 1.12 *Irritant:* Desquamation, lichenification and post-inflammatory hyperpigmentation are seen on both the palmar (**a**) and dorsal (**b**) aspects of the hands of this man who had been repeatedly exposed to floor wax stripper. Patch tests to screening allergens were negative. There were no vesicles.

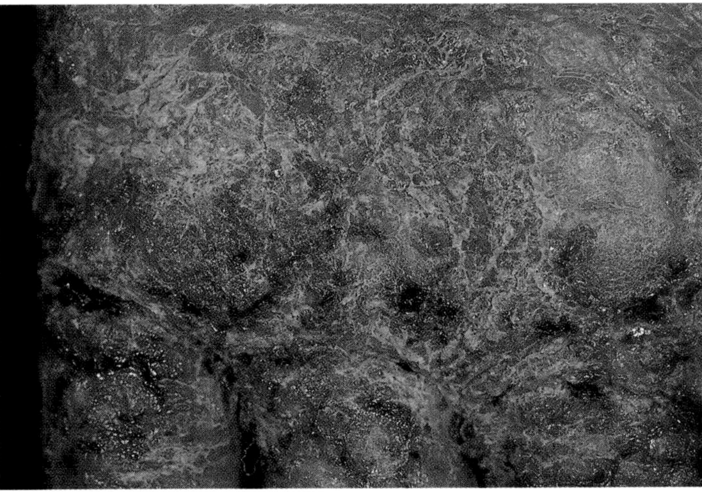

Figure 1.13 *Allergic:* Different morphological patterns of dermatitis may coexist in a single individual, as is seen in this picture of the same patient as seen in Figure 1.5. Scaling and hyperkeratosis to the point of fissuring are more typical of chronic contact dermatitis. At times, chronic contact dermatitis can resemble papulosquamous disorders more than eczematous conditions.

SEQUELAE OF CONTACT DERMATITIS

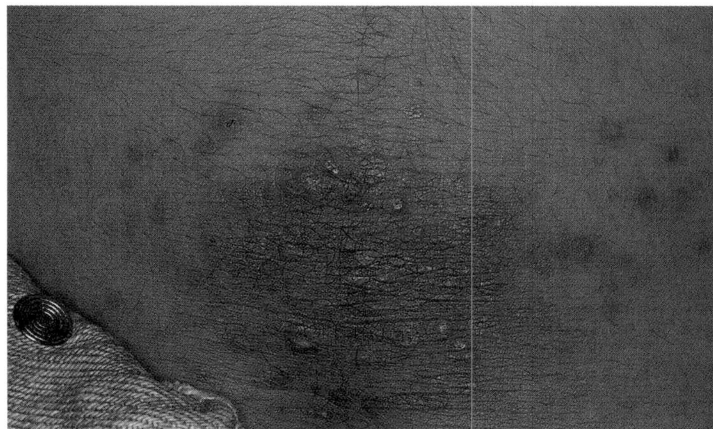

Figure 1.14 This 31-year-old woman with post-inflammatory hyperpigmentation had an antecedent nickel dermatitis due to a jeans button.

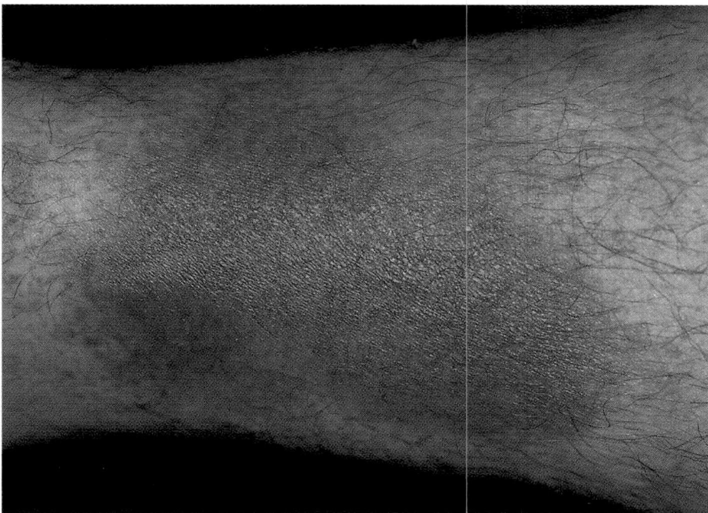

Figure 1.15 Hyperpigmentation may be the sequela of many forms of dermatitis; in this example the initial eruption was stasis dermatitis.

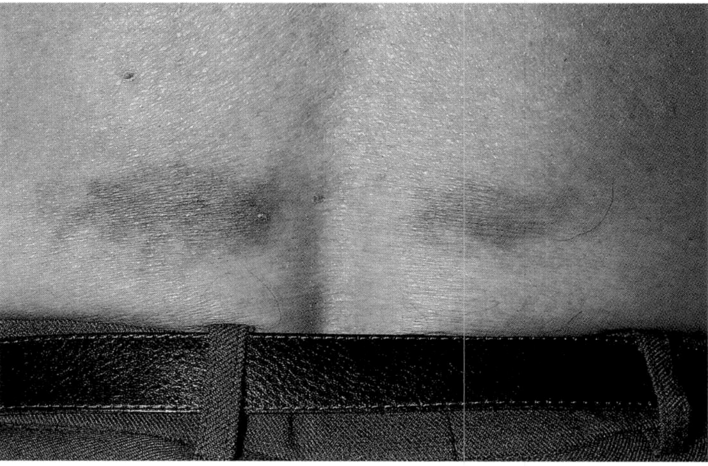

Figure 1.16 This is a 76-year-old man with post-inflammatory hyperpigmentation following mechanical dermatitis from his belt.

PUSTULAR IRRITANT REACTIONS

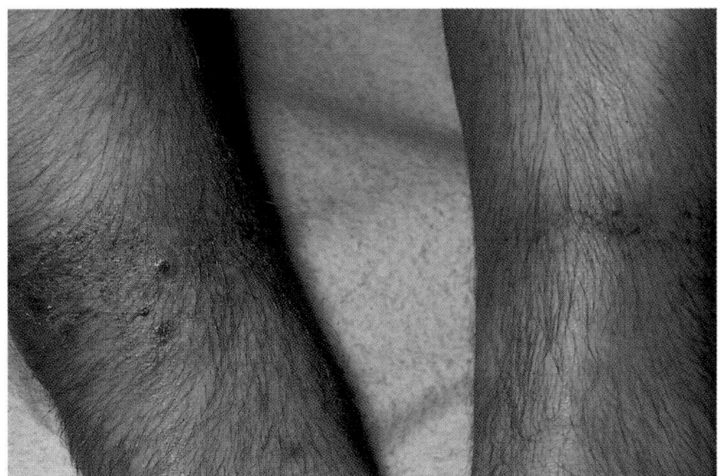
(a)

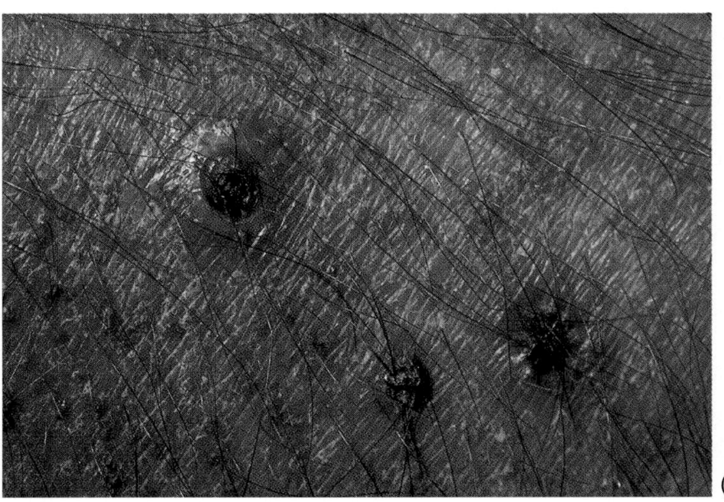
(b)

Figure 1.17 Pustular reactions that are not due to infection, but rather to external contactants, are deemed to be irritant reactions. (**a**) This morphological variant of irritant contact dermatitis was due to hexafluorosilicate, which is a pustulogen. (**b**) This shows a closer view of the pustules.

EPIDEMIOLOGY

The prevalence of contact dermatitis among women (13–14%) is about twice as high as for men (5–9%) in Scandinavian studies, while in the USA prevalence is about the same for the two sexes (Coenraads and Smit, 1995, p.141). Prevalence studies conducted in various parts of the world indicate that age and sex are not, in themselves, important risk factors for contact dermatitis. The higher prevalence among women is due to exposure patterns rather than gender. Exposure at work and in the home to environmental agents is much more important. One example of this is allergic contact dermatitis caused by poison ivy or poison oak. In certain parts of the USA, 80% of the population are sensitized to urushiols in these plants – a prevalence not seen anywhere else in the world. This example shows that if a population is exposed to a sufficiently potent allergen, most individuals will become sensitized. Strong irritants can likewise precipitate irritant contact dermatitis in most persons if the exposure is sufficiently intense. This is sometimes the case in industrial settings when protective measures are inadequate.

Of all types of contact dermatitis, hand dermatitis has been studied most extensively, and the point prevalence of hand eczema among 20 000 adult Swedes has been shown to be 5.5% for women and 3.7% for men, with irritant contact dermatitis being the most common type of hand dermatitis (Meding, 1990). The incidence of occupational skin disease is approximately 0.5 cases per 1000 workers per year. Skin disease ranks as one of the most common occupational diseases in studies carried out in several centres (Coenraads and Smit, 1995, p.146).

With regard to the prognosis of contact dermatitis, interest has also focused on hand dermatitis. One study showed the mean duration of irritant hand dermatitis to be 10 years, compared with 12 years for allergic hand dermatitis (Meding, 1990). The duration was the same for occupational and for non-occupational hand dermatitis. Although occupational hand dermatitis does not necessarily clear following a change of job (Shah et al, 1996), the severity of the dermatitis may be reduced. Over a period of years, approximately 25% of cases of occupational hand dermatitis clear and 50–75% improve (Keczkes et al, 1983; Halkier-Sørensen, 1996).

It is difficult to assess the cost of occupational skin diseases. In Denmark, with a population of five million, the total costs have been estimated to be DKK 600 million (US$ 85 million) per year (Halkier-Sørensen, 1996).

BIOLOGY AND IMMUNOLOGY

Contact dermatitis

The stratum corneum of the epidermis, which is composed of corneocytes and intercellular lipids, is a very effective barrier against irritants. Damage to the stratum corneum is followed by loss of water, causing the surface of the skin to become dry and cracked, thus making it easier for irritants to penetrate. The irritants themselves then increase both barrier damage and the number of antigen-presenting cells. This can result in irritant contact dermatitis as illustrated in Figure 1.18(a).

Haptens normally have a molecular weight of less than 1000 daltons. They can penetrate even an intact stratum corneum and epidermis; damage to this barrier facilitates such penetration.

Epidermal Langerhans cells may bind haptens via class II MHC molecules coded for in the HLA-D region of the human genome and then present the haptens to naive T cells after migration to the regional lymph nodes. Once a person has acquired specific sensitization to a hapten, re-exposure and presentation by the Langerhans cells will attract specifically sensitized T cells, initiating the release of a cascade of cytokines. The resulting inflammation will be clinically expressed as contact dermatitis (Keczkes et al, 1983) (see Figure 1.18b). Although sensitized T cells carry a high specificity for a particular allergen, the profiles of cytokine release and the dermal and epidermal inflammation seen in irritant and allergic contact dermatitis are very similar. This may, in part, explain why it is difficult to distinguish clinically and histologically between allergic and irritant contact dermatitis (Hoefakker et al, 1995; Rietschel, 1997).

Sensitization to most haptens persists indefinitely, but may weaken if the sensitized person is not re-exposed for a period of years. Tolerance may alter the immunological response, and it is possible to induce tolerance experimentally in a sensitized person by repeated oral or intravenous administration of the hapten. Sensitization may even be prevented by similar administration of the hapten prior to cutaneous exposure. Suppressor cells are probably involved in this process.

The immunology of photoallergic contact dermatitis is very similar to that of allergic contact dermatitis. The difference between the two is that exposure to ultraviolet light is a prerequisite for the formation and presentation of the antigen in photoallergic contact dermatitis.

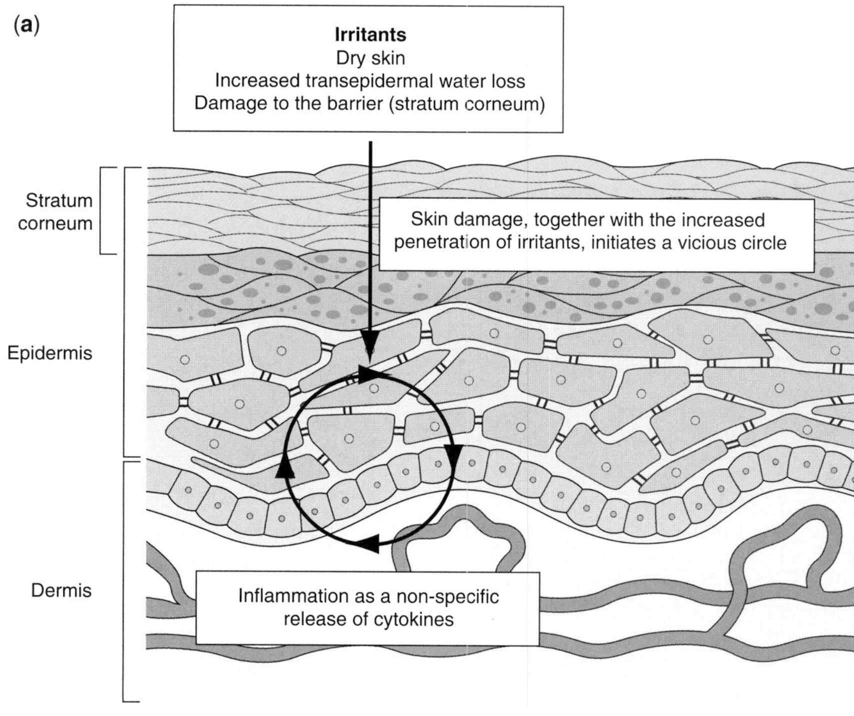

(**a**) In **irritant contact dermatitis** (ICD), the primary event is barrier damage, especially of the stratum corneum. The increased penetration of irritants causes skin damage with increased transepidermal water loss. This is followed by inflammation due to cytokine release, which, in turn, eases the penetration of irritants – a vicious circle has appeared.

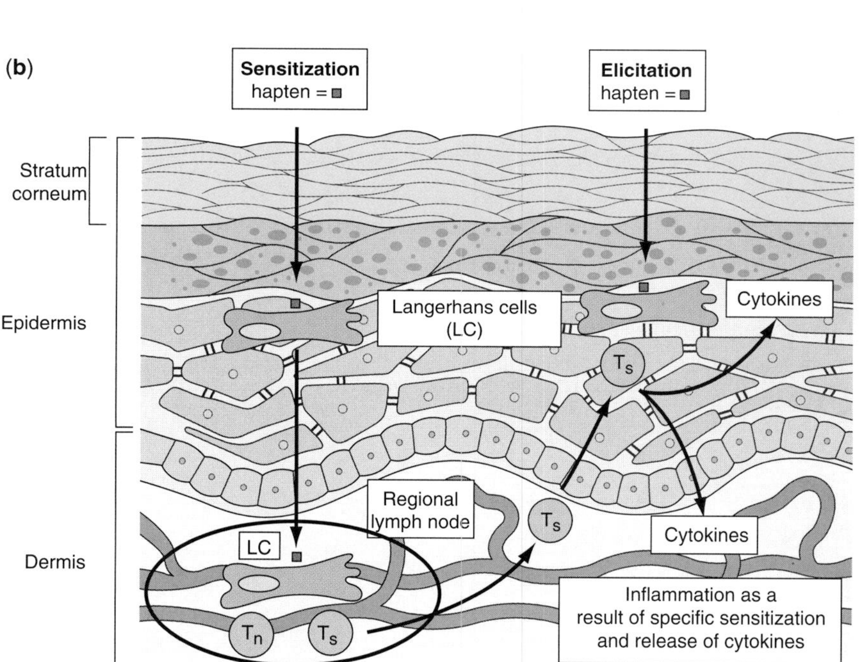

(**b**) In **allergic contact dermatitis** (ACD), the primary event is specific sensitization to a low-molecular-weight hapten. Sensitization occurs in the regional lymph node. When sensitized individuals are re-exposed to the same hapten, sensitized T lymphocytes are recruited via chemo-attractants, and cytokines are released. This causes an inflammatory response much like that seen in ICD. T_n = naive T lymphocytes; T_s = specifically sensitized T lymphocytes.

Figure 1.18 The mechanisms of (**a**) irritant and (**b**) allergic contact dermatitis.

Contact urticaria

Immunological contact urticaria is an immediate-type reaction to circulating, specific IgE antibodies. Histamine and other mediators are released as a consequence of the antigen–antibody reaction, thus causing the pruritic, urticarial reaction. In non-immunological contact urticaria, similar mediators are released owing to the direct action of the offending substance on, for example, mast cells.

Immunological and non-immunological contact urticaria are clinically indistinguishable. A long list of substances can cause non-immunological contact urticaria. These include caterpillars, jellyfish, benzaldehyde and sorbic acid. Immunological contact urticaria is caused by latex protein, animal dander, the amniotic fluid of cows, and a number of plants, including fruits and vegetables (Lahti and Maibach, 1990).

Proteins in food items handled by cooks cause eczematous immediate-type reactions known as protein contact dermatitis (see section on 'Contact urticaria and protein contact dermatitis' in Chapter 5).

Allergens that are known to cause immediate-type reactions may also cause delayed-type reactions, as demonstrated by positive patch tests. This has been studied in detail in patients with atopic dermatitis, particularly in relation to house dust mite antigens (Lahti, 1995).

HISTOPATHOLOGY

Histologically, acute contact dermatitis is characterized by acanthosis and spongiosis in the epidermis, possibly with confluence of the spongiotic areas into vesicles. In the dermis there is vasodilatation and a perivascular infiltrate with histiocytes and lymphocytes. In chronic contact dermatitis spongiosis is less prominent. There is hyperkeratosis, the epidermis thickens, and it may develop a psoriasiform appearance. The perivascular dermal inflammatory infiltrate becomes more subtle, and consists of histiocytes and lymphocytes (Figures 1.19 and 1.20).

While histological examination can help to identify various etiologies of eczematous dermatitis, it is histologically impossible to distinguish between allergic and irritant contact dermatitis (Lever and Schaumburg-Lever, 1990).

RISK FACTORS FOR THE DEVELOPMENT OF IRRITANT CONTACT DERMATITIS

Individual factors

Present or previous atopic dermatitis is perhaps the most important risk factor for developing irritant contact dermatitis. Approximately half of patients with severe atopic dermatitis in childhood develop hand dermatitis as adults (Rystedt, 1985).

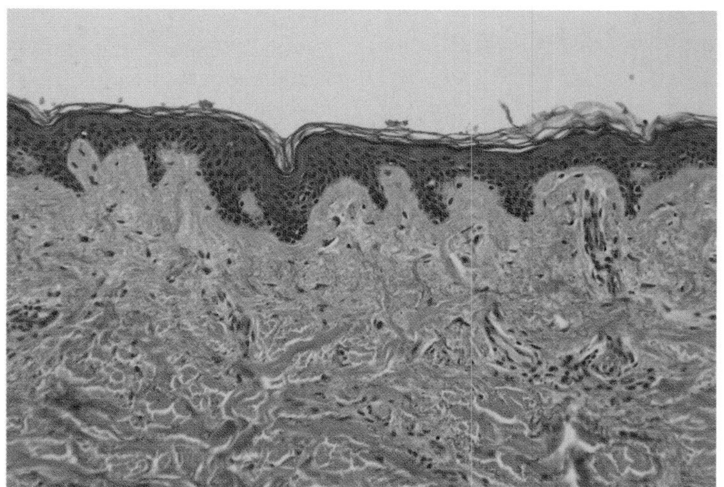
(a)

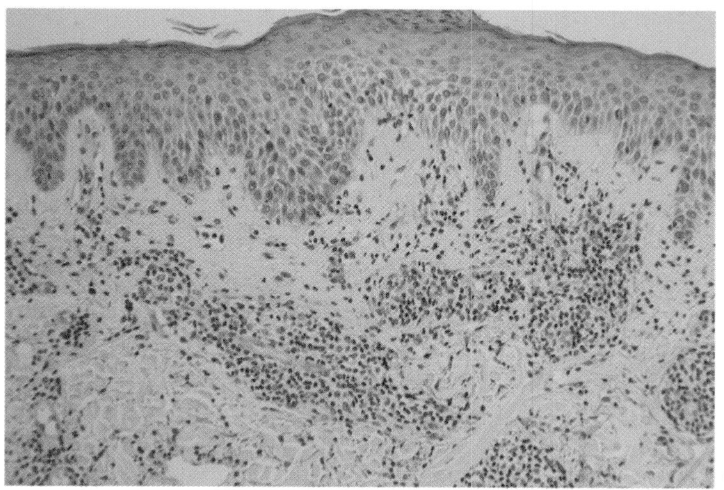
(b)

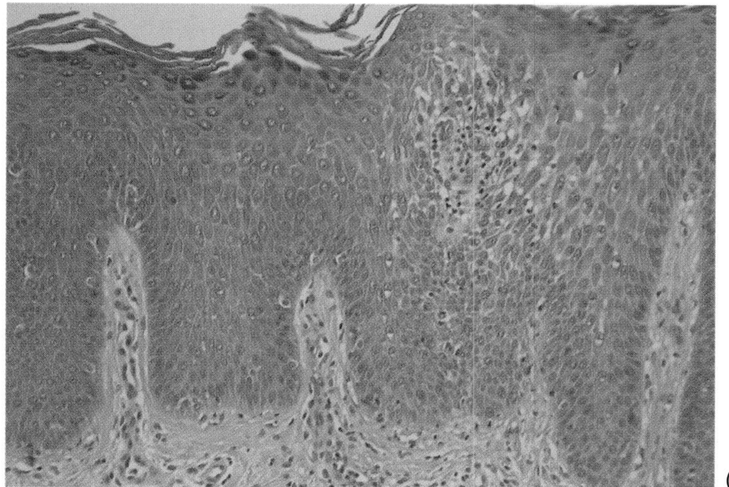
(c)

Figure 1.19 (**a**) Histopathology of normal skin. (**b**) Histopathology of subacute contact dermatitis. There is spongiosis in the epidermis and a rather dense perivascular inflammatory infiltrate. (**c**) Histopathology of chronic contact dermatitis. There is thickening of the epidermis and spongiosis in some areas. (a–c, ×100 hematoxylin–eosin stain). (Courtesy of Eva Spaun, Aalborg Hospital, Aalborg, Denmark.)

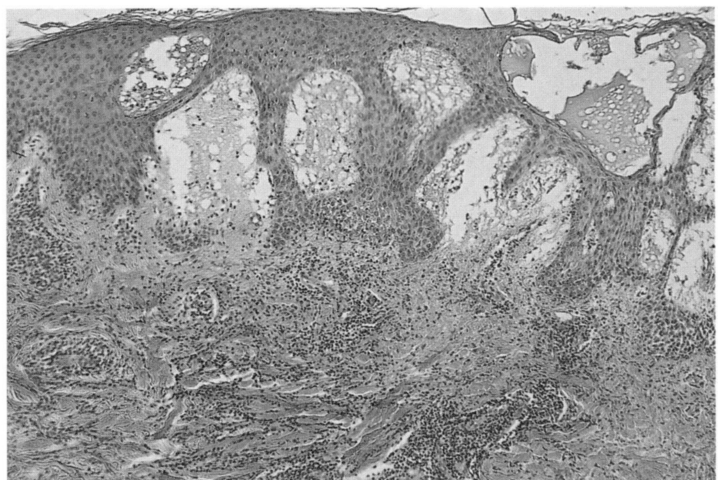

(a)

Figure 1.20 (**a**) Histological picture of acute allergic contact dermatitis showing more pronounced spongiotic vesiculation of the epidermis than shown in Figure 1.19, with exocytosis of mononuclear cells and intercellular oedema. (**b**) At higher magnification. In general, it is not possible to use histology to distinguish between allergic and irritant contact dermatitis.

(b)

Environmental factors

If an irritant is sufficiently strong, anyone can develop irritant contact dermatitis. For men, the most important irritants are found in the metal industry, and include oils, solvents and soluble cutting oils. For women, soaps and detergents play a significant role. Differences in exposure patterns probably explain why twice as many women as men have hand dermatitis. Mechanical trauma increases the risk of irritant contact dermatitis from chemicals, and mechanical trauma can, in itself, cause irritant contact dermatitis. Low environmental humidity, as seen in winter in temperate climates and in dry working environments, lowers the threshold for the development of irritant contact dermatitis.

RISK FACTORS FOR THE DEVELOPMENT OF ALLERGIC CONTACT DERMATITIS

Individual factors

A genetic disposition to the development of contact sensitization has been demonstrated in animal experiments as well as in human family studies. The specific locus for this genetic disposition has not been identified, and population studies indicate that, in comparison with exposure pattern, heredity plays a minor role for contact sensitization. Atopic dermatitis may decrease the risk of contact sensitivity, as do diseases known to impair immune response. Age and sex are not in themselves significant risk factors.

Environmental factors

More than 3000 sensitizing chemicals have been identified. Chemical compounds vary from virtually non-sensitizing, such as iron salts, to extremely sensitizing, such as the urushiols found in poison ivy and poison oak. For strong sensitizers, a single exposure may be sufficient to sensitize. Massive exposure can turn even a moderate sensitizer into a major problem. This is true, for example, for nickel in women. The application of a topical medicament under occlusion, for example neomycin under bandages for the treatment of leg ulcers or in intertriginous areas, can make even this moderate sensitizer a common cause of allergic contact dermatitis. The sensitizing capacity of an individual chemical compound is related to some aspects of its chemical structure as well as to its concentration.

Exposure patterns vary in different parts of the world. The most common contact allergens are included in regional standard series such as the European Standard Patch Test Series and the North American Contact Dermatitis Group Standard Series (see Appendix). Many allergens are the same in the two series.

RISK FACTORS FOR THE DEVELOPMENT OF CONTACT URTICARCIA/PROTEIN CONTACT DERMATITIS

Individual factors

Pre-existing hand dermatitis enhances the penetration of high-molecular-weight proteins, which can become allergens for immediate-type reactions. This is why persons with chronic hand dermatitis commonly develop secondary protein contact dermatitis. Important risk factors for contact urticaria of the hands from latex protein include atopy and the presence of hand dermatitis (Turjanmaa, 1994; Taylor and Praditsuwan, 1996).

Environmental factors

The amount of free latex protein in latex items can vary considerably (Boyer, 1995). In occupations such as sandwich making, where there is extensive contact with raw food items, there is an increased risk of developing secondary protein contact dermatitis.

PREVENTION OF CONTACT DERMATITIS

Primary prevention (the prevention of the induction of contact dermatitis) can include prohibiting the use of certain chemicals, substituting certain chemicals with less noxious substances, using strong sensitizers and irritants only in closed systems or automated work processes, and individual training, as well as the use of individual protective measures.

Secondary prevention (the prevention of relapses in persons with previous contact dermatitis) includes educating the patient about irritants and allergens and the use of individual protective measures, as well as other means of regulating exposure.

Preventive measures already taken include prohibition of the use of persulfate as a flour improver in the 1950s. Up until that time, persulfate was a common contact allergen among bakers. Likewise, the addition of ferrous sulfate to cement to reduce hexavalent chromates to less-sensitizing trivalent chromium salts has reduced the prevalence of occupational hand dermatitis in the building industry (Avnstorp, 1992). Requirements for the use of protective clothing and the education of workers exposed to epoxy products has decreased the rate of epoxy sensitization.

The pre-employment identification of persons at risk of developing contact dermatitis based on their medical history, possibly in combination with patch and/or prick testing, is, theoretically, a means of reducing the incidence of occupational dermatoses in certain high-risk occupations. The value of such screening is debatable and controversial, since those rejected are likely to be measurably less employable.

REFERENCES

Avnstorp C (1992) Cement eczema. An epidemiological intervention study. *Acta Derm Venereol (Stockh)* Suppl 179:1–22.

Belsito DV (1997) The rise and fall of allergic contact dermatitis. *Am J Contact Dermatitis* **8**:193–201.

Boyer EM (1995) The effectiveness of a low-chemical, low-protein medical glove to prevent or reduce dermatological problems. *J Dent Hyg* **69**:67–73.

Coenraads P-J, Smit J (1995) Epidemiology. In: *Textbook of Contact Dermatitis*, 2nd edn (Rycroft RJG, Menné T, Frosch PJ, eds). Berlin: Springer-Verlag: 133–50.

Halkier-Sørensen L (1996) Occupational skin diseases. *Contact Dermatitis* **35**:Suppl 1: 1–120.

Hoefakker S, Caubo M, van't Erve EHM et al (1995) In vivo cytokine profiles in allergic and irritant contact dermatitis. *Contact Dermatitis* **33**:258–66.

Keczkes K, Bhate SM, Wyatt EH (1983) The outcome of primary irritant hand dermatitis. *Br J Dermatol* **109**:665–8.

Lahti A (1995) Immediate contact reactions. In: *Textbook of Contact Dermatitis*, 2nd edn (Rycroft RJG, Menné T, Frosch PJ, eds). Berlin: Springer-Verlag: 62–74.

Lahti A, Maibach HI (1990) Immediate contact reactions. In: *Exogenous Dermatoses: Environmental Dermatitis* (Menné T, Maibach HI, eds). Boca Raton, FL: CRC Press: 21–35.

Lever WF, Schaumburg-Lever G (1990) *Histopathology of the Skin*, 7th edn. Philadelphia: WB Saunders: 106–10.

Meding B (1990) Epidemiology of hand eczema in an industrial city. *Acta Derm Venereol (Stockh)* Suppl 153: 1–43.

Rietschel RL (1997) Mechanisms in irritant contact dermatitis. *Clin Dermatol* **15**:557–9.

Rystedt I (1985) Hand eczema and long-term prognosis in atopic dermatitis. Dissertation. Department of Occupational Dermatology, National Board of Occupational Safety and Health and Karolinska Hospital, Karolinska Institute, Stockholm: 1–59.

Shah M, Lewis FM, Gawkrodger DJ (1996) Prognosis of occupational hand dermatitis in metalworkers. *Contact Dermatitis* **34**:27–30.

Taylor JS, Praditsuwan P (1996) Latex allergy. Review of 44 cases including outcome and frequent association with allergic hand eczema. *Arch Dermatol* **132**:265–71.

Turjanmaa K (1994) Update on occupational natural rubber latex allergy. *Dermatol Clin* **12**:561–7.

2

Patch Test and Prick Test Techniques

Patch Test Technique

When patch tests are to be carried out, a number of precautions must be taken in order to obtain a correct result.

First, a detailed clinical history of the patient should be prepared, emphasizing current occupation, place of work and products handled. Previous occupations and products handled then are also important, since these could cause latent sensitization. In addition to occupation, it is important to identify hobbies and materials handled in connection with these, and, finally, what, if any, medications or folk or herbal remedies are used.

Once the background of a patient is known, a complete examination should be carried out. Even though lesions may be on the face or hands, it is essential to examine the entire skin surface, including mucous membranes.

Once the history and examination of the patient have been completed, there are three options:

- It is not necessary to patch test.
- Patch testing should be postponed because:
  - the patient is in an acute phase; there is a widespread outbreak of dermatitis or dermatitis in the patch test area;
  - the patient is taking medication that could cause false-negative reactions (e.g. corticosteroids, immunosuppressants);
  - the patient is pregnant (some physicians believe that patch testing should be postponed until after delivery).
- Patch testing should be carried out.

If the decision is made to carry out patch testing, a standard series of well-known allergens prepared for this purpose is used (see Appendix on the European and US Standard Patch Test Series). Additional testing can be carried out with substances related to the patient's occupation or specific products handled in the workplace or at home. In some cases, the patient may bring a set of substances with which he or she wishes to be patch-tested. Because of the risk of irritating or sensitizing the patient, these non-standard substances should not be used for patch testing unless their exact composition, pH and other properties are known. A patient's own products can be diluted in petrolatum, water or other solvents after consulting the literature to determine the correct dilution for patch testing. If the non-standard substances are not described in the literature, control testing of healthy persons should be carried out.

Patch testing should be done on the back by persons trained in the application of such tests. The patches should be removed after two days for the first reading, and the patient should be asked to return for a final reading after three or four days after the initial application. A range of two to five days after removal of patches is common practice in most countries for the delayed readings. Non-standard tests should be labelled and applied to the back at a site separate from the site of standard tests. The patient should be informed that if the tests cause a great deal of discomfort, they can be removed before the two days have passed.

The reading after two days serves as a guide, and, in many cases, non-specific reactions to the tape used, sweat, etc. may be observed, so the reading should be taken 30 minutes or more after the patches are removed. Generally, patches are applied on a Monday, so that the first reading can be taken on Wednesday (two days) and the second and final reading on Thursday or Friday (after three or four days).

The reading after three or four days gives more specific information. Patients should be asked to report any reactions in the test area observed after a week, since these unusually delayed reactions may be significant.

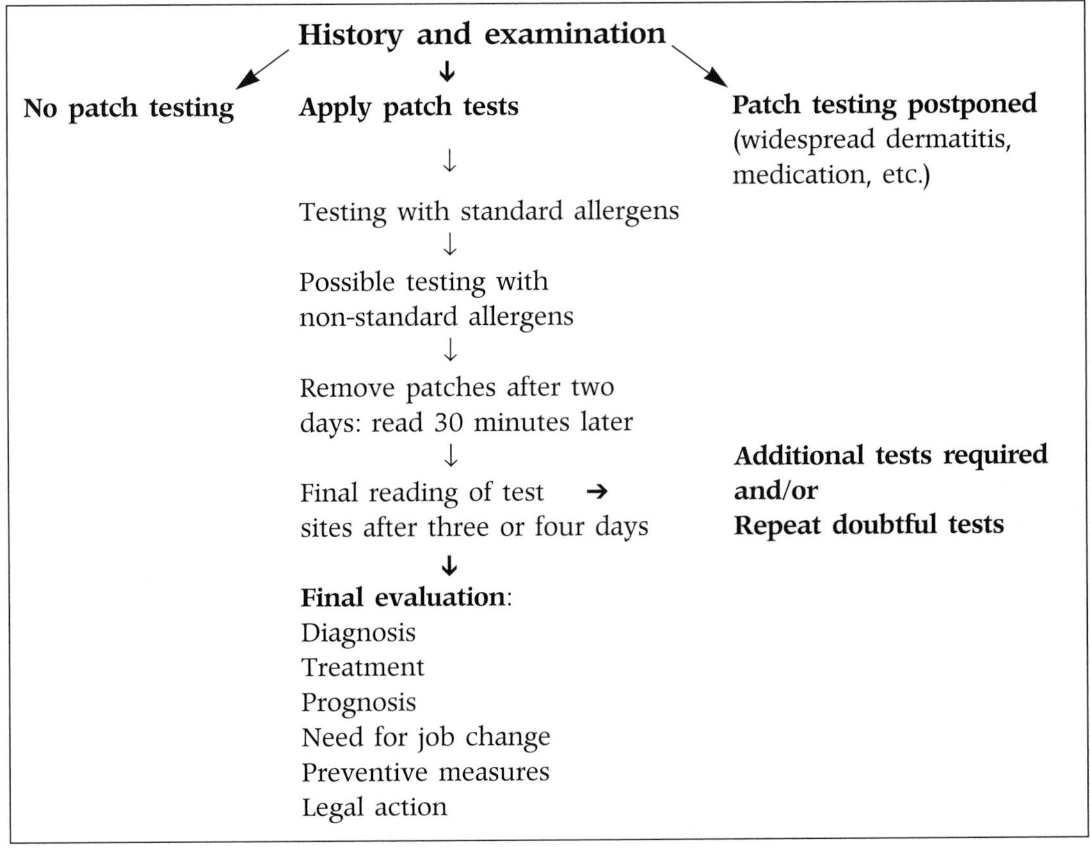

Once the tests have been evaluated, they can be used to determine a diagnosis, treatment, possible prognosis, the need for a change of job, preventive measures (items and substances to be avoided) as well as possible legal compensation.

The above procedure is summarized in the flow diagram (Conde-Salazar and Guimaraens, 1986).

PATCH TEST SYSTEMS

Several systems are currently used to patch test patients. The TRUE test system is the simplest to use, since the allergens are already on the application tape. Chamber systems, comprising a series of circular chambers made of aluminium or plastic, require the insertion in each chamber of the appropriate amount and type of each allergen prior to application. While TRUE test allergens are suspended in hydrophilic gel, the allergens in chamber systems are suspended in petrolatum or aqueous vehicles. Both methods of testing are biological, and although no two systems give exactly the same results (Wilkinson et al, 1990), the two methods are generally accepted as being equivalent (TRUE Test Study Group, 1989).

The type of test substances used and their concentrations have been validated to ensure a maximum number of true-positive reactions and as few false-positive and false-negative reactions as possible. Those allergens that most commonly produce positive reactions have been incorporated into the European Standard Patch Test Series (see Appendix).

Non-standard substances should be used for patch testing only after consulting the literature to ensure that the proper dilution has been made. It may be necessary to use a series of dilutions, and it is important to have an adequate number of controls. Great care must be exercised in the interpretation of test results, since false-positive and false-negative reactions are common when testing with non-standard substances.

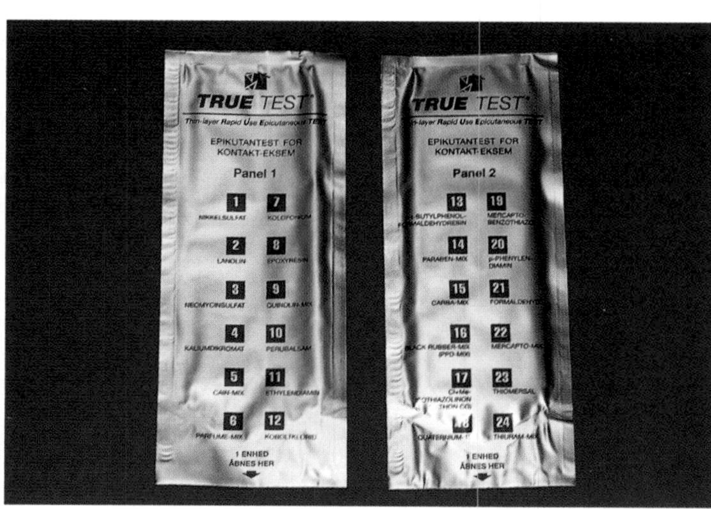

Figure 2.1 The main advantage of the TRUE test system is its ease of application. The two foil packages contain the two panels of allergens. The system comes complete with patient instructions about the individual allergens.

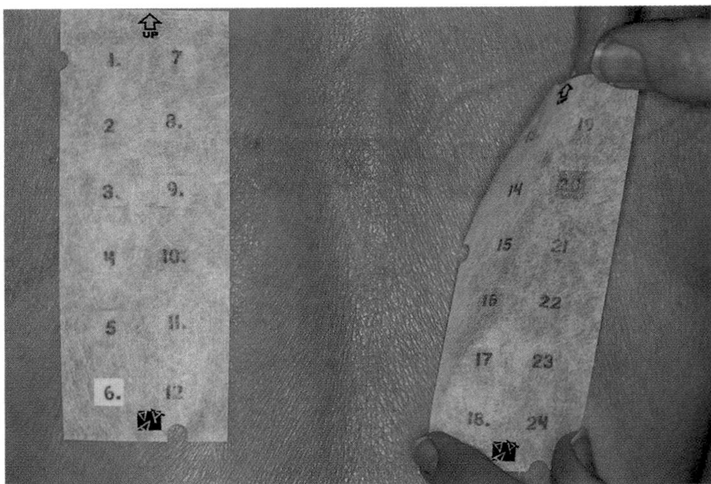

Figure 2.2 The panels are applied as shown. The disadvantage of this convenient system is a higher price and the inclusion of only a limited number of allergens. This system is suitable for use by dermatologists who test only a limited number of patients.

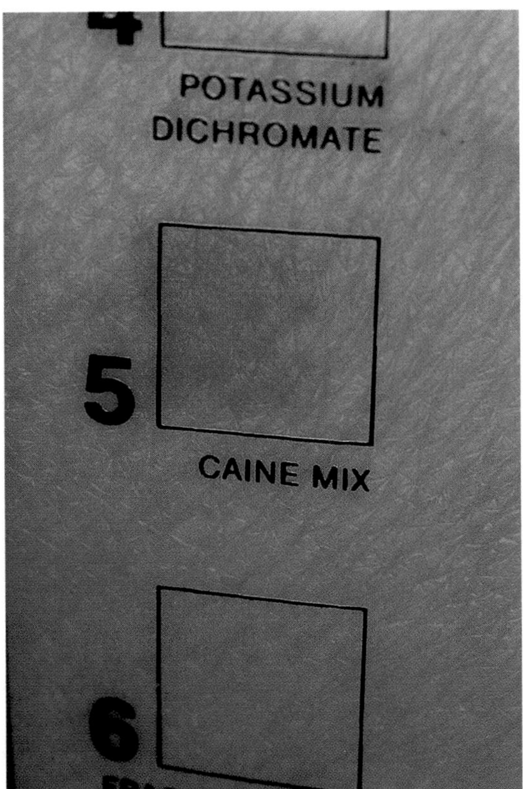

Figure 2.3 A clear plastic template that allows identification of the allergen is supplied by the manufacturer.

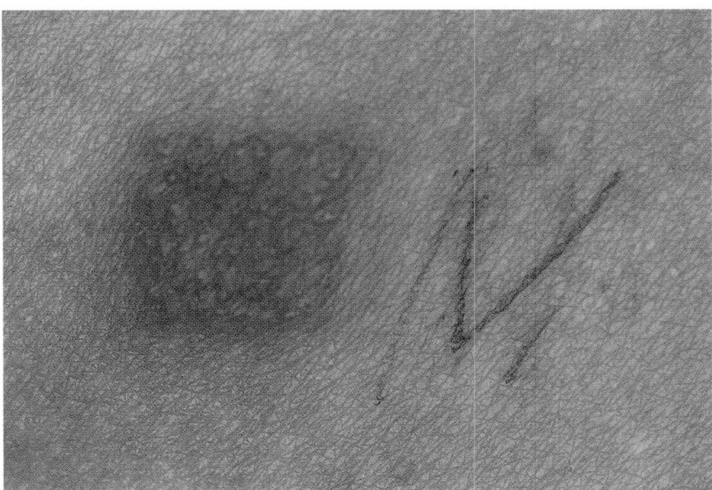

Figure 2.4 Positive reactions with the TRUE test are square, in contrast to those with the circular Finn chambers.

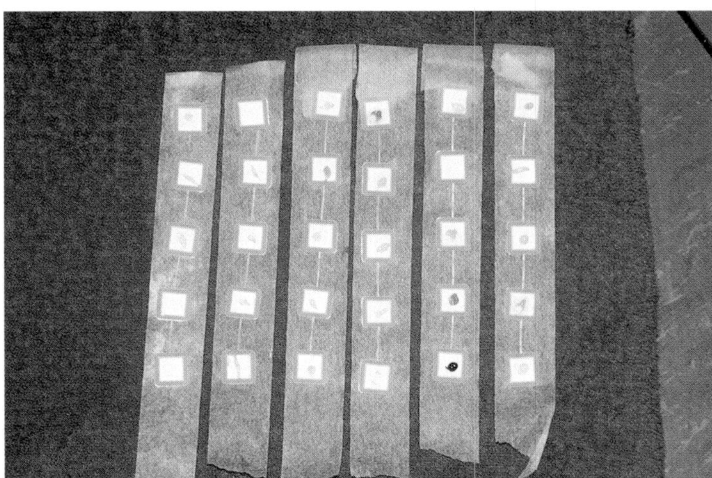

(**a**)

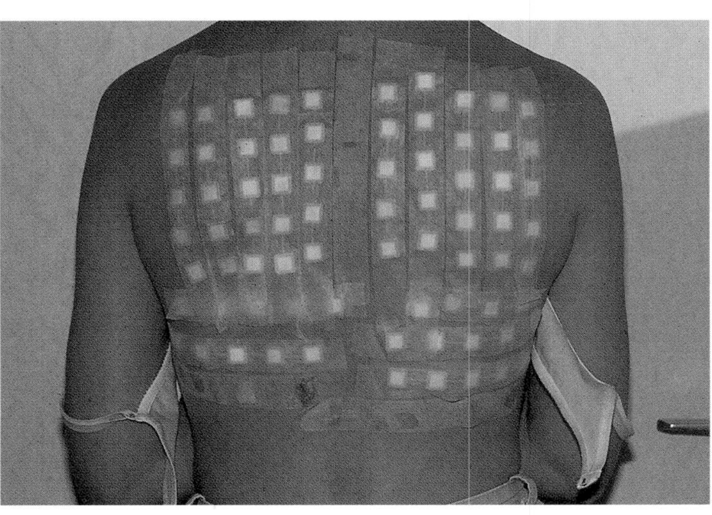

(**b**)

Figure 2.5 (**a**) Square chambers are available from van der Bend, and can be secured with Micropore tape (3M, Minneapolis/St Paul, MN) as seen in (**b**).

(a)

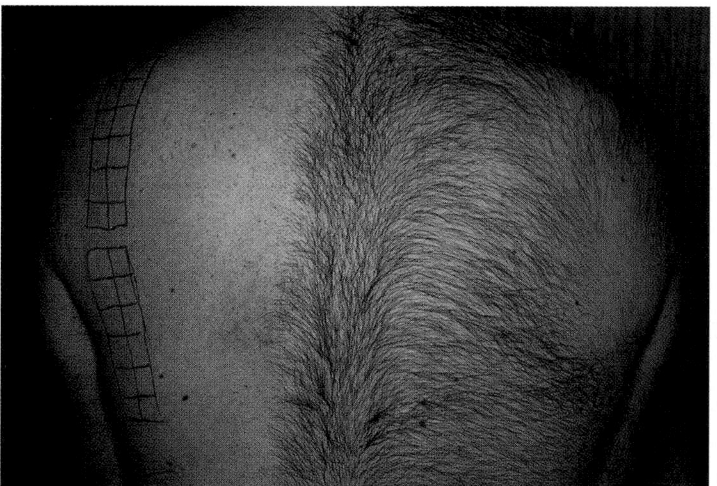

(b)

Figure 2.6 The application of a patch test to the upper back requires the back to be free of dermatitis. (**a**) This example shows a back with multiple lesions, a condition which makes patch testing difficult. (**b**) Similarly, if the back is hairy, it must be shaved.

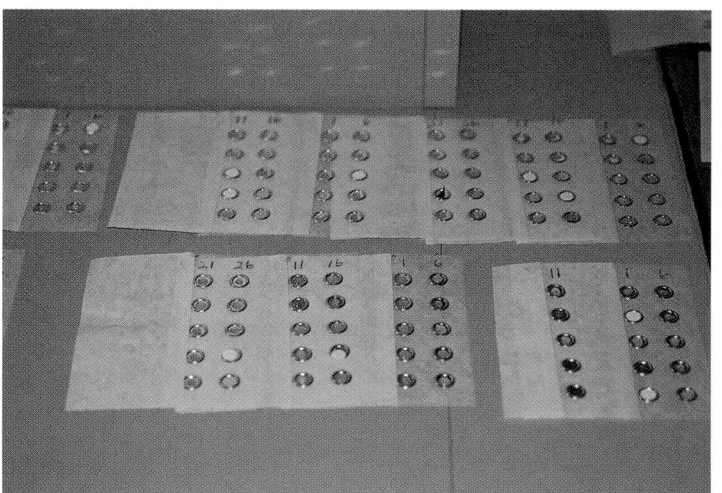

Figure 2.7 Petrolatum-based allergens can be applied to Finn chambers prior to the arrival of the patient for testing. Aqueous-based allergens must be applied to the chambers immediately before application to the patient's back.

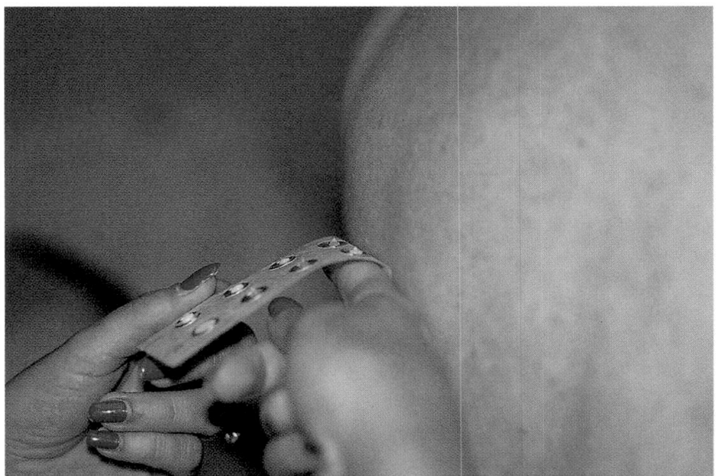

(**a**)

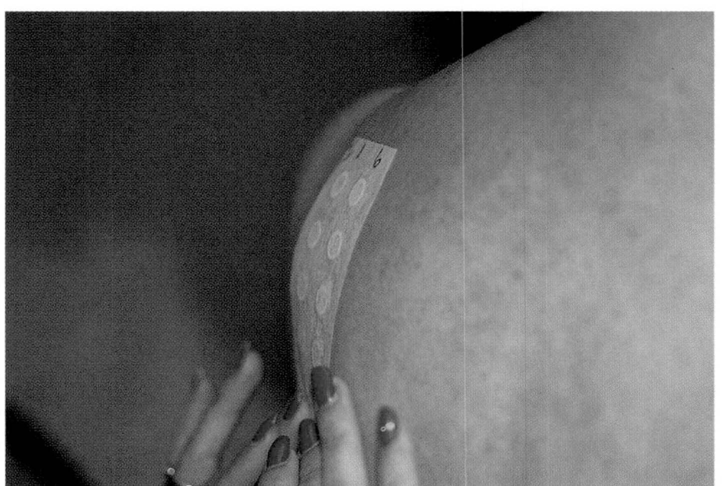

(**b**)

Figure 2.8 Finn chambers are applied to the back starting at the bottom of the panel (**a**) and working upwards (**b**).

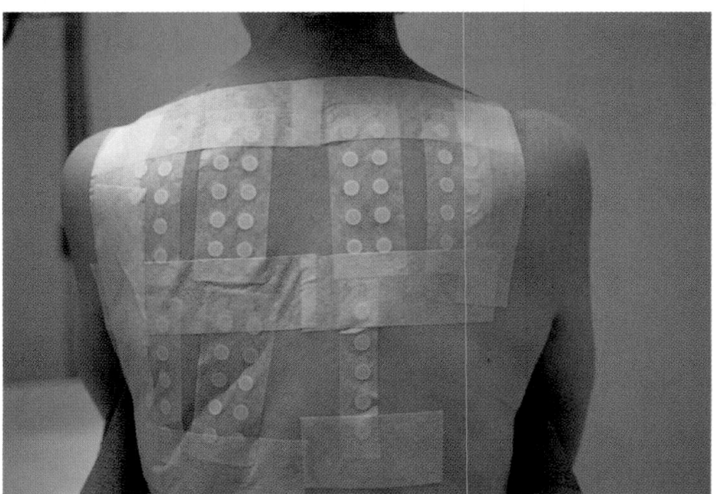

Figure 2.9 Finn chambers are pre-mounted on Scanpor tape (Norgesplaster, Kristiansand). Extra Scanpor tape is used to secure the patches against inadvertent removal.

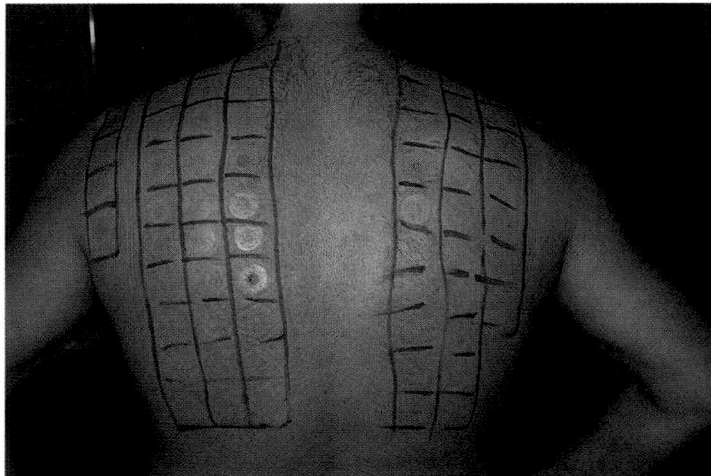

Figure 2.10 One method of keeping track of patch test locations is the use of various inks, as seen here. A Pilot Spotlighter pen is another marking device. The ink is visible under black light examination, but almost invisible otherwise.

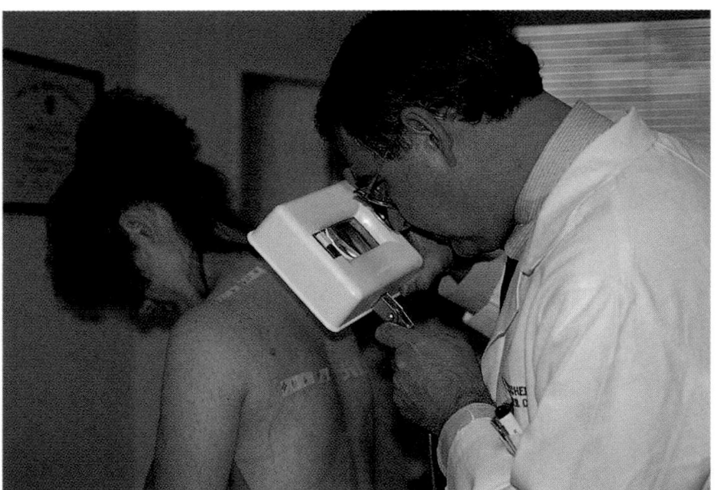

Figure 2.11 This shows the use of a black light device to check the location of specific patch tests. Patch tests are commonly read on day 2 and at various times after day 2 ranging from day 3 to day 7 (Rietschel et al, 1988).

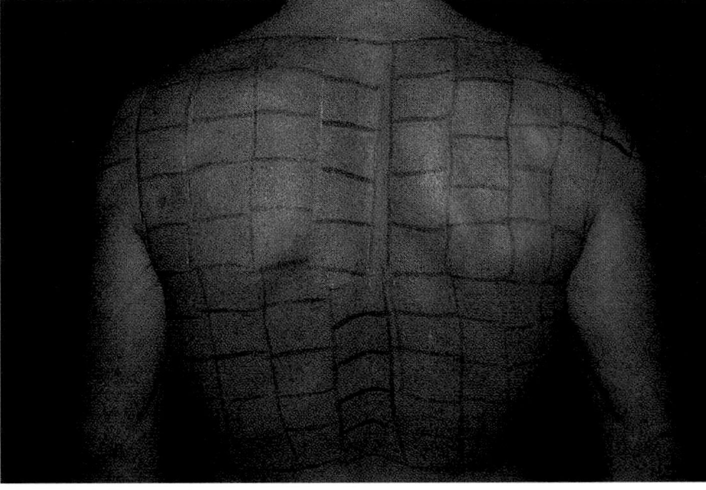

Figure 2.12 Reflex erythema is observed in some patients after carrying out the tests, but it disappears in a few hours.

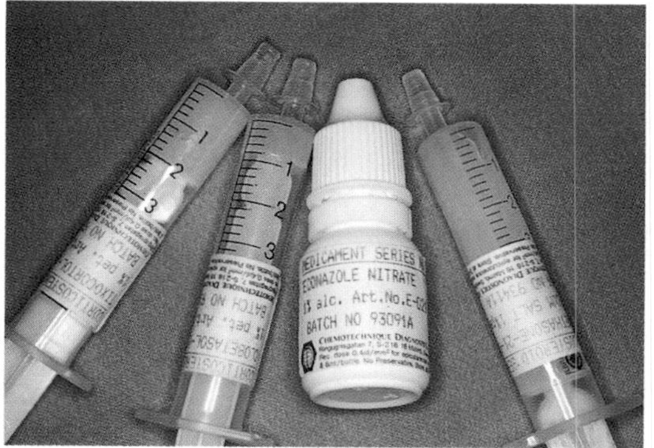

Figure 2.13 Various allergens prepared in petrolatum jelly, water or oil. The syringes and vessels should not contain contaminants.

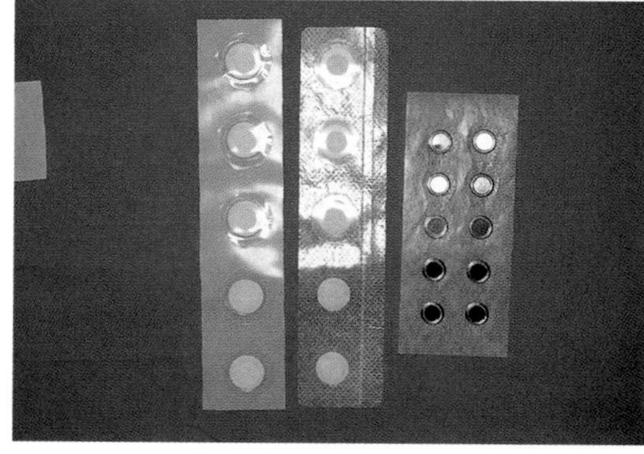

Figure 2.14 Various types of patches on which the allergen is placed.

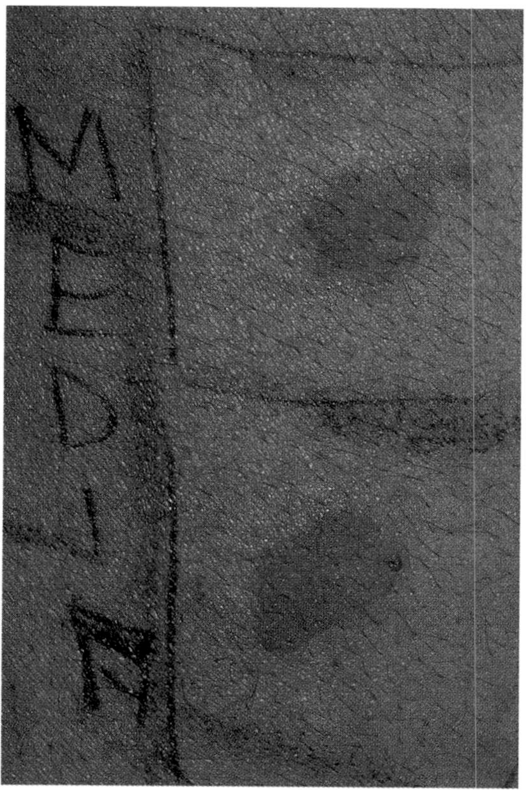

Figure 2.15 Patch test reaction confirming sensitization to disperse yellow and disperse orange, these being the dyes present in a stocking.

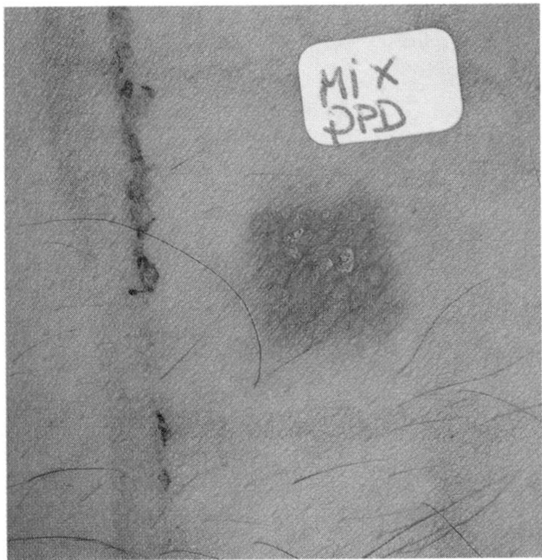

Figure 2.16 This positive reaction was scored a 1–2 plus. Positive reactions are scored 1, 2 or 3-plus, with 1 being a mild, 2 a moderate and 3 an extreme reaction. While morphological descriptions have been assigned to these numbers, it is clear that even experienced dermatologists do not apply these numbers in a uniform manner (Bruze et al, 1995).

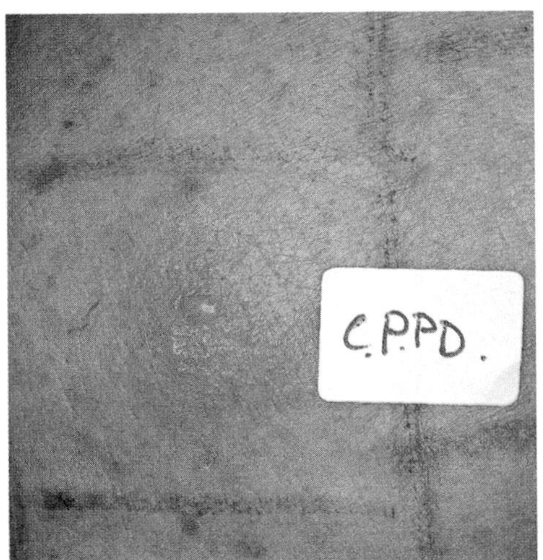

Figure 2.17 A 2-plus reaction.

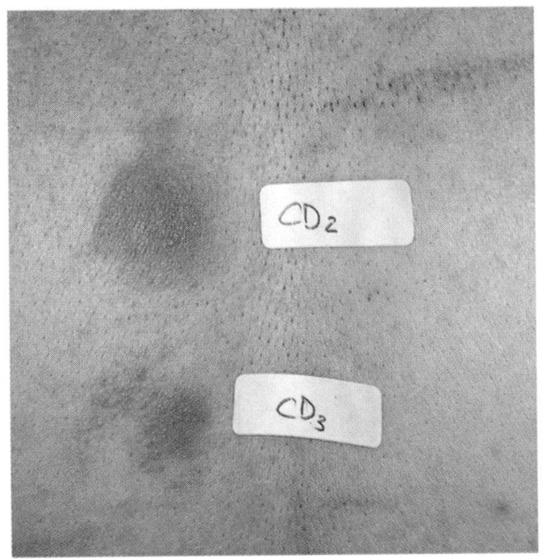

Figure 2.18 A 3-plus reaction.

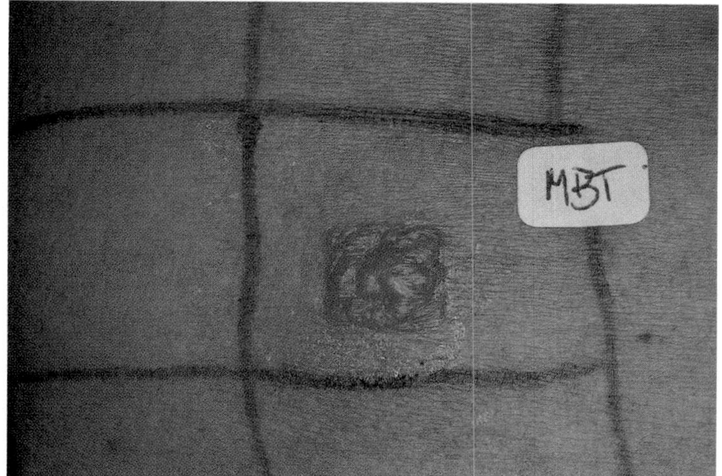

Figure 2.19 Patch test reaction to the allergen mercaptobenzothiazole, which was found to be present in the rubber cover of a suction device used by an amputee.

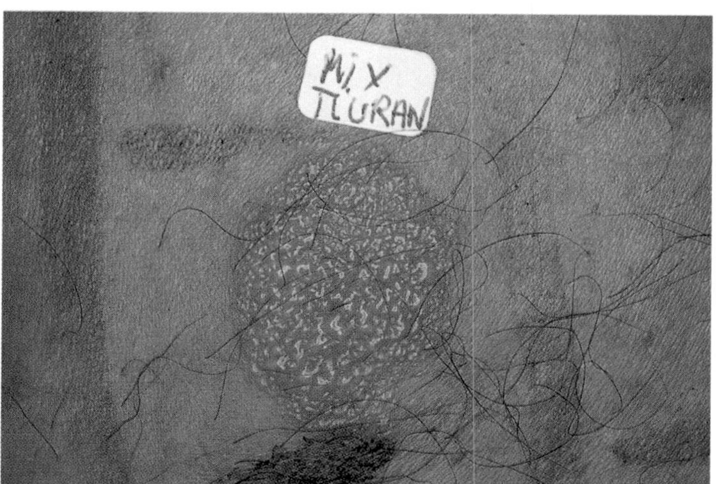

Figure 2.20 Patch test confirming allergy to thiuram mix.

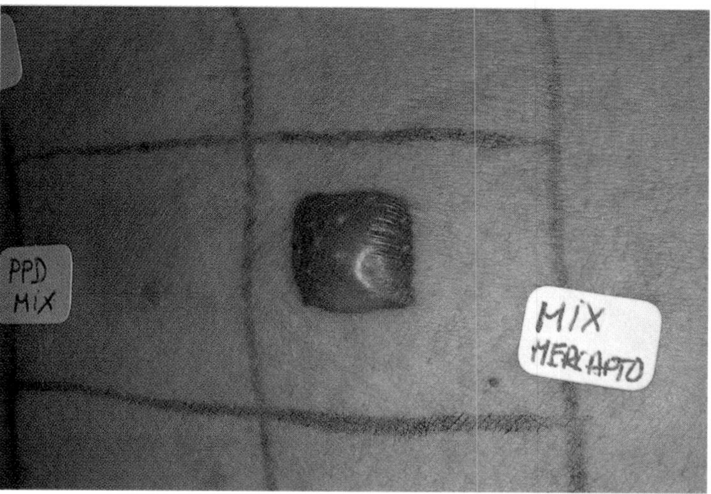

Figure 2.21 A bullous 3-plus reaction.

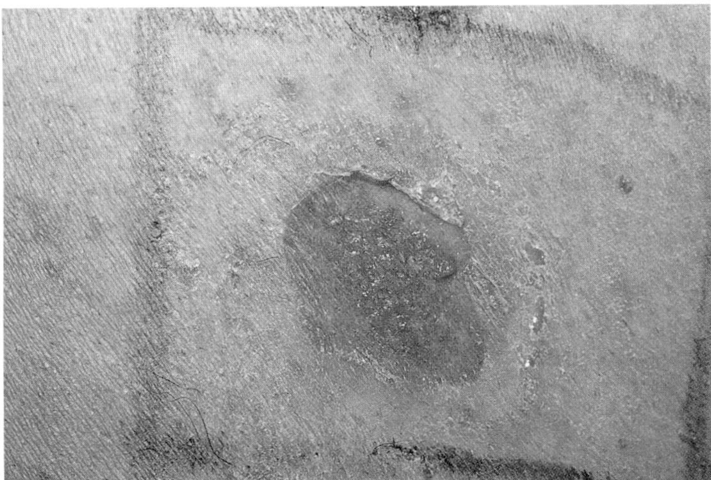

Figure 2.22 It is important to recognize artefacts and false information. This is an irritant reaction.

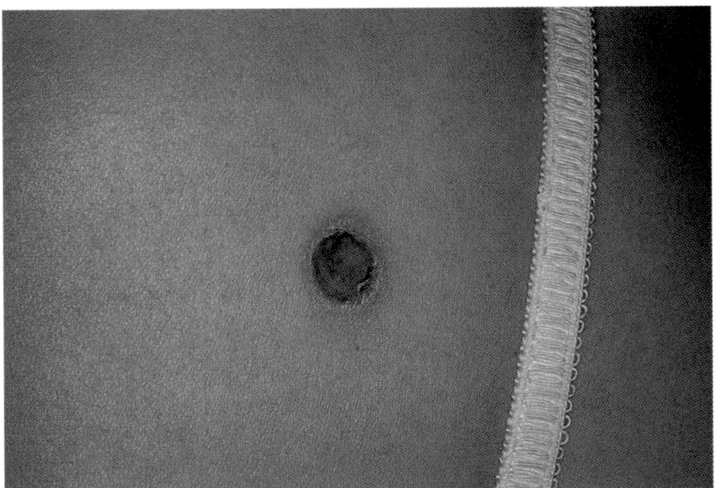

Figure 2.23 This is a gross irritant reaction to a non-standard allergen prepared by an inexperienced physician.

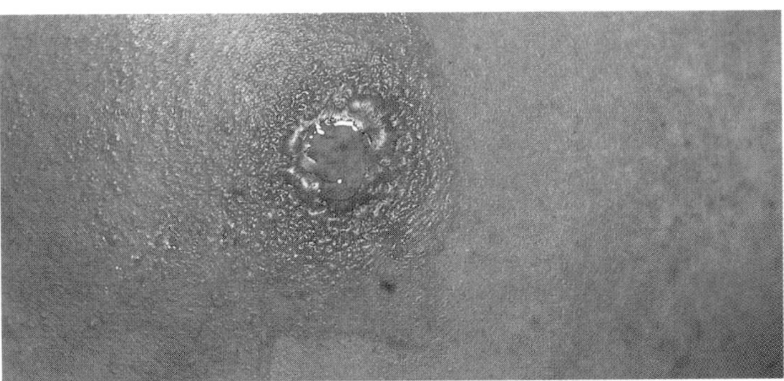

Figure 2.24 Sometimes a combined irritant and allergic patch test reaction can be observed. This chlorocresol-sensitive patient was tested with too high a concentration of this preservative agent.

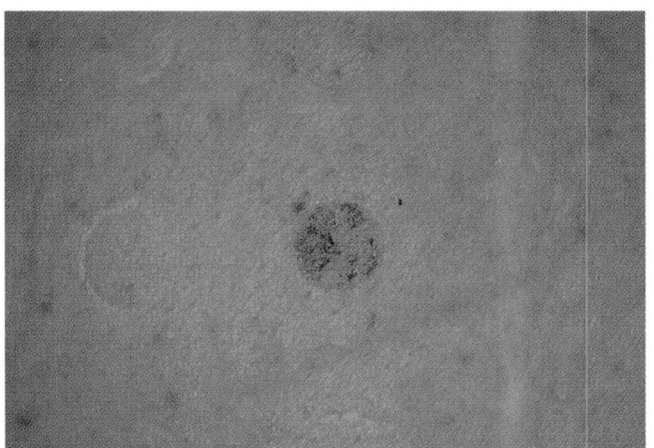

(**a**)

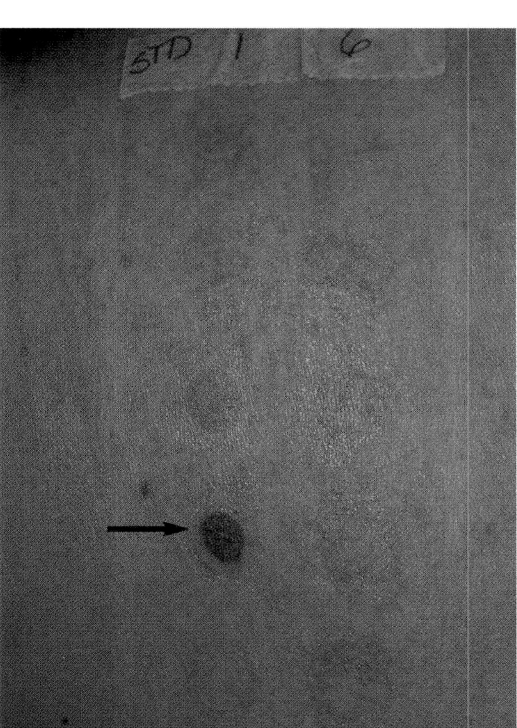

(**b**)

Figure 2.25 Staining of the skin can occur from some of the commonly tested substances. These are not signs of allergy: (**a**) shows a stain from balsam of Peru, which is occasionally seen; (**b**) shows the stain of paraphenylenediamine, which is expected and can be helpful in identifying patch test locations (arrow).

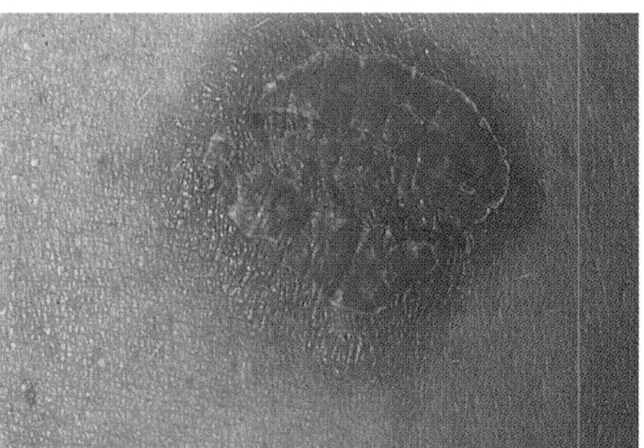

Figure 2.26 When testing new allergens, it is possible to encounter substances so allergenic that the patch test itself sensitizes rather than just eliciting allergy. Such was the case with this very reactive pharmaceutical intermediate, 3,4,6-trichloropyridazine. This is called primary sensitization.

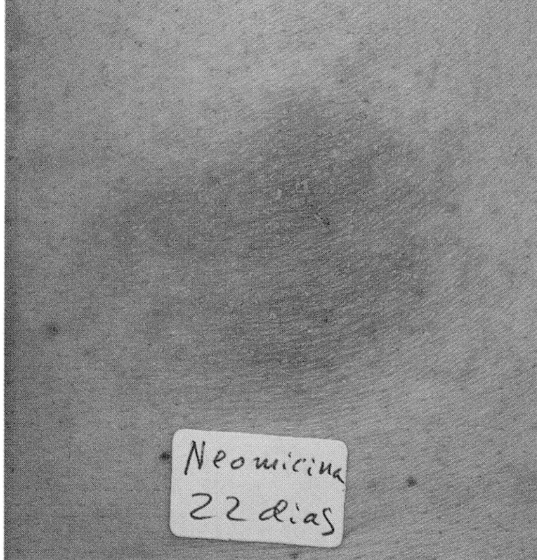

Figure 2.27 Primary sensitization by standard screening allergens is rare, but can occur, as seen here. This neomycin reaction occurred 22 days after the patch test was placed. Induction of new allergy generally takes 10–14 days. Patch test reactions that develop more than two weeks after the test was placed are usually considered examples of primary sensitization.

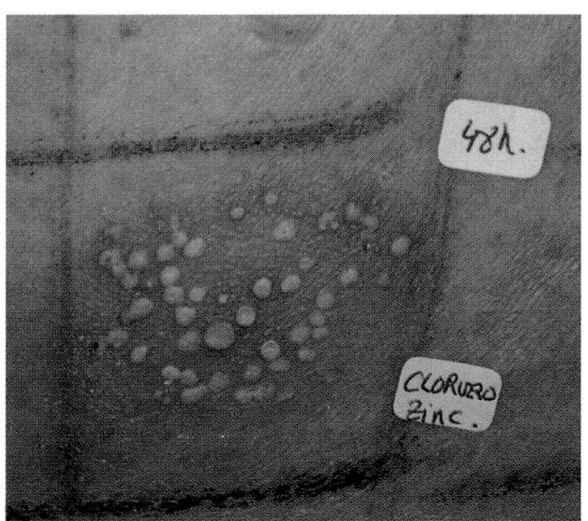

Figure 2.28 Pustular reactions are not a sign of allergy.

(**a**)

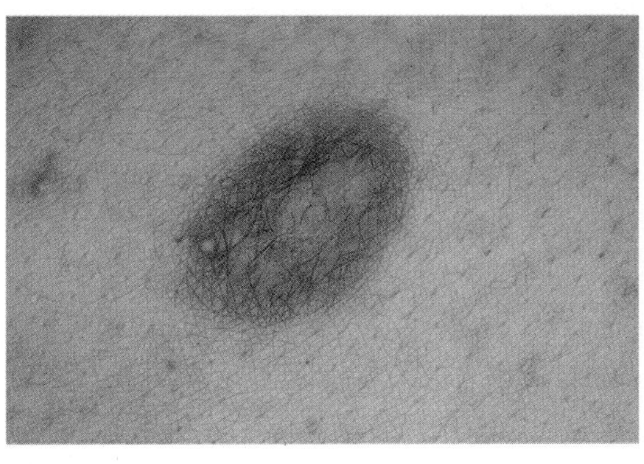

(**b**)

Figure 2.29 Complications of patch testing with standard screening series are rare: (**a**) post-inflammatory hypopigmentation; (**b**) a keloid that occurred at the site of the positive patch test.

Prick Test Technique

Patch testing is designed for the diagnosis of delayed-type hypersensitivity to substances that can penetrate the skin. Prick tests detect immediate-type hypersensitivity to allergens, usually proteins, with molecules that are often so large that it is necessary to damage the surface of the skin with the prick of a lancet to facilitate penetration of the allergen.

Allergens used for the prick test are dispersed in glycerol, and a drop is placed on the skin. Tape designed for this purpose is used as a template for the tests. A 1 mm lancet is then used to prick the skin through the drop of allergen in glycerol. For control purposes, a histamine prick test (10 mg/ml) and a saline prick test, both containing 50% glycerol, are made at the same time. Ideally, the histamine prick test will be positive and the saline prick test negative. Positive reactions to the allergens are read after 15–20 minutes, and are measured in relation to the histamine prick test in HEP (histamine-equivalent prick). A reaction measured to be 1 HEP is thus the size of the corresponding histamine prick test. This reaction is equal to the reactivity of the average patient sensitive to the allergen in question.

Prick tests are used primarily to detect the causes of respiratory allergy, but the tests are also relevant for dermatologists. Grass-allergic children with atopic dermatitis can experience aggravation of plantar dermatitis when playing on grass in bare feet. Facial dermatitis can follow contact with animal dander. Adults with atopic dermatitis who have positive prick tests to the yeast *Pityrosporum ovale* may exhibit 'head and neck dermatitis' (Kieffer et al, 1990). Repeated eruptions of contact urticaria may result in protein contact dermatitis, indistinguishable from other forms of chronic dermatitis. The latter is typically seen in food handlers and farmers (Hjorth and Roed-Petersen, 1976; Kanerva et al, 1996; Kanerva and Estlander, 1997). It is also a common complication of chronic hand dermatitis.

Typical inhalant allergens and typical food allergens are listed in the box on the following page.

In suspected occupational immediate-type hypersensitivity, a prick may be made through the suspected cause and then the skin.

A scratch-chamber test, possibly carried out at the site of the dermatitis, may be used to detect protein contact dermatitis. Such tests are difficult to read and should be interpreted with caution. A number of controls should be tested as well as the patient.

Typical inhalant allergens	Typical food allergens
Alternaria	Beef
Artemisia	Cod
Birch pollen	Egg
Cat dander	Milk
Dog dander	Oats
Grass pollen	Pork
Horse dander	Potato
House dust mites:	Rye flour
Dermatophagoides pteronyssimus	Wheat flour
Dermatophagoides farinae	
Pityrosporum ovale	

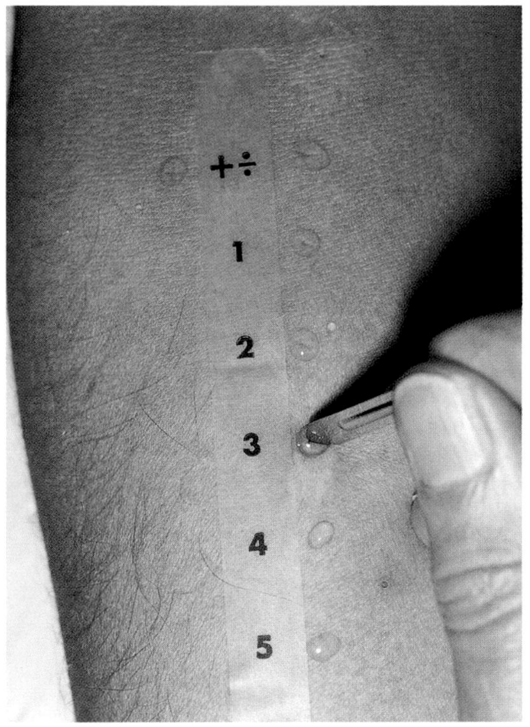

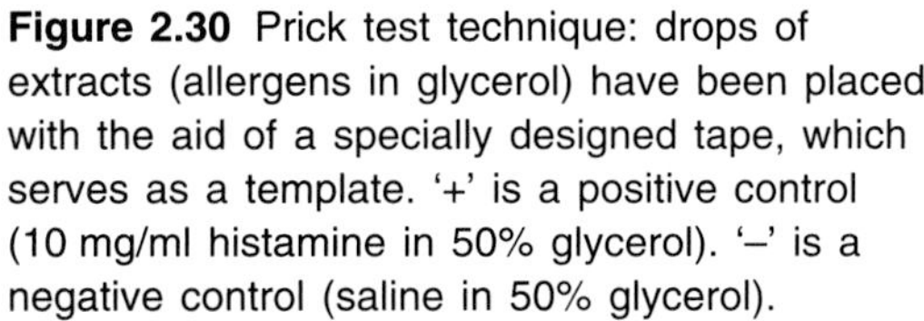
Figure 2.30 Prick test technique: drops of extracts (allergens in glycerol) have been placed with the aid of a specially designed tape, which serves as a template. '+' is a positive control (10 mg/ml histamine in 50% glycerol). '–' is a negative control (saline in 50% glycerol).

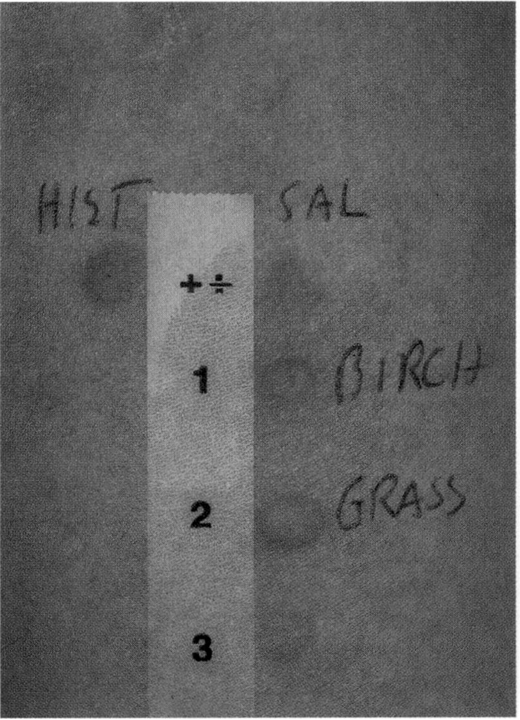

Figure 2.31 A positive histamine control and a negative saline control, and positive reactions to birch and grass pollen.

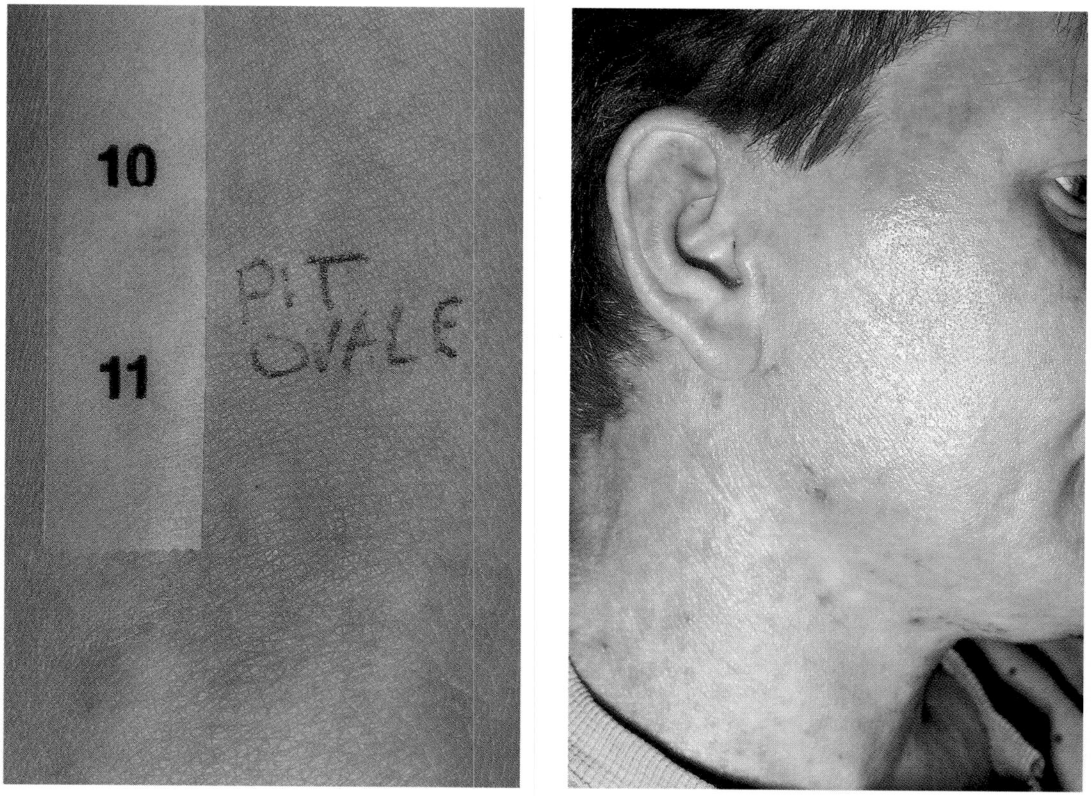

(a) (b)

Figure 2.32 (**a**) A positive prick test to *Pityrosporum ovale.* (**b**) An adult patient with atopic dermatitis and a head-and-neck pattern.

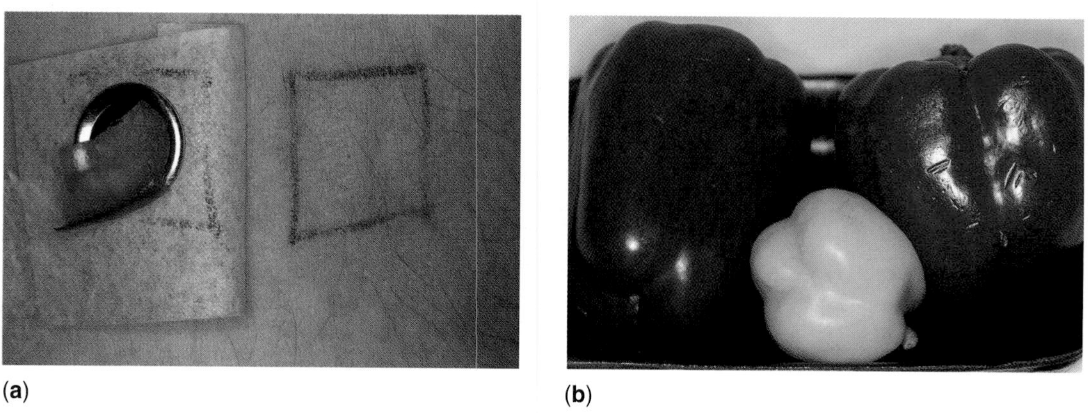

(a) (b)

Figure 2.33 (**a**) A positive scratch-chamber test to green pepper; (**b**) but not to other peppers.

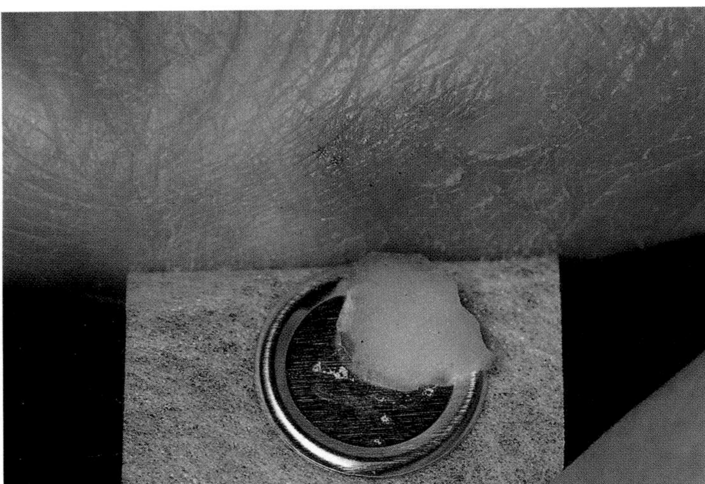

Figure 2.34 A scratch-chamber test with cod in a patient with protein contact dermatitis of the hands from cod. The test site is a finger with dermatitis.

REFERENCES

Bruze M, Isaksson M, Edman B et al (1995) A study on expert reading of patch test reactions: inter-individual accordance. *Contact Dermatitis* **32**:331–7.

Conde-Salazar L, Guimaraens D (1986) Pruebas epicutaneas. *Piel* **1**:45–50.

Hjorth N, Roed-Petersen J (1976) Occupational protein contact dermatitis in food handlers. *Contact Dermatitis* **2**:28–42.

Kanerva L, Estlander T (1997) Immediate and delayed skin allergy from cow dander. *Am J Contact Derm* **8**:167–9.

Kanerva L, Toikkanen J, Jolanki R, Estlander T (1996) Statistical data on occupational contact urticaria. *Contact Dermatitis* **35**:229–33.

Kieffer M, Bergbrant IM, Faergemann J et al (1990) Immune reactions to *Pityrosporum ovale* in adult patients with atopic and seborrheic dermatitis. *J Am Acad Dermatol* **22**:739–42.

Rietschel RL, Adams RM, Maibach HI et al (1988) The case for patch test readings beyond day 2. Notes from the lost and found department. *J Am Acad Dermatol* **18**:42–5.

TRUE Test Study Group (1989) Comparative multicenter studies with TRUE test and Finn chambers in eight Swedish hospitals. *J Am Acad Dermatol* **21**:846–9.

Wilkinson JD, Bruynzeel DP, Ducombs G et al (1990) European multicenter study of TRUE test, panel 2. *Contact Dermatitis* **22**:218–25.

3

Management of Contact Dermatitis

As in other fields of medicine, a correct diagnosis is required in order to establish a correct treatment plan. Irritant and allergic contact dermatitis share a common treatment strategy, namely avoidance of the irritant or allergen coupled with anti-inflammatory measures appropriate to the intensity of the dermatitis. Patch testing is done to establish the diagnosis of allergic contact dermatitis, and negative patch test results are a key component in the diagnosis of irritant contact dermatitis. Intentional patch testing with known irritants is not recommended, and proves nothing of value for either the patient or physician. Identification of an allergen can lead to proper protection, allergen substitution or allergen avoidance. Allergen substitution means identifying the offending chemical for a patient, such as a metalworking fluid that contains a biocide to which the patient reacts, and recommending an alternative fluid that contains a different biocide to which the patient is not sensitive.

In some cases of allergic contact dermatitis, such as that due to poison ivy, the diagnosis is not generally confirmed by patch testing, partly because of the lack of an available standard allergen, the possibility that a diagnostic test with this material is so potent that a non-sensitized individual may be sensitized by the diagnostic test, and the ease with which this diagnosis can usually be made without further testing. As most poison ivy cases are acute and self-limited, a distinction needs to be made between the management of this type of case and that of chronic or subacute cases.

ACUTE CONTACT DERMATITIS

Intense vesiculo-bullous dermatitis is usually accompanied by pruritus and actual oozing of serum through the inflamed areas. Laymen frequently assume that this fluid is capable of spreading the dermatitis, but this is not the case. Acute poison ivy dermatitis, for example, evolves over a period of 7–10 days, giving rise to the impression that the rash is 'spreading'. In fact, the area of greatest exposure or absorption of the allergen reacts first, and areas of lesser exposure develop into dermatitis more gradually. Physicians who are not familiar with this acute stage of contact dermatitis frequently assume the oozing to be a sign of infection. Secondary infection of contact dermatitis can occur, but is usually marked by purulence rather than clear serous drainage.

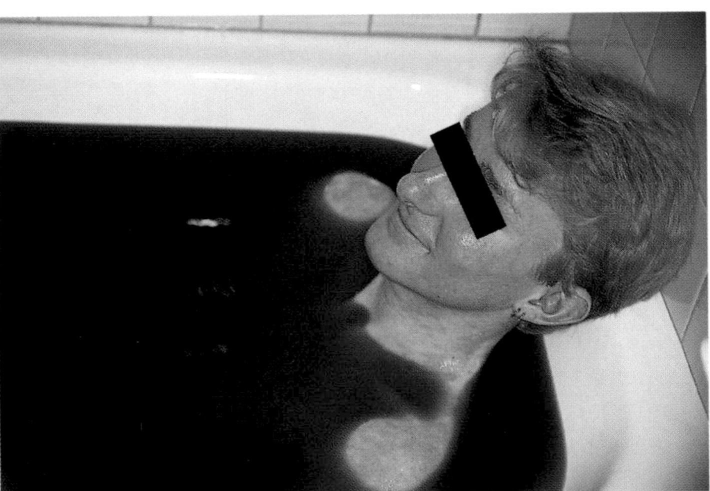

Figure 3.1 A 16-year-old boy with widespread acute dermatitis, in a potassium permanganate bath.

Oedema and erythema accompany the vesicles and bullae, and this inflamed area is warmer than the surrounding skin. Microscopically, vasodilatation is seen, and transudation of inflammatory cells into the dermis and subsequently the epidermis occurs. The release of mediators of inflammation by these cells leads to the vesiculation that is seen macroscopically. This pathophysiological change can be addressed with a very simple and inexpensive treatment: the compress. The basis for a compress is the removal of heat by the process of evaporation. Heat is required to convert water from the liquid to the gaseous state. This heat comes from the skin, leaving it cooler and triggering vasoconstriction, which in turn decreases the transudation of cells and serum from the cutaneous vasculature. A porous cloth is dampened and placed over the inflamed area and the water is allowed to evaporate. Tapwater compresses are the least expensive, but frequently Burow's solution (1 part to 20 parts water) is used. Burow's solution is based on aluminium subacetate, and has antiseptic and astringent properties. Compresses are repeated three or four times a day for several days or until the surface of the skin is no longer oozing. Other such solutions, such as potassium permanganate (1:10 000) may also be used. Potassium permanganate oxidizes protein and acts as a disinfectant. It can be used in bath water, but may stain the tub (Figure 3.1). Shake lotions such as calamine lotion produce evaporative cooling, and contain a powder to absorb the transudate.

Topical corticosteroids are generally inadequate for the management of acute contact dermatitis, and systemic corticosteroids are the drugs of choice. This is in large part due to the self-limiting nature of the condition. Poison ivy left untreated usually lasts for three or four weeks. If the area of exposure is small, and the symptoms mild, it is appropriate to use the most potent topical corticosteroids, but if the area is extensive, or involves the eyelids or other areas where normal function is compromised, a better treatment is prednisone (or an equivalent corticosteroid) in a dose of 1 mg/kg for 3–7 days, tapered over a period of 7–14 days.

Acutely, intramuscular corticosteroids may be added to the above treatment to provide a more rapid onset of action. Antihistamines do not decrease the inflammation of acute contact dermatitis, but the soporific effect of some older antihistamines can be helpful at bedtime, when pruritus is more bothersome.

SUBACUTE AND CHRONIC CONTACT DERMATITIS

Although systemic corticosteroids are useful in acute disease, they are to be avoided in chronic disease as much as possible, since unwelcome side-effects are likely in this setting. Patch testing and other diagnostic tests are critical to proper management of these cases. Cool compresses are of limited value here, since the dermatitis may be dry and scaly, and further drying with compresses will only increase pruritus and perpetuate the dermatitis. Generally, compresses will only be needed if the condition is subacute.

Topical corticosteroids are the backbone of treatment, coupled with avoidance of all known irritants or allergens. The selection of a proper topical corticosteroid is based on the intensity of the dermatitis, the body site to be treated, and possible allergy to the vehicle ingredients or the corticosteroid itself. Lotions, solutions or spray forms of corticosteroids are used for the scalp, but many of these preparations contain alcohol and can sting when applied to open or excoriated dermatitis. The face is generally treated with non-fluorinated, low-potency corticosteroids to avoid such side-effects as steroid rosacea or cutaneous atrophy. Similar selections are made for flexural sites such as the axillae or inguinal regions, where striae are another possible complication of over-aggressive corticosteroid use.

Dermatitis on the hands commonly requires potent corticosteroids. This is due to both the intensity of exposure to which the hands are subjected and the thickness of the stratum corneum in this location. A common problem seen on the palmar surfaces of the hands and fingers in chronic contact dermatitis is fissuring. This produces pain rather than pruritus. A simple treatment that can rapidly reduce this pain is to place a small drop of cyanoacrylate glue into the fissure. This provides a tough layer of protection and immediate relief of pain. The skin expels the glue in a few days. The skin on the dorsum of the hands is much more prone to atrophy from long-term corticosteroid use than palmar skin. It is thinner, and is exposed to other atrophogens, such as the sun. Some patients have the habit of spreading excess topical corticosteroid all over the hands by rubbing them together after application of the preparation to the area of dermatitis. This practice should be discouraged when the patient is instructed about the treatment (Figure 3.2).

The selection of a cream or ointment vehicle for the corticosteroid may be based on patient preference if allergy to vehicle ingredients is not a concern. Creams contain preservatives, which may be an issue if patch testing has not been performed to evaluate the possibility of allergy, whereas ointments do not require preservatives and generally have simpler formulas. However, the greasy

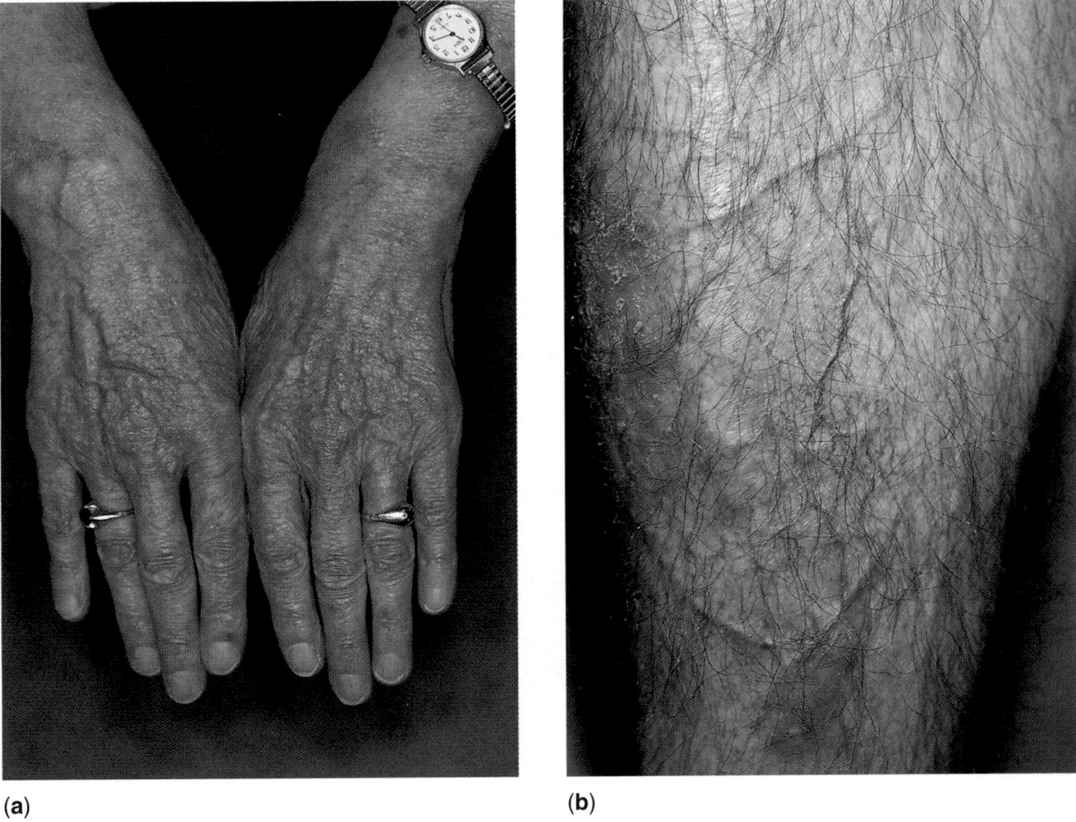

(a) (b)

Figure 3.2 (**a**) Atrophy of the skin of the dorsal aspects of the hands after misuse of topical corticosteroids. (**b**) Atrophy of the skin of the lower legs after long-term use of a high-potency topical corticosteroid.

nature of ointments may be intolerable in certain job settings. Propylene glycol may be added to some ointments to increase potency by increasing steroid solubility, and this may be of concern in patients where this allergen is under consideration as part of the problem. Ointments are less likely to cause stinging than creams, and are a better choice for dry, fissured dermatitis, particularly hand and foot dermatitis. Creams have a more-soothing effect when rubbed on dermatitis, and this may be a deciding factor. For practical reasons, creams or fatty creams can be used during the day, and ointments at bedtime.

Enhanced potency of the topical corticosteroid may be necessary for resolution of refractory areas of dermatitis. This can be achieved by an occlusive plastic wrap applied overnight on top of the corticosteroid. This warms and moisturizes the skin, leading to enhanced absorption. Plastic gloves are available for this purpose when the hands require a boost in treatment potency. Table 3.1 provides some examples of corticosteroids and their common uses, and Table 3.2 shows the classification of topical corticosteroids.

Table 3.1 Examples and common uses of corticosteroids

Setting	Comments	Corticosteroid
Face, axilla, groin	Low-potency drugs preferred	Aclometasone dipropionate; hydrocortisone base, acetate, valerate or butyrate; desonide
Torso, extremities, but not face or flexors	Maintenance therapy	Triamcinolone acetonide, fluocinolone acetonide, betamethasone valerate, desoxymethasone, fluandrenolone
Body or hand dermatitis	Subacute therapy	Fluocinonide, halcinonide, amcinonide, betamethasone dipropionate, clobetasone butyrate
Body or hand dermatitis	Acute therapy, resistant dermatitis, short-term treatment	Clobetasol propionate, diflorasone diacetate, augmented betamethasone dipropionate, diflucortolone valerate

IRRITANT CONTACT DERMATITIS

The backbone of the treatment of irritant contact dermatitis can be summed up as maintaining cutaneous integrity. The goal is to restore the barrier function of the stratum corneum by elimination of those irritants that caused disruption in the first place, and promotion of healing, often by maintaining proper stratum corneum hydration. Frequent exposure to moisture can macerate the stratum corneum, leading to chapping and allowing minor irritants, solvents, soaps or detergents to enter the epidermis and trigger inflammatory events.

Protection with gloves may be effective if the glove selected can actually keep the offending substance from contacting the skin. Common notorious allergens such as nickel, paraphenylenediamine and the acrylates will readily pass through rubber gloves. If a specific irritant is identified, industrial hygiene texts provide information on the protection afforded by gloves of differing composition. Glove wearing should be as brief and targeted as possible, to prevent moisture buildup within the glove and subsequent maceration. Cotton liners to assist with moisture retention are favoured by some physicians, but it should be remembered that cotton is absorbent and may absorb and hold onto an offending substance, leading to counterproductive effects (Rietschel, 1984).

Table 3.2 Classification of topical corticosteroids

Level of potency	Preparations
Low potency	Hydrocortisone, hydrocortisone acetate, hydrocortisone valerate
Moderate potency	Aclometasone dipropionate, clobetasone butyrate, hydrocortisone buteprat (Europe), hydrocortisone butyrate, triamcinolone acetonide
High potency	Betamethasone dipropionate, betamethasone valerate, desoximethasone, diflucortolone valerate, diflurasone diacetate (Europe), fluocinolone acetonide, fluocinonide, fluticasone propionate, mometasone furoate
Extra-high potency	Augmented betamethasone dipropionate, clobetasone dipropionate, diflorasone diacetate ointment (USA), halcinonide (Europe), halobetasol propionate (USA)

Barrier creams may promote hygiene, and as such they may provide limited benefit in circumstances where dirt, grit or soil are thought to be the primary irritants. The notion that barrier creams can function as invisible gloves is not supported by scientific study. When barrier products have been successful, this has generally been when a specific product was used for a very specific irritant or even allergen. Such is the case for quaternium 18-bentonite and poison ivy (Marks et al, 1995) or for 10% ascorbic acid for chromate (Valsecchi and Cainelli, 1984).

Moisturizers can assist in the restoration of the stratum corneum and the maintenance of plasticity, which is key to avoiding chapping. Glycerol-based moisturizers are well tolerated and generally effective. Buffered lactic acid- or urea-containing products are effective, but may irritate already inflamed skin.

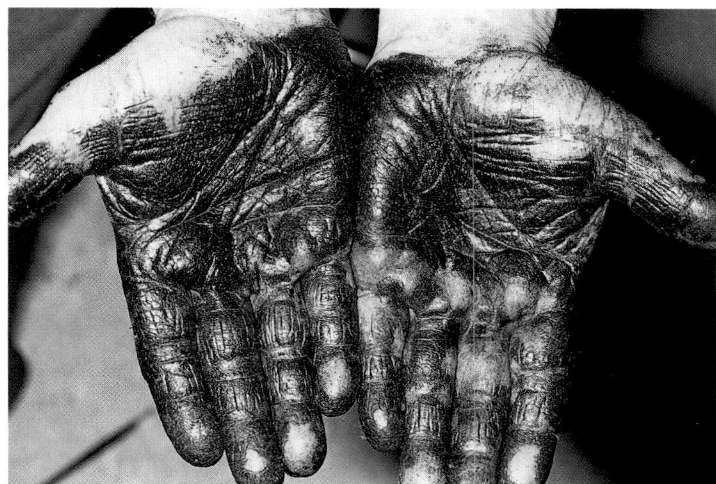

Figure 3.3 Crude coal tar used to treat chronic palmar dermatitis in a 57-year-old man. Such treatment is best suited to in-patients.

The role of corticosteroids in irritant contact dermatitis has been studied, since it has been questioned whether their anti-inflammatory activity is helpful (Van de Valk and Maibach, 1989). One study found that simultaneous application of irritant with triamcinolone acetonide showed the ability of the corticosteroid to diminish the irritant reaction (Rietschel, 1985). This study involved grossly visible irritant reactions. Much of the literature challenging the benefit of corticosteroids is based on irritant reactions of such mild intensity that instrumentation is necessary to evaluate the invisible to barely visible reactions. This type of study is helpful for understanding basic mechanisms, but does not address the same problem as encountered in the clinic. Nevertheless, a recent study found benefit to betamethasone 17-valerate in the treatment of experimentally induced irritant reactions (Ramsing and Agner, 1995).

NON-CORTICOSTEROID MANAGEMENT

Tar ointments have a modest anti-inflammatory effect. Crude coal tar is effective for chronic dermatitis, but it stains and smells (Figure 3.3).

Grenz ray treatment is very effective for chronic dermatitis of allergic or endogenous origin. Its benefit for irritant dermatitis has been questioned (Lindelöf and Lindberg, 1987). The treatment is palliative rather than curative, but may induce remissions lasting several months. One treatment schedule is 2 Gray, repeated weekly for two to three weeks. Grenz ray machines are not commonly found in dermatologists' clinics today, but photochemotherapy with PUVA is more widely available and also useful (Rosen et al, 1987). PUVA does not have as strong a stigma as X-ray therapy for benign conditions, but it is more cumbersome than Grenz ray treatment. The oral medication used in PUVA, 8-methoxypsoralen, can cause nausea and transient photosensitivity, which is not encountered with Grenz ray treatment, and PUVA requires frequent maintenance therapy. In selected cases this treatment option may eliminate the need for systemic corticosteroid treatment. As PUVA is generally administered in a physician's clinic, travel, sick leave and inconvenience are issues in the decision to offer a patient this treatment. Also, outdoor occupations or activities can limit the use of PUVA as a treatment option. Topical PUVA tends to be disappointing for these individuals.

REFERENCES

Lindelöf B, Lindberg M (1987) The effects of Grenz rays on the expression of allergic contact dermatitis in man. *Acta Derm Venereol (Stockh)* **67**:128–32.

Marks JG Jr, Fowler JF Jr, Sheretz EF, Rietschel RL (1995) Prevention of poison ivy and poison oak allergic contact dermatitis by quaternium-18 bentonite. *J Am Acad Dermatol* **33**:212–6.

Ramsing DW, Agner T (1995) Efficacy of topical corticosteroids on irritant skin reactions. *Contact Dermatitis* **32**:293–7.

Rietschel RL (1984) Role of socks in shoe dermatitis. *Arch Dermatol* **120**:398.

Rietschel RL (1985) Irritant and allergic response as influenced by triamcinolone in patch test materials. *Arch Dermatol* **121**: 68–9.

Rosen K, Mobacken H, Swanbeck G (1987) Chronic eczematous dermatitis of the hands: a comparison of PUVA and UVB treatment. *Acta Derm Venereol (Stockh)* **67**:48–54.

Valsecchi R, Cainelli T (1984) Chromium dermatitis and ascorbic acid. *Contact Dermatitis* **10**:252–3.

Van der Valk PGM, Maibach HI (1989) Do topical corticosteroids modulate skin irritation in human beings? Assessment by transepidermal water loss and visual scoring. *J Am Acad Dermatol* **21**:519–22.

4

Contact Dermatitis by Specific Body Region

Contact dermatitis can be confined to specific anatomical regions because of the nature of the intended use of a product or by unintentional transfer from the hands to another anatomical site (Dooms-Goossens et al, 1986; Veien, 1995). This section of the Atlas is intended to give the reader a flavour of the patterns encountered based on location as well as on the nature and intensity of the elicited reaction. A statistical correlation has been found between some contact allergens and certain body sites. Fragrance mix correlated with axillary dermatitis, balsam of Peru with facial dermatitis, and lanolin and neomycin with dermatitis of the lower legs (Dooms-Goossens, 1993).

CORRELATION BETWEEN SENSITIZATION SOURCE AND SITE OF CONTACT DERMATITIS LESIONS

Contact allergens may reach the skin in several ways (Dooms-Goossens et al, 1986; Dooms-Goossens, 1993):

- by intentional application of the allergen;
- by direct contact with an allergenic or allergen-contaminated surface;
- by exposure to gases, droplets or particles in the atmosphere, which results in 'airborne' dermatitis;
- by contact with spouses, partners, friends or colleagues who convey the allergens, to cause 'connubial' or 'consort' dermatitis;
- by transfer from other sites on the body, generally the hands, to more sensitive areas such as lips or eyelids, which is called 'ectopic' dermatitis;
- by systemic exposure in previously sensitized patients, the result being a flare-up reaction on a previously affected site or elsewhere, as is the case with vesicular hand eczema;
- in combination with exposure to the sun, as is the case with photoallergens;
- moreover, id-like spreads of a contact dermatitis reaction may occur elsewhere on the body.

In general, the contact dermatitis occurs in the area of the skin that is in direct contact with the causal substance, and, if it is allergic, generally extends beyond the specific limits of the application of the allergen.

Table 4.1 Main sources of contact dermatitis by body region

Scalp
- Hair-care products, including the instruments used, such as brushes and hair curlers

Face and eyelids
- In general: cosmetics, cosmetic appliances, topical pharmaceutical products
- Forehead: head coverings, hair-care products, sweatbands
- Eyebrows: protective masks, swimming goggles, eyebrow tweezers, eyebrow pencils
- Upper eyelids: eye make-up, eyelash curlers, hair-care products
- Lower eyelids: eye make-up, topical pharmaceutical products, contact lens solutions
- Bridge of the nose: spectacle frames, face masks, goggles
- Cheeks: cosmetics, shaving products, protective masks, pillows
- Nostrils and area under the nose: nasal medication, drugs, snuff, handkerchiefs (perfumed), depilatory agents
- Lips: lipstick, topical and oral pharmaceutical products, foods, drinks (and their packaging), spices, tobacco, any object that can be put into the mouth (e.g. pacifiers and toys), dental products, masks and probes, mouthpieces of musical instruments
- Chin: shaving products, hat straps, chin rests

Ears
- In general: hair-care products, pharmaceutical products
- Helix: hairdressing products, hearing aids, telephone receivers, helmets
- Auditory meatus: ear plugs, matches, pins, paper clips
- Behind the ears: spectacle earpieces, hearing aids, perfumes, fur collars
- Ear lobe: earrings, perfume

Neck
- Cosmetic products, perfumes, shaving products, clothes, accessories such as jewellery and scarves

Trunk and axillae
- Clothing and clothing accessories containing formaldehyde, resins, rubber and nickel; personal hygiene products (e.g. deodorants and antiperspirants); perfumes

Arms
- Clothing (especially in the elbow flexures), elbow rests, table surfaces (e.g. plasticized cloth)

Extremities and genitalia
- Clothing (especially in elbow flexures), stockings, elbow rests, table surfaces (e.g. plasticized cloth)
- Condoms, personal hygiene products (e.g. deodorants and sanitary towels), spermicidal preparations, medicaments, seminal fluid, substances on the hands transferred to the genitals

Hands
- Gloves, occupational chemicals, plants, skin-care products, solvents

Nails
- Nail-care products, occupational chemicals

Feet
- Footwear, medicaments, socks

In occupational dermatitis, it is important to relate the specific occupational exposure and the topography of the lesions to each other (for example, tool handling involves specific areas of the palms of the hands). Nevertheless, there are situations where the allergic contact dermatitis does not occur at the actual contact site. Thus the lesion topography can be strongly influenced by factors that influence the penetration of the allergen. For example, a hand dermatitis caused by liquids or powders is often located on the backs of the hands and the lower arms, but not on the palms, which have a particularly thick corneal layer. In the same way, even though an allergen may be manipulated by the hands, the allergic dermatitis may occur only on the face or specifically on the upper eyelids, where the skin is particularly delicate. This is typical for an allergy to nail polish, but it is also seen with allergies to chemicals that are handled in an occupational context.

Airborne dermatitis (see Chapter 5) is characterized by the occurrence of the dermatitis on areas exposed to the air, which often makes it difficult to differentiate from photodermatitis, and often by symmetry (e.g. eyelids, neck, backs of the hands). However, reactions to remote body sites (id-like spread), as well as 'endogenous' contact dermatitis reactions caused by systemic exposure to the allergen, are also often symmetrical.

The main sources of contact dermatitis reactions for specific regions of the body are given in Table 4.1.

Face and Scalp

The face is among the most common sites of contact dermatitis. It is exposed to airborne allergens and irritants, and is a typical site of photocontact dermatitis. Skin-care products and cosmetics are the most frequent causes of contact dermatitis of the face, together with many substances (e.g. occupational and plant allergens) transferred from the hand to the face. Studies have found the fragrance and preservative ingredients of cosmetics to be the chief causes of allergic contact dermatitis, while the causes of irritant contact dermatitis include cleansers, astringents, acne medications and rejuvenating creams. Although a less common site of contact dermatitis, the scalp may also be affected. The most common allergens are given in the box below.

Allergens

Cosmetics
Fragrances
Hair colour
Permanent wave chemicals
Preservatives

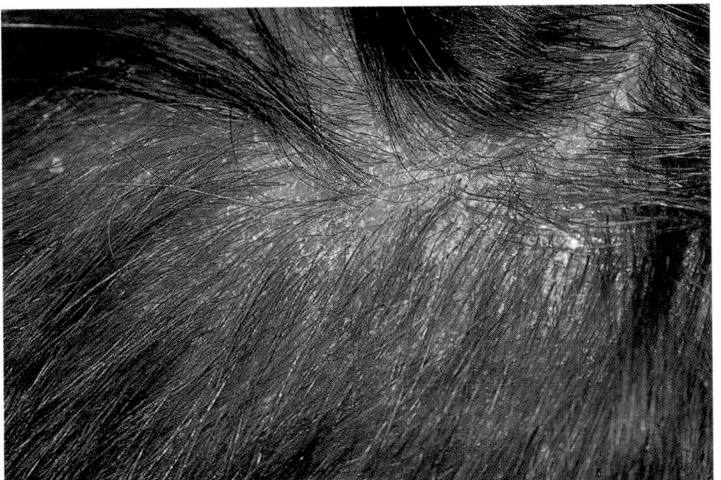

(**a**)

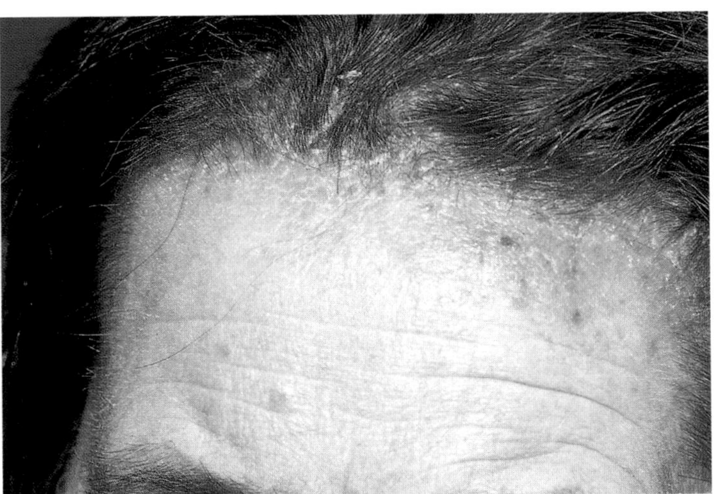

(**b**)

Figure 4.1 Cases of (**a**) severe contact dermatitis and (**b**) allergic contact dermatitis of the scalp, both caused by hair dye containing paraphenylenediamine.

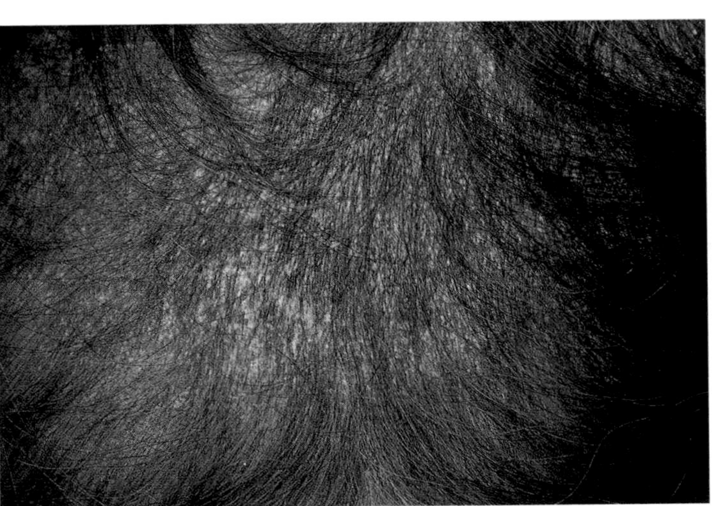

Figure 4.2 Tinea amiantacea-like dermatitis (severe desquamation and hair loss), caused by a setting lotion.

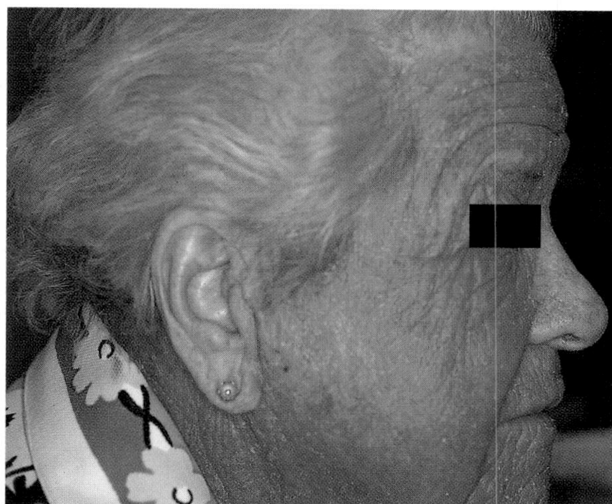

Figure 4.3 The face may react with an even intensity, as seen in this reaction due to the preservative in a popular facial moisturizer. The even distribution is due in part to even and intentional application to the face. No areas of enhanced or diminished reactivity are seen. Cosmetics are common causes of facial dermatitis (Edman, 1985).

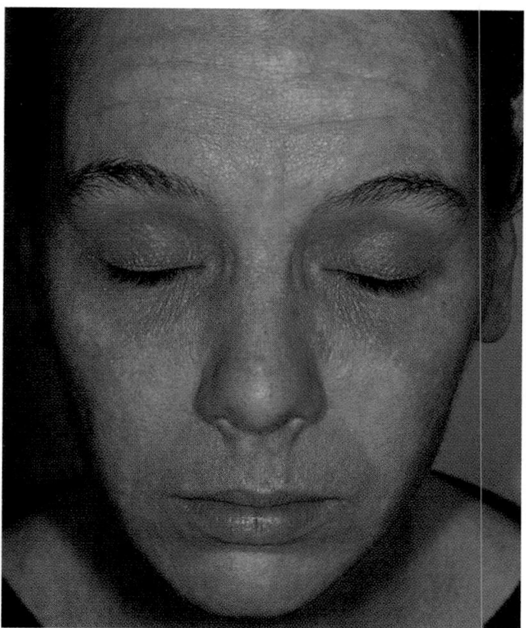

Figure 4.4 In contrast to Figure 4.3, a different level of reactivity is seen across the face, even though the application of a lanolin-containing cosmetic was made to the entire face. A greater degree of reactivity is seen around the eyelid skin, to a lesser degree the perioral skin, and the facial creases. A positive patch test to lanolin identified the source of this eruption.

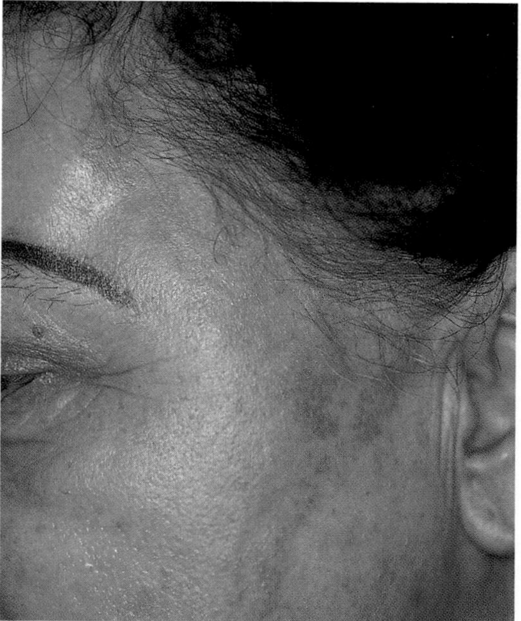

Figure 4.5 At times, the face erupts from contact with items applied intentionally to other body regions. This eruption near the hairline occurred in a 66-year-old woman who dyed her hair, and presented with pruritus, erythema and dermatitis of the scalp and adjacent hairline. Patch testing showed a reaction to the hair dye, paraphenylenediamine.

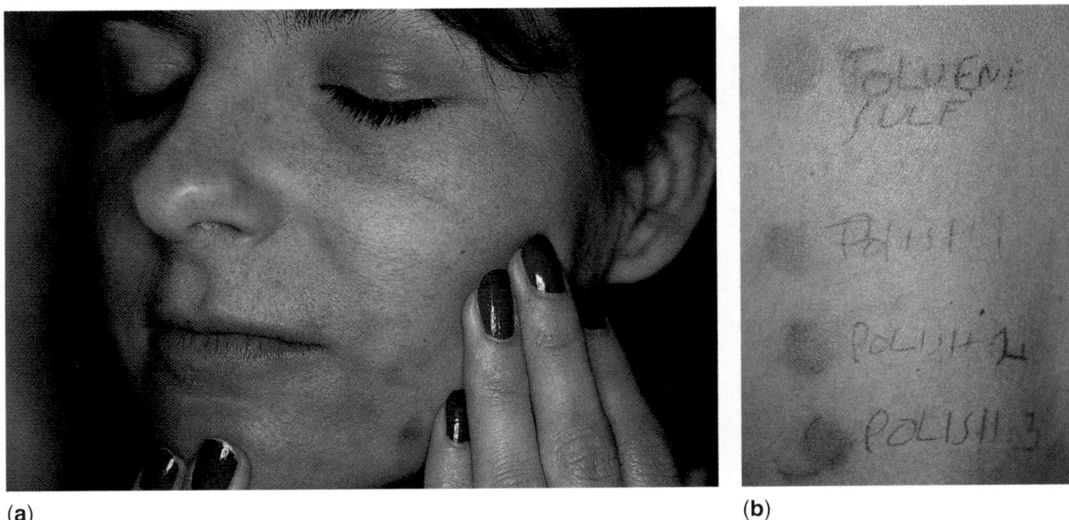

(a) (b)

Figure 4.6 Facial dermatitis and eyelid dermatitis may be caused by allergens in nail polish that do not cause dermatitis of the periungual area. If carefully applied, the nail polish does not necessarily produce dermatitis on the thicker skin of the fingers. When the fingers touch the skin of the face and eyelids, however, dermatitis may develop in these areas. (**a**) An example is seen in this 28-year-old woman, who was sensitive to toluenesulfonamide–formaldehyde resin (this product has recently been renamed tosylamide–formaldehyde resin). Her positive patch test reactions are seen in (**b**). The ectopic nature of this dermatitis can easily lead to misdiagnosis and prolonged morbidity. In a Swedish study of 18 patients with this form of contact dermatitis, it was seen that 9 of the 18 were placed on sick leave for a period of time ranging from two weeks to seven months, 2 changed jobs thinking their dermatitis was work related, 4 were hospitalized and 2 lost their jobs – all because of misdiagnosis (Liden et al, 1993).

EYELIDS

Dermatitis of the eyelids is commonly, but not always, due to contact dermatitis (Nethercott et al, 1989; Valsecchi et al, 1992). At times, only the upper eyelid is dermatitic, and an upper eyelid dermatitis syndrome (UEDS) has been proposed (Rietschel and Fowler, 1995, p.307). The differential diagnosis of the UEDS includes psoriasis, atopic dermatitis, contact urticaria, secondary effects of conjunctivitis or blephritis, irritant reactions, allergic contact dermatitis, collagen-vascular disease, low-grade streptococcal infection, photoirritation due to oral medication, dermatitis secondary to repeated rubbing, and finally, idiopathic reaction. The most common contact allergens are given in the box on the following page.

Allergens

Cosmetics
Fingernail polish
Medications
Nickel or rubber on eyelash curlers

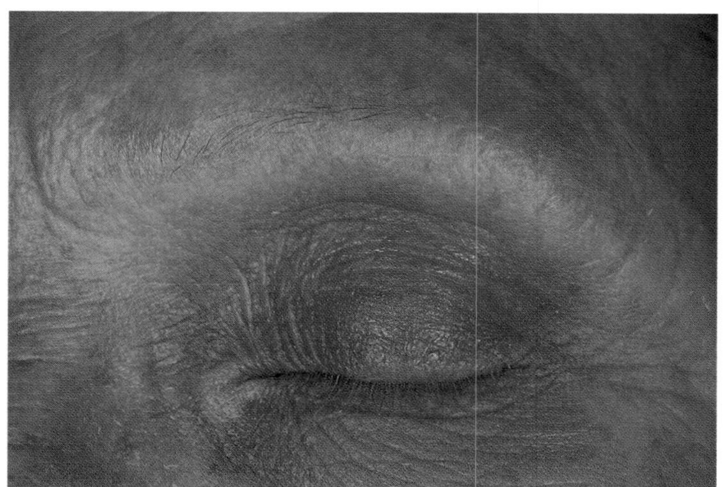

(**a**)

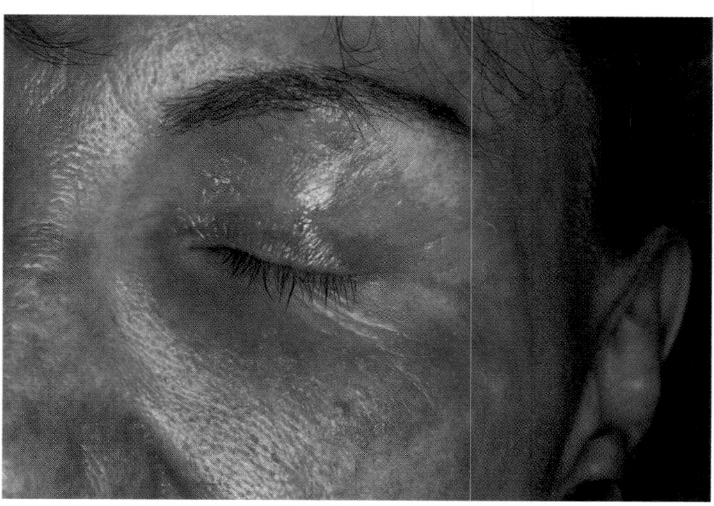

(**b**)

Figure 4.7 (**a**) The mild inflammation seen on the upper eyelid is typical of the upper eyelid dermatitis syndrome (UEDS). In this case, patch tests were negative, and atopic dermatitis was the suspected cause. (**b**) In contrast to (**a**), this dermatitis involved both upper and lower eyelids, and was traced to a mascara used by the patient.

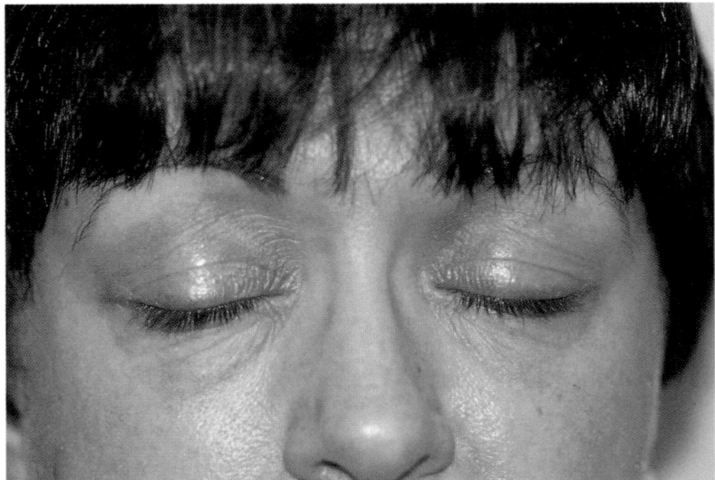

Figure 4.8 Eyelid dermatitis is not always due to materials applied intentionally to the eyelids. This dermatitis was due to allergic contact dermatitis from the rubber component of eyelash curlers. The patch test was positive to thiuram. Other allergens found in eyelash curlers include nickel and rubber antioxidants derived from paraphenylene-diamine (McKenna and McMillan, 1992).

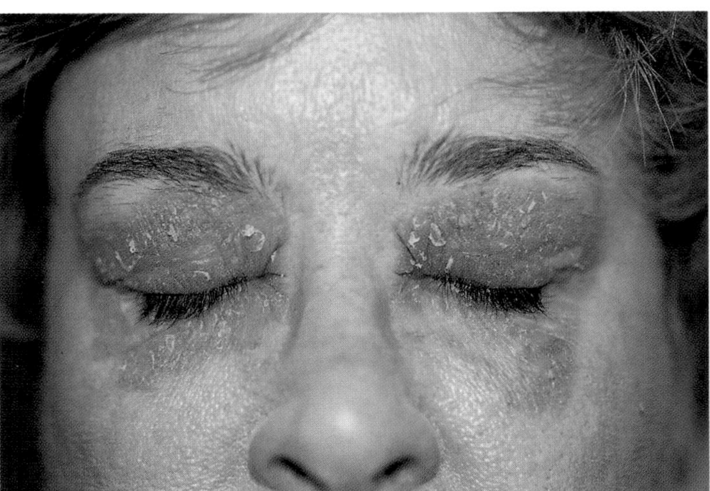

(**a**)

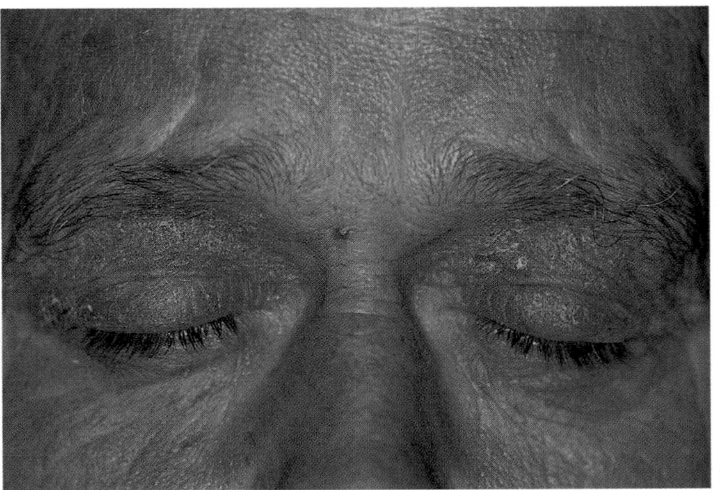

(**b**)

Figure 4.9 (**a**) This eyelid dermatitis occurred after wearing special eyelid make-up as part of a Halloween costume. The patient and physician suspected the make-up, but patch tests showed the culprit to be thiuram present in the foam sponges used to apply the make-up. Patch tests to the make-up were negative. (**b**) A differential diagnosis is psoriasis as a Koebner phenomenon. In this case it was occupational, and irritated by rockwool fibres. The pruritus from the fibres was followed by eye rubbing.

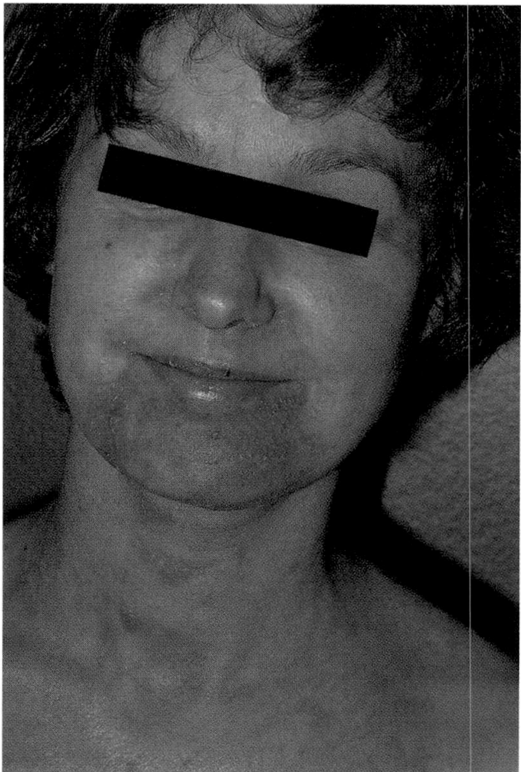

Figure 4.10 This is another example of ectopic dermatitis caused by fingernail polish, resulting in an eyelid eruption and mild erythema of the cheeks, showing where the patient has touched her face. The allergen was toluenesulfonamide–formaldehyde resin (tosylamide–formaldehyde resin). No dermatitis was present on the fingers.

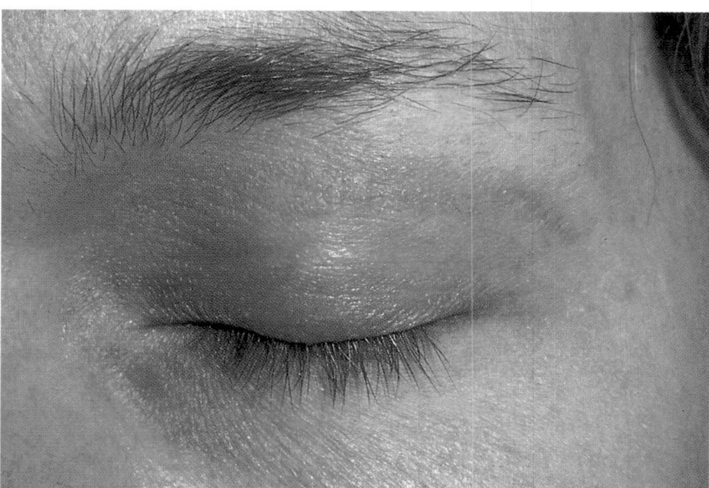

Figure 4.11 This eyelid dermatitis was caused by wearing swim goggles. The allergen was not identified, but the construction of the goggles suggested that a plastic allergen was probable.

LIPS AND MOUTH

Cheilitis and stomatitis can be caused by irritants in food and cosmetics, as well as by a number of allergens. The most important contact allergens are given in the box.

Allergens

Dental materials:
- Metals
- Acrylates
- Eugenol

Lipstick ingredients

Oral hygiene products:
- Flavouring/fragrance chemicals

Sesquiterpene lactones

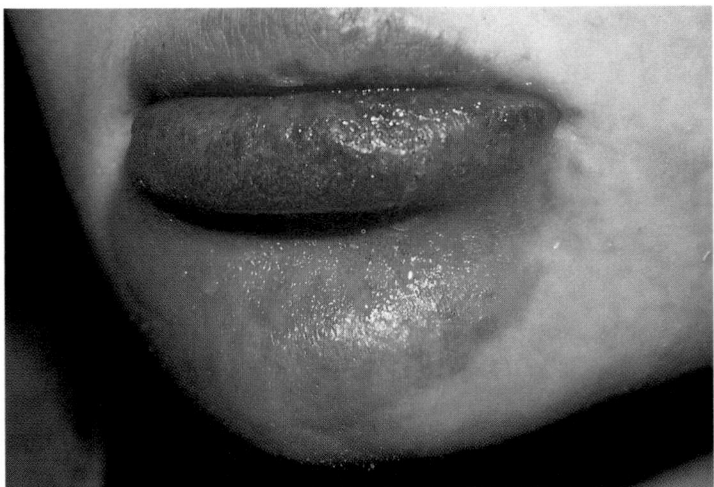

(**a**)

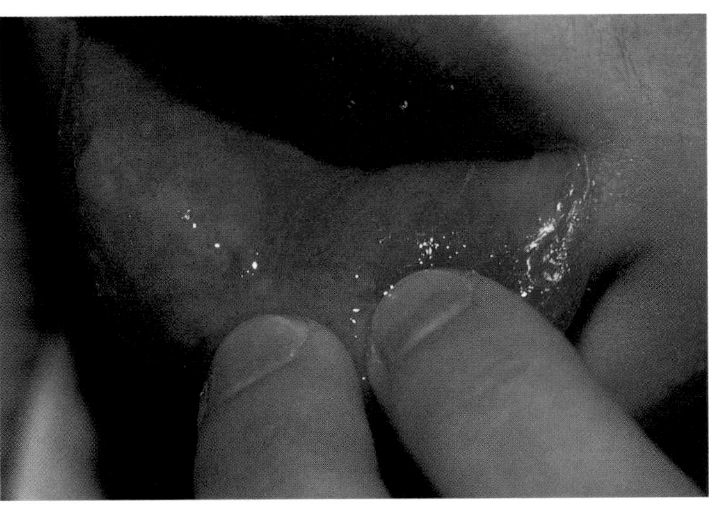

(**b**)

Figure 4.12 (**a**) Cheilitis may be accompanied by dermatitis of the adjacent non-mucosal skin. This is an example of allergic contact dermatitis to tromantadine, which is used for the treatment of herpes simplex infections. This antiviral agent is derived from amantadine and may cross-react with it (Patruno et al, 1990). (**b**) In this example of contact dermatitis due to tromantadine, the reaction is also on the mucosal surface.

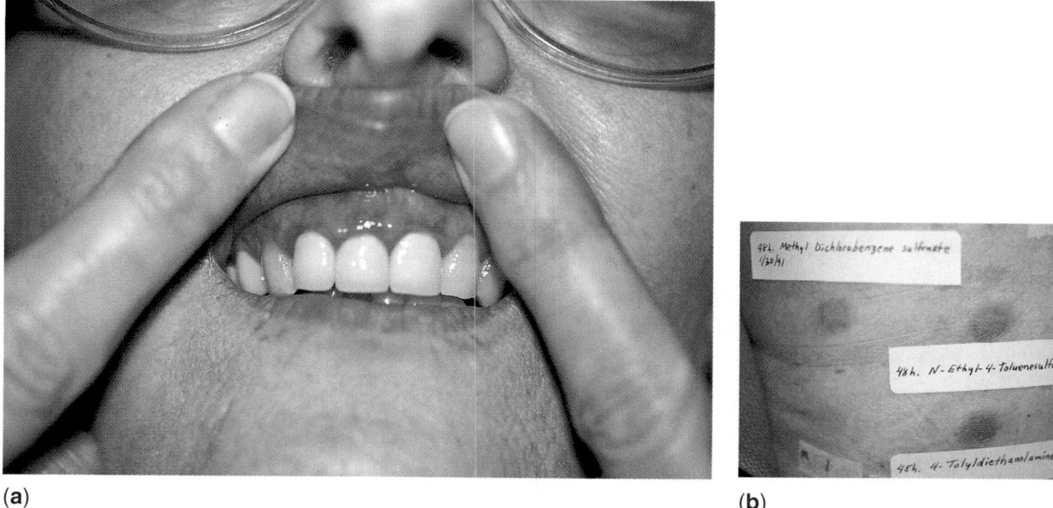

(**a**) (**b**)

Figure 4.13 (**a**) Intraoral reactions can occur, and are usually localized to the mucosa adjacent to the substance. The inflammation of the gums adjacent to the three central teeth in this photograph is due to a reaction to material used to bond these crowns in place. (**b**) The patch test reactions.

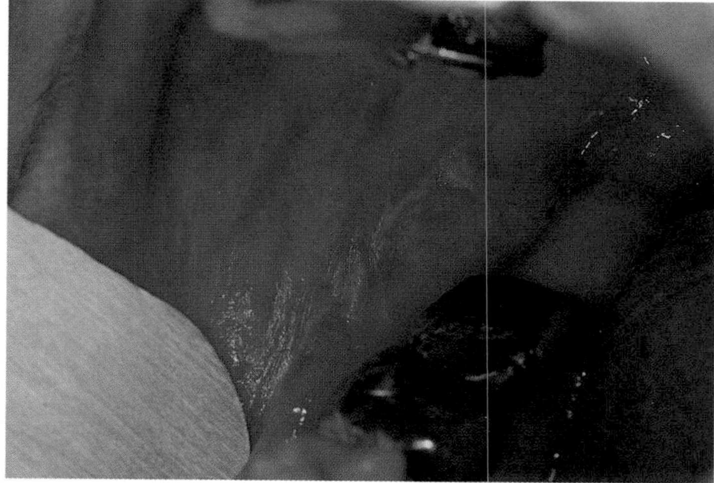

Figure 4.14 This 67-year-old woman was sensitive to mercury, and had lichen planus-like stomatitis on the buccal mucosa adjacent to amalgam dental fillings (Ophaswongse and Maibach, 1995).

Ears

Dermatitis of the ears is commonly due to medications intentionally applied to treat an external otitis. The active ingredient or vehicle components may be the cause. It can also be caused by foreign objects inserted into the external auditory canal to remove ear wax. Nickel-containing objects such as bobbypins are a prime example. Dermatitis of the ear lobe is classically associated with allergy to nickel-containing jewellery and topical medicaments (Goh, 1989). However, when patch tests are negative in the setting of ear lobe dermatitis, the likely correct diagnosis is atopic dermatitis (McDonagh et al, 1992). A retro-auricular fissure also indicates atopic dermatitis. Common contact allergens are given in the box.

Allergens

Fragrances
Lanolin
Topical medicaments

Jewellery:
Nickel
Cobalt
Gold

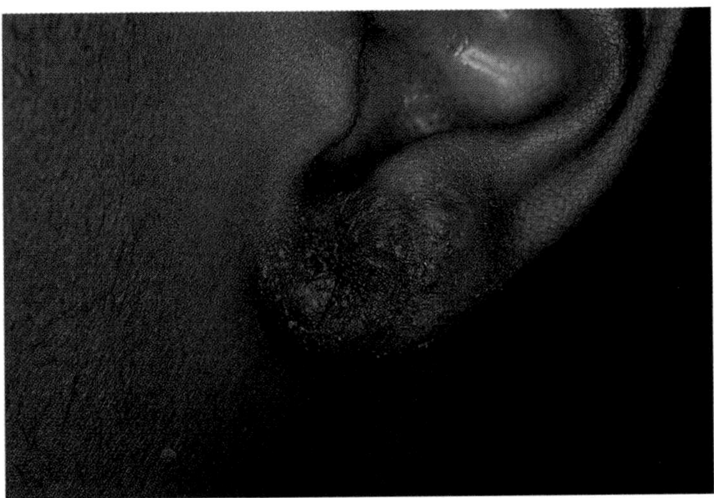

Figure 4.15 Dermatitis of the ear lobe is most commonly due to nickel-containing jewellery, as was the case in this individual. The chronic nature of the eruption and the dark complexion led to prominent post-inflammatory hyperpigmentation.

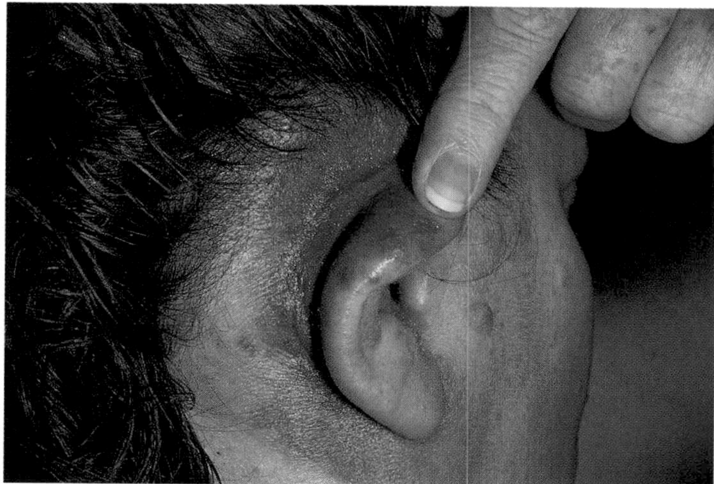

Figure 4.16 Dermatitis involved the external auditory canal, pinna and post-auricular sulcus due to the use of a neomycin-containing medication applied to all affected areas. Cellulitis was suspected by the physician, who prescribed both topical and systemic antibiotics, but after several weeks of progressive worsening, the correct diagnosis of allergic contact dermatitis to neomycin was made.

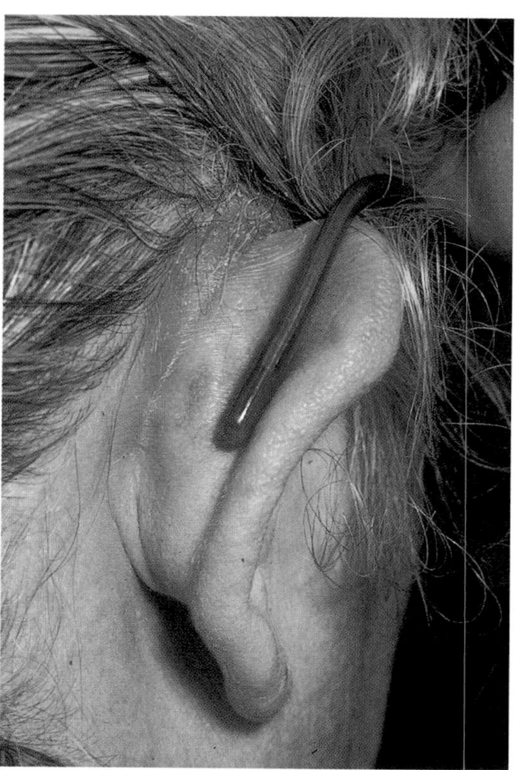

Figure 4.17 Retro-auricular allergic contact dermatitis was caused by an anthraquinone dye in the plastic spectacle frames worn by this patient. Other components of plastic spectacle frames that have caused allergic contact dermatitis include cellulose acetate (Jordan and Dahl, 1972), tricresyl phosphate (tritolyl phosphate) and triphenyl phosphate (Pegum, 1960), resorcinol monobenzoate (Calnan, 1975) and epoxy resin (Fisher, 1976).

Trunk and Axillae

This section considers the causes of dermatitis from the neck down to the thighs. Clothing, metal objects and personal hygiene products are the primary causes of contact dermatitis in this body region (Hatch and Maibach, 1985, 1986; Fowler et al, 1992). Common contact allergens are given in the box.

Allergens

- Carbamates
- Cobalt
- Formaldehyde
- Fragrances
- Mercaptobenzothiazole
- Naphthol AS
- Nickel
- Resins in clothing
- Textile dyes

CLOTHING

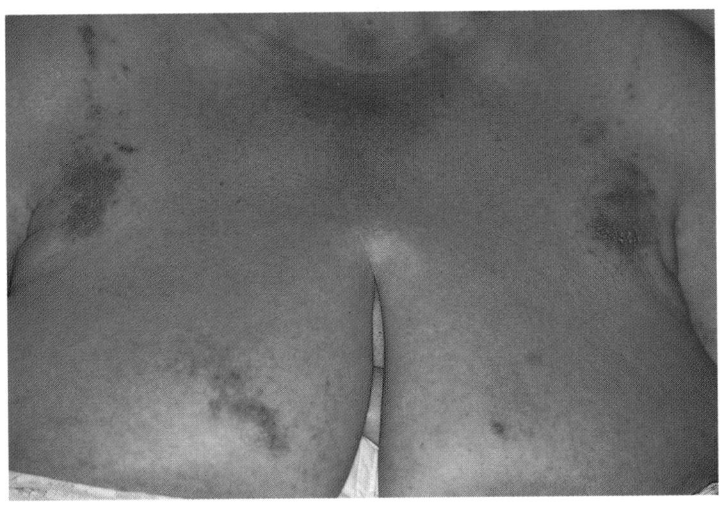

Figure 4.18 The elastic in the brassiere of this 73-year-old woman was the cause of this dermatitis, which follows the outline of her garment. In this case, the specific rubber chemical responsible was not identified.

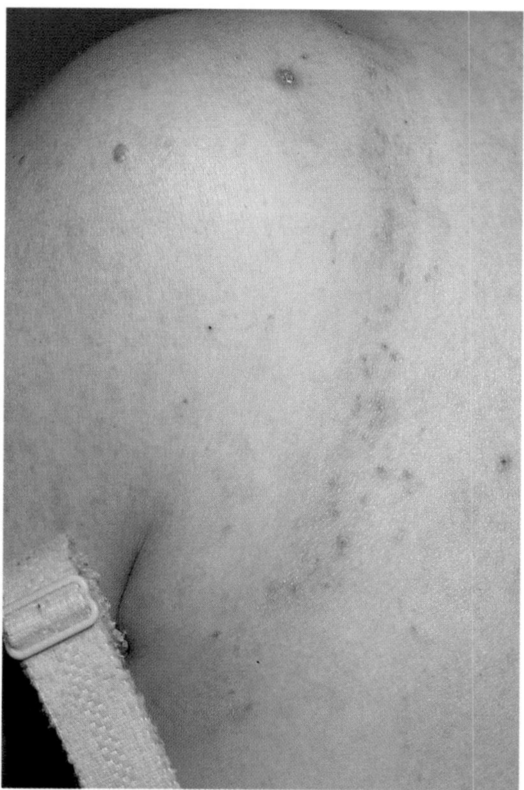

Figure 4.19 The dermatitis of this 58-year-old woman followed the outline of the elastic in her brassiere. She was patch-test positive to carba mix.

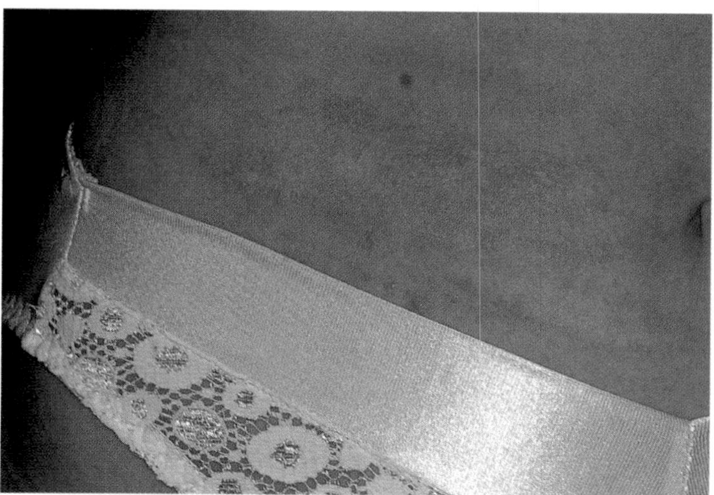

Figure 4.20 Pruritic dermatitis occurred around the waist of this 26-year-old woman who was allergic to mercapto-benzothiazole present in the elastic waistband of her underwear.

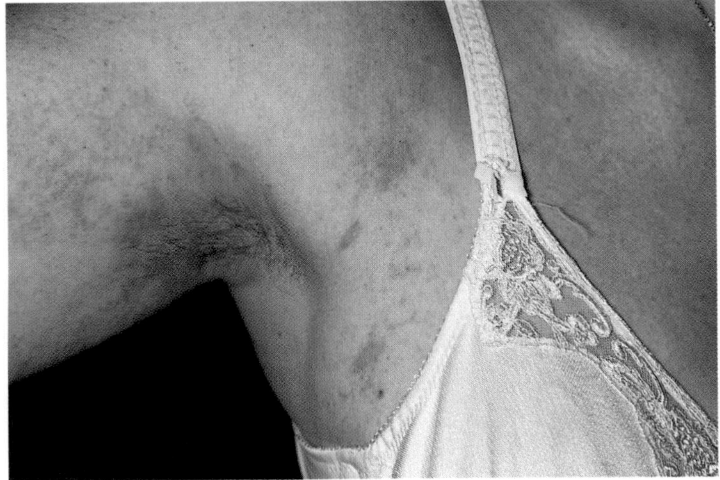

Figure 4.21 A 48-year-old woman with a positive patch test to the perfume mixture developed contact dermatitis after changing to a strongly scented detergent. Dermatitis of the axillary folds and the adjoining areas is a pattern of dermatitis commonly caused by clothing or by detergents or fabric softeners.

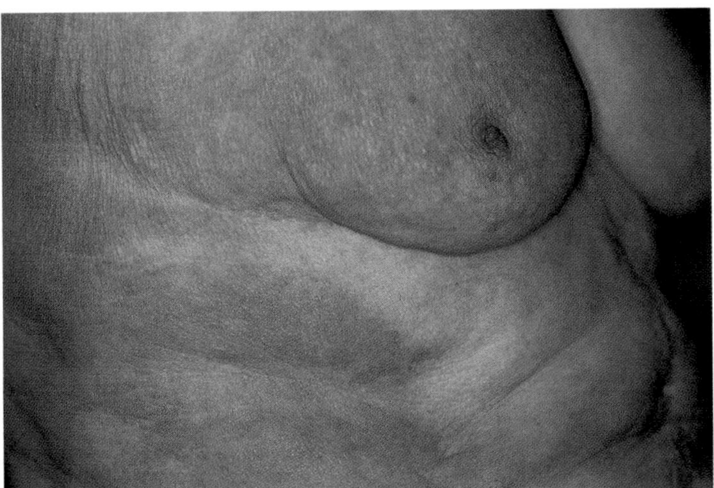

Figure 4.22 The dermatitis on the trunk of this 75-year-old woman was caused by a washing detergent. Note that there is dermatitis only where her clothing touched the skin, but there is no dermatitis in the deep skin folds or below the breast.

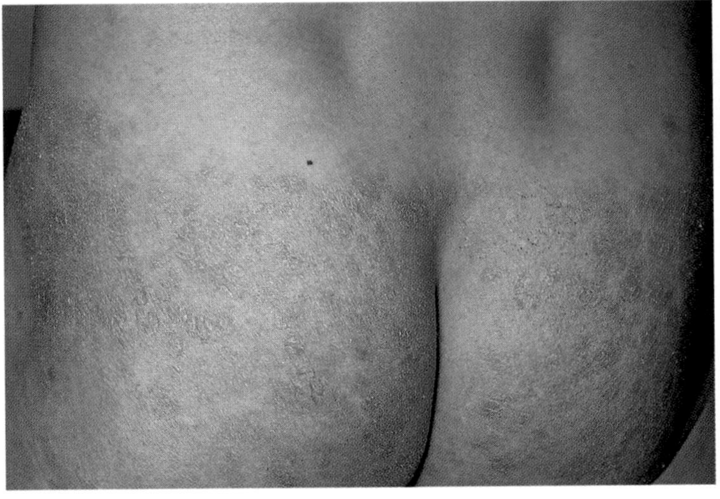

Figure 4.23 Another pattern of irritant contact dermatitis caused by clothing or detergents may be seen under tightly fitting underwear, as in this 41-year-old man.

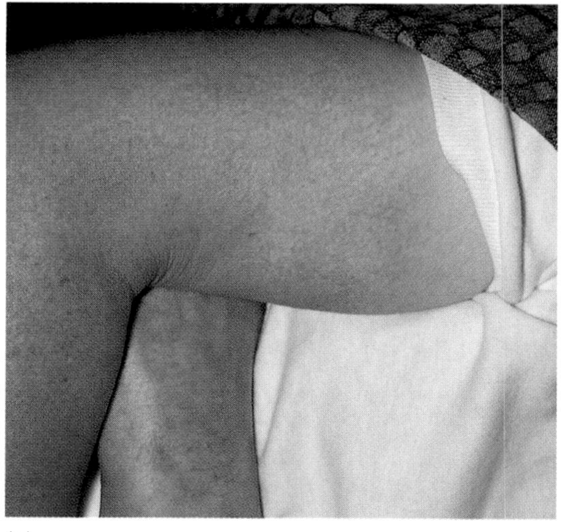

(a)

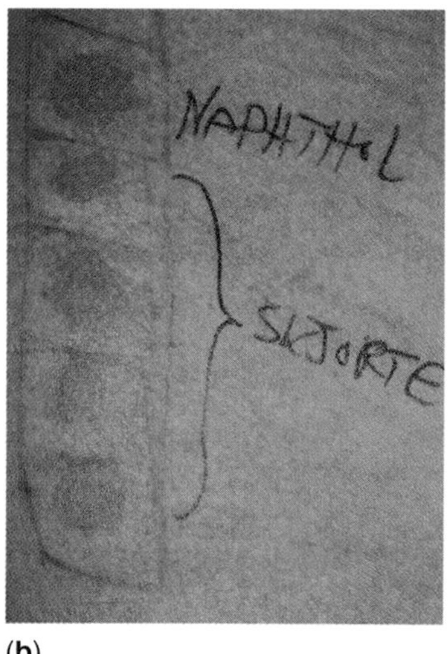

(b)

Figure 4.24 (**a**) A particular pattern of clothing dermatitis is caused by the coupling agent Naphthol AS, used to bind colours in printed fabric (Ancona-Alayon et al, 1976; Roed-Petersen et al, 1990). For example, brightly coloured fabrics with only light colours on the inside can cause severely pruritic dermatitis at the sites of contact with the shirt, as seen on the legs of this patient. (**b**) The patch test reaction.

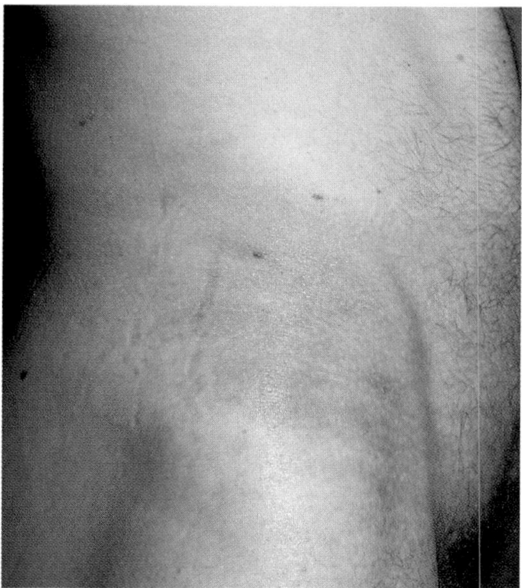

Figure 4.25 Hyperpigmentation during active, pruritic dermatitis is a characteristic of allergic contact dermatitis caused by Naphthol AS.

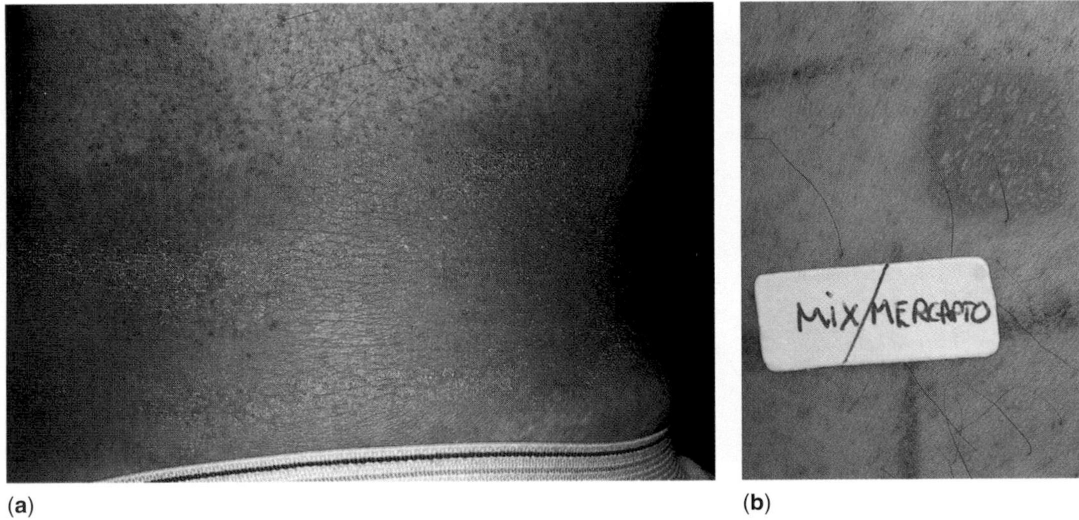

(a) (b)

Figure 4.26 (a) Elastic in clothing can cause contact dermatitis due to components such as rubber accelerators or antioxidants. An example of waistband dermatitis is seen here. (**b**) The offending agent in this waistband dermatitis was found to be mercaptobenzothiazole.

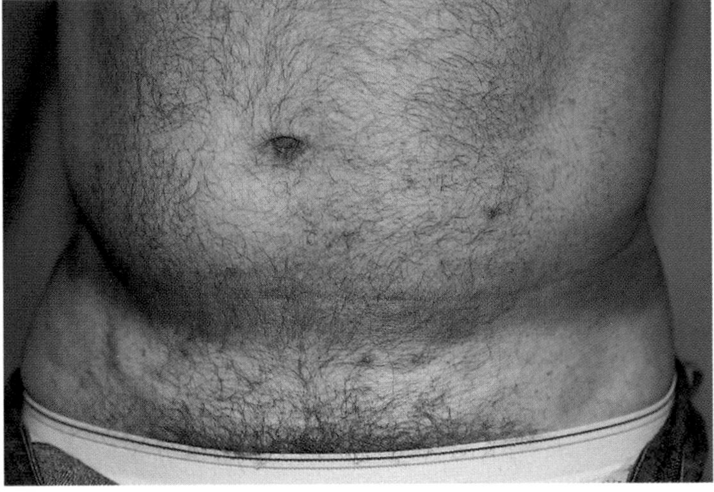

Figure 4.27 The same type of waistband dermatitis can occur owing to an interaction between bleach and some forms of elastic during the washing process. In these cases the standard screening allergens for rubber-induced dermatitis will be negative, since the offending agent is *N*,*N*'-dibenzylcarbamyl chloride (Jordan and Bourlas, 1975).

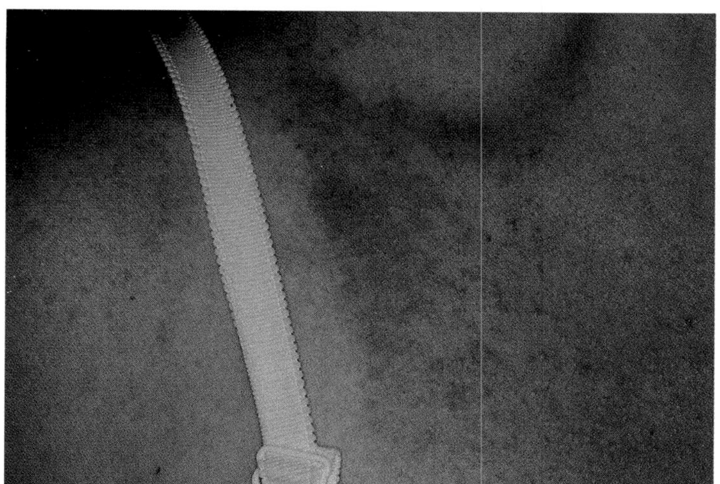

(a)

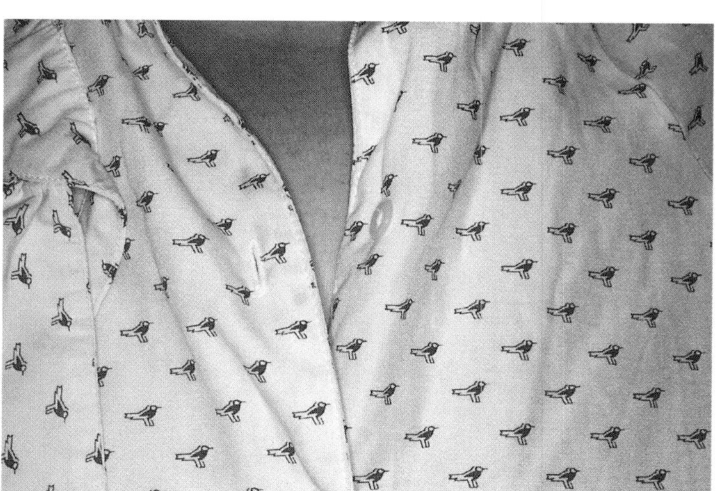

(b)

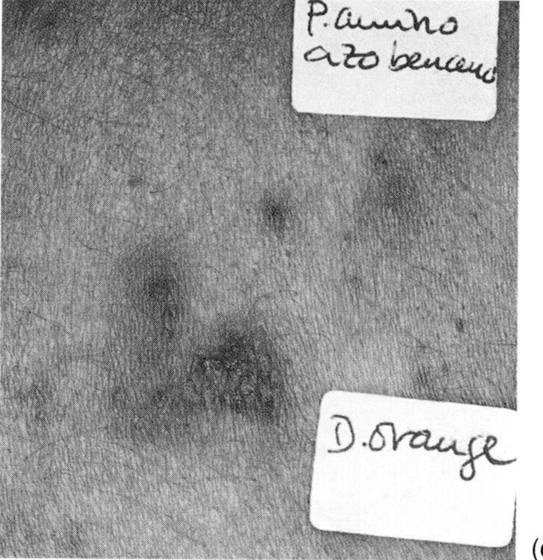

(c)

Figure 4.28 (**a**) A uniform worn by a supermarket cashier resulted in dermatitis that did not occur under her bra strap. (**b**) The offending agent was found to be a textile dye (disperse orange). (**c**) The patch test reaction.

METALS

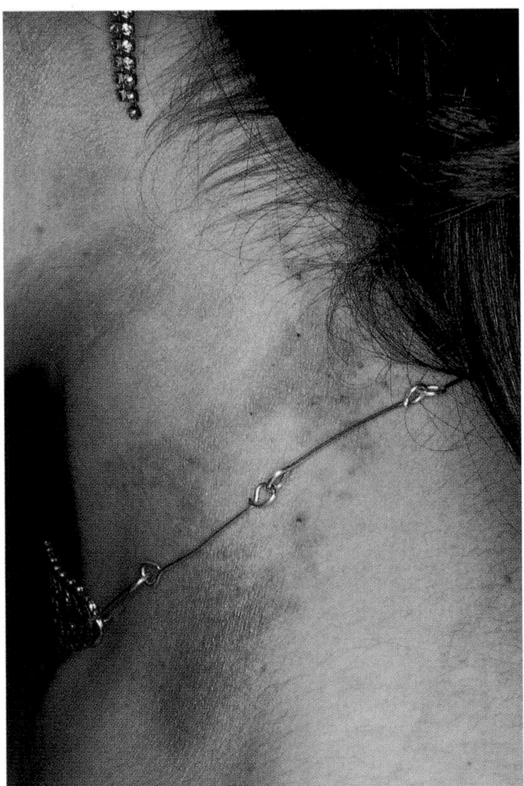

Figure 4.29 In women, the most common allergen found with the standard patch screening series is nickel. Nickel in the necklace seen here caused dermatitis of the neck, which extended to the clavicles.

Figure 4.30 Zippers can cause dermatitis, as in this theatrical artist who developed dermatitis from the zipper in a costume.

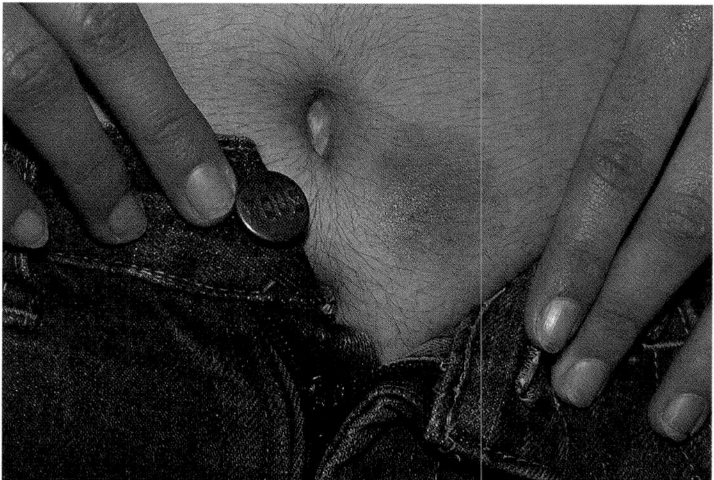

Figure 4.31 Fasteners made of metal can cause discrete areas of contact dermatitis, as caused by the button on these denim jeans.

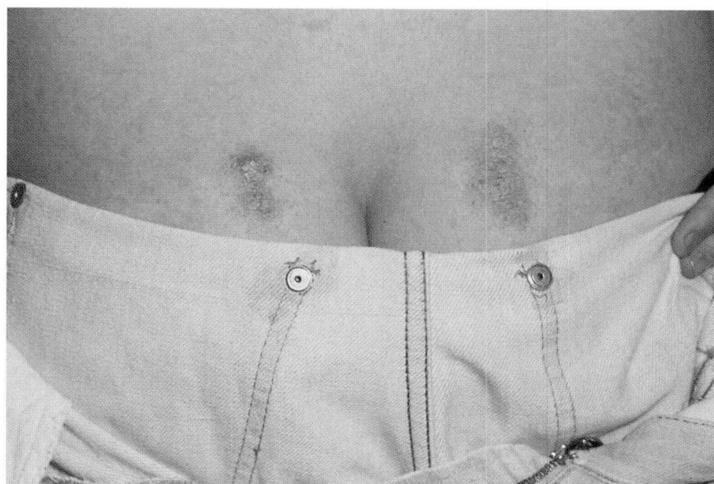

Figure 4.32 Metal rivets on blue jeans are another source of nickel dermatitis, as seen in this woman.

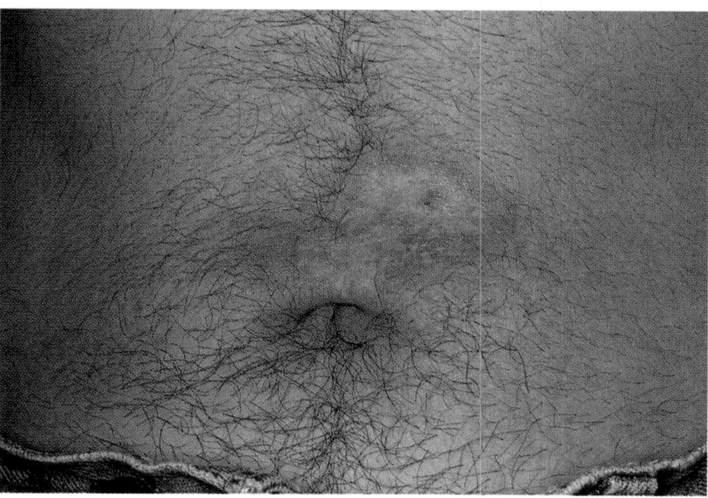

Figure 4.33 Residual post-inflammatory pigment alteration can occur after metal contact dermatitis due to buttons, rivets and other objects.

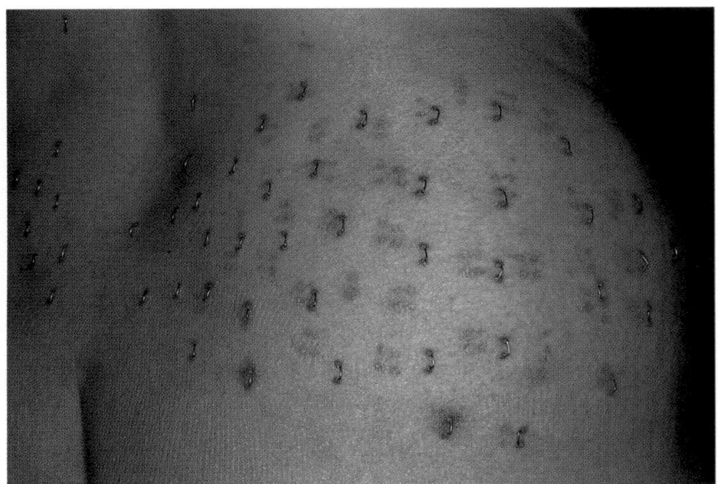
(**a**)

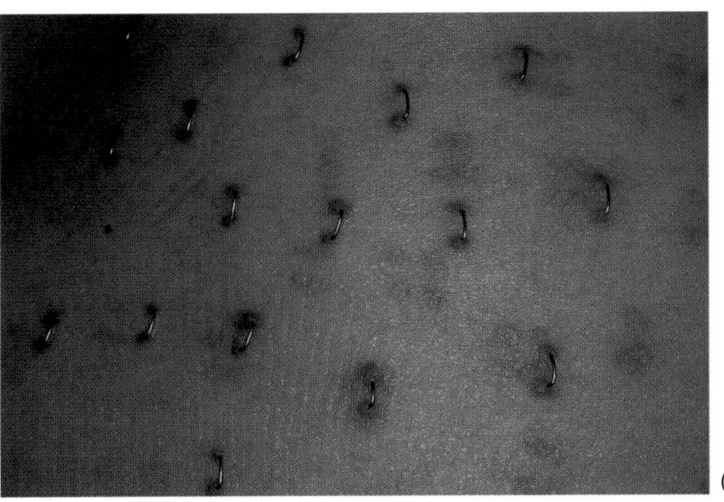
(**b**)

Figure 4.34 (**a**, **b**) The patient seen here had acupuncture staples placed, as shown. Unfortunately, the staples had a high nickel content. The patient was nickel-sensitive and developed dermatitis around the staples.

PERSONAL HYGIENE PRODUCTS

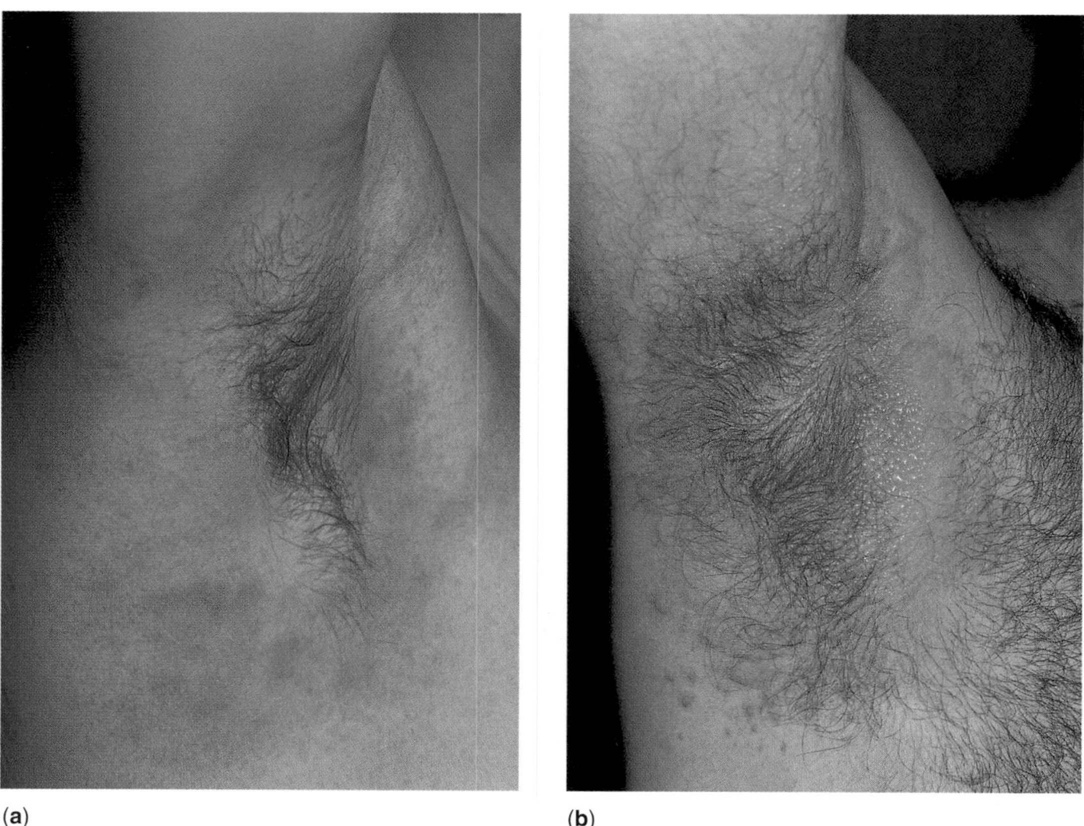

(a) (b)

Figure 4.35 Axillary vault dermatitis is usually due to underarm deodorants or antiperspirants. (**a**) A spice-scented underarm antiperspirant caused this dermatitis due to isoeugenol. Seborrhoeic dermatitis and intertrigo are differential diagnoses; (**b**) shows a patient who was suffering from both a seborrhoeic dermatitis and contact allergy to musk in a deodorant.

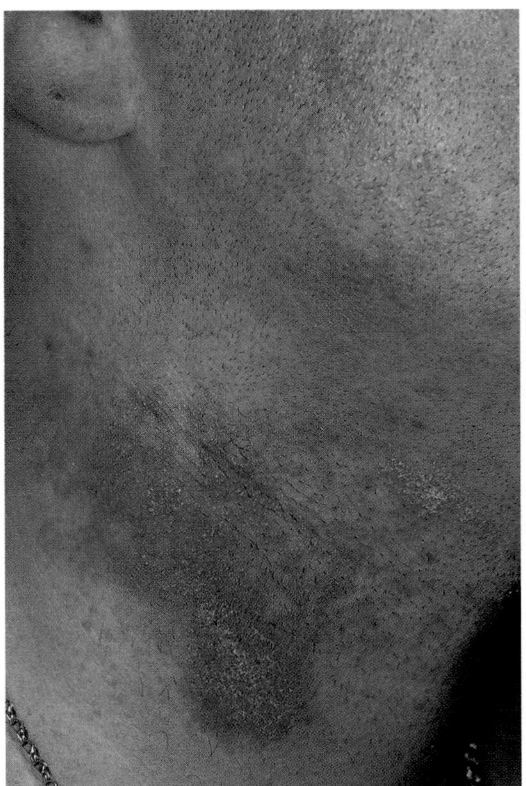

Figure 4.36 After using a new aftershave for one to two weeks, this 22-year-old man developed dermatitis on his neck. Patch testing with the European Standard Patch Test Series of allergens showed a strong reaction to the fragrance mixture. The dermatitis faded when he discontinued use of the offending aftershave.

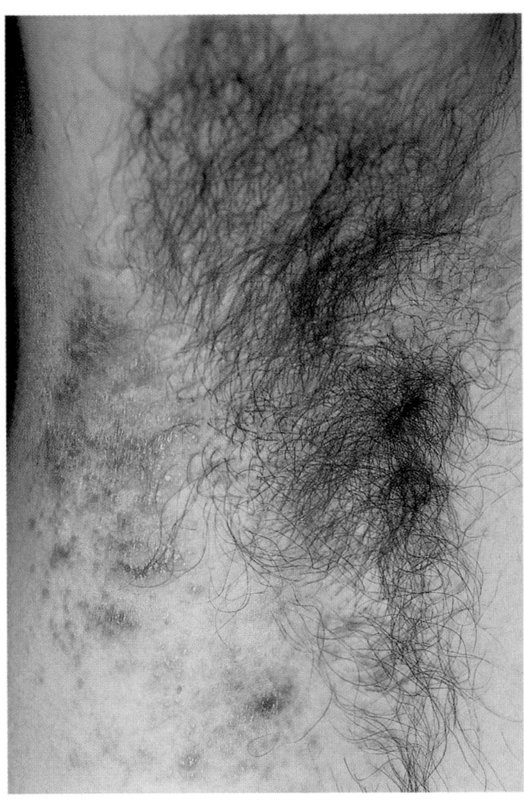

Figure 4.37 Antiperspirant dermatitis is often more pronounced along the axillary folds, as seen here along the posterior axillary fold. This can be confused with clothing contact dermatitis.

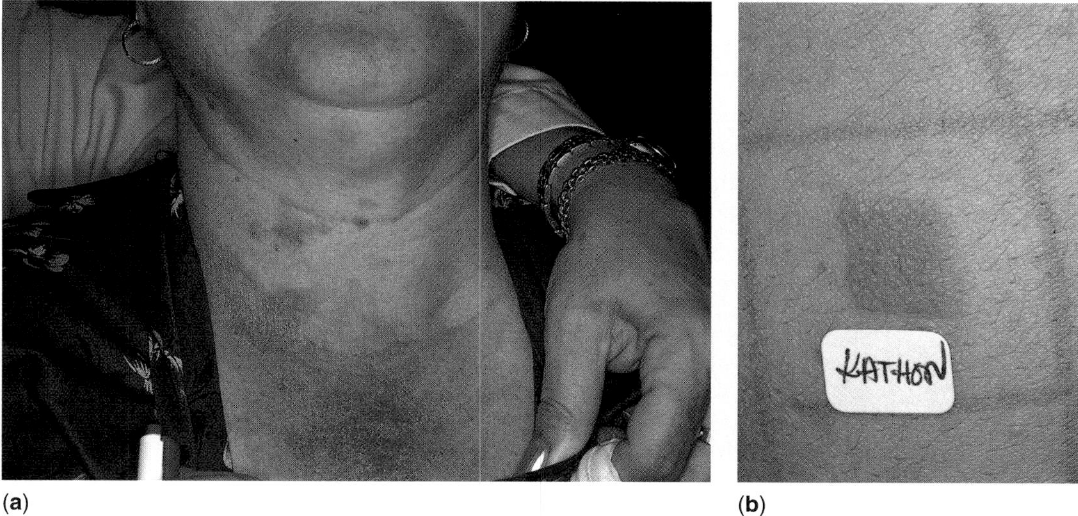

(**a**) (**b**)

Figure 4.38 (**a**) A body lotion containing the preservative methylchloroisothiazolinone–methylisothiazolinone (Kathon CG) was applied to the chest of this woman, resulting in contact dermatitis. (**b**) The patch test reaction at four days.

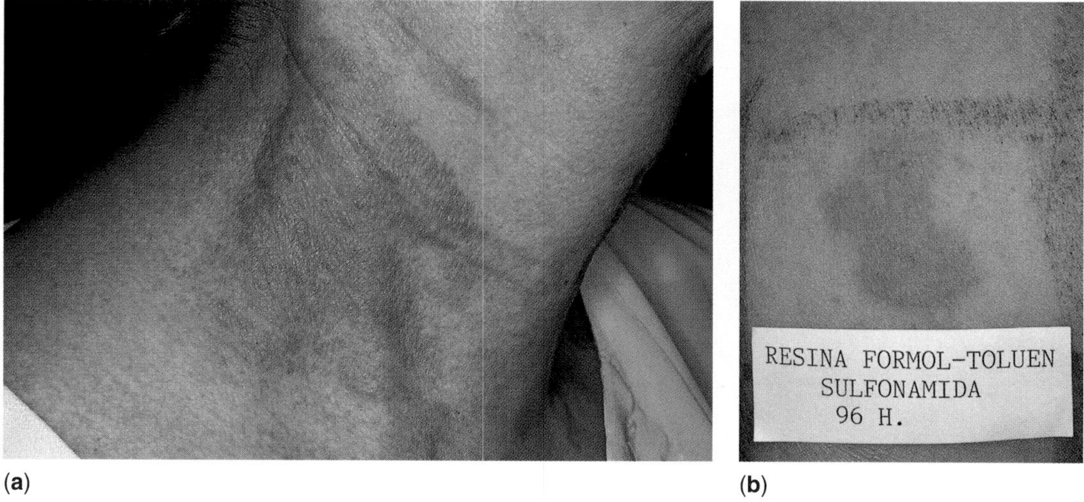

(**a**) (**b**)

Figure 4.39 Dermatitis of the neck can be ectopic – that is, caused by allergens applied to distant body parts that do not manifest the reaction (Rietschel and Fowler, 1995, p.66). The eyelids are most frequently associated with ectopic contact dermatitis, but the same principle applies to the neck, as seen in this example (**a**), caused by nail polish. (**b**) The ingredient in nail polish responsible for this dermatitis is toluenesulfonamide–formaldehyde resin (tosylamide–formaldehyde resin, INCI).

Extremities and Genitalia

The extremities come in contact with similar objects as the trunk and axillae do: metal objects and products are common contactants. Other objects unique to an individual's occupation or hobbies can readily affect the arms or legs. Common contact allergens are given in the box.

Allergens

Fragrances
Mercaptobenzothiazole
Nickel
Potassium dichromate
Preservatives:
- Parabens
- Kathon CG
- Formaldehyde

Textile dyes
Thiurams
Topical medications:
- Neomycin
- Clioquinol
- Lanolin

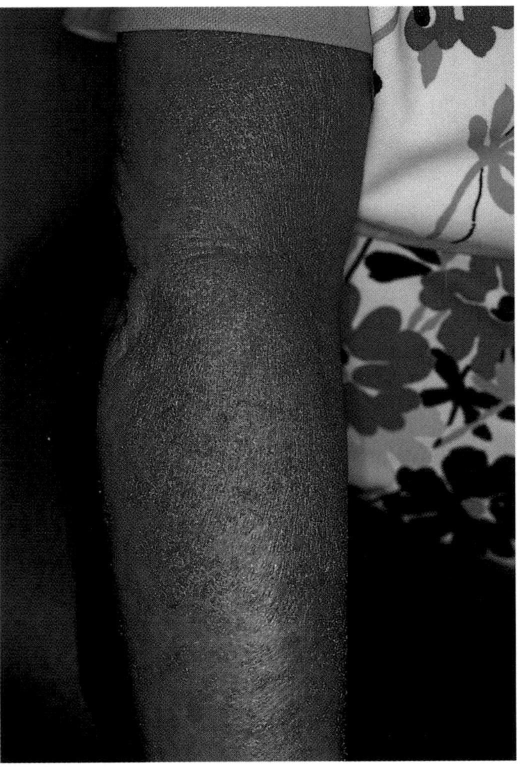

Figure 4.40 Substances intentionally applied to the skin of the extremities can produce confluent dermatitis, as seen in this patient who applied a moisturizer to her arms. The preservative was the cause of the dermatitis.

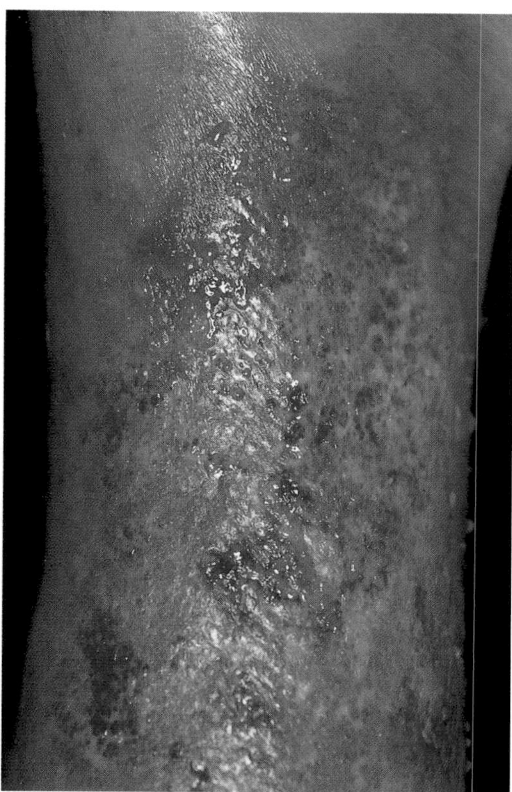

Figure 4.41 Application of contact allergens can occur iatrogenically (Jenni and Zala, 1980). This dermatitis on the lower legs was due to topical medications used under occlusive dressings. This 84-year-old woman had a positive patch test to lanolin, and had been treated with a topical corticosteroid containing lanolin.

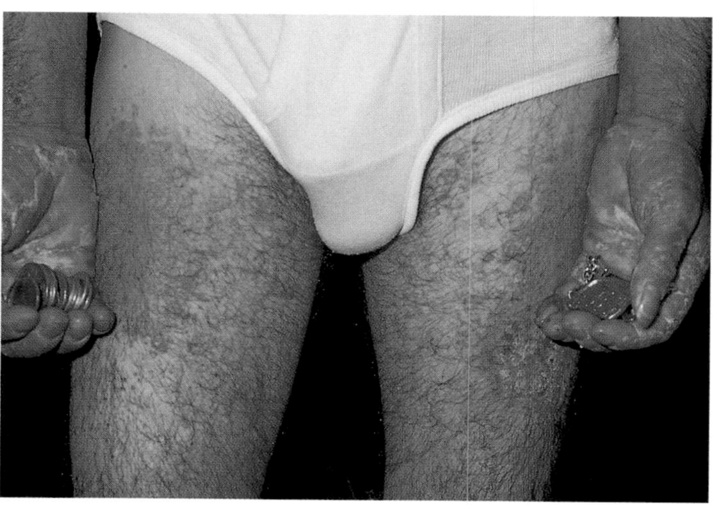

Figure 4.42 Objects carried in the pockets can cause contact dermatitis. This construction worker was sensitive to chromium, cobalt and nickel. He had hand dermatitis due to his work with cement, but on the anterior of both thighs he had dermatitis due to coins and keys that he habitually carried in his trouser pockets.

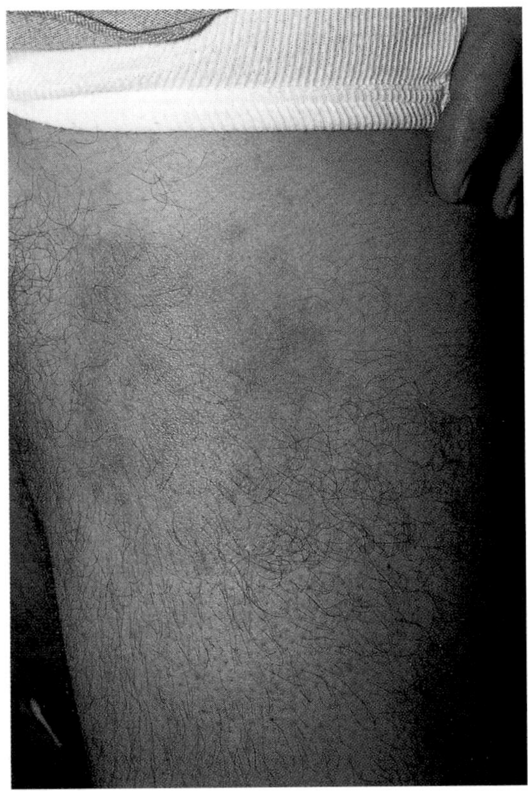

(**a**)

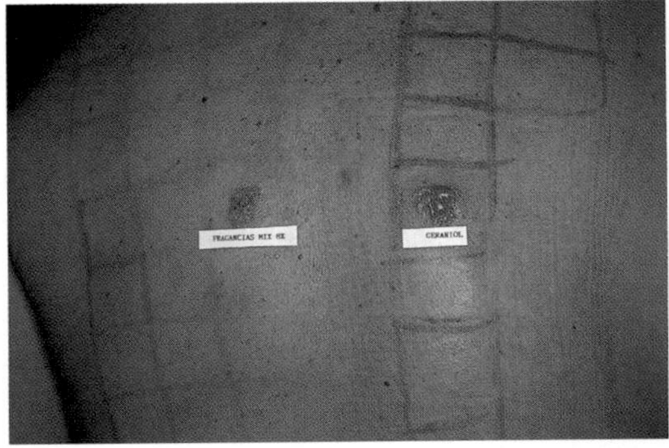

(**b**)

Figure 4.43 (**a**) Fragrance was applied to a handkerchief carried in the pocket, leading to this dermatitis. (**b**) The cause was determined to be geraniol, as seen by the patch test reaction. Geraniol is a component of the fragrance mixture in the standard patch test series.

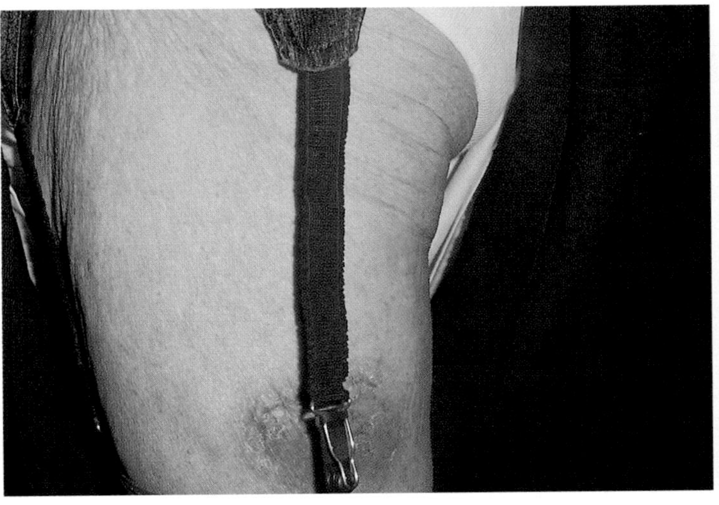

(**a**)

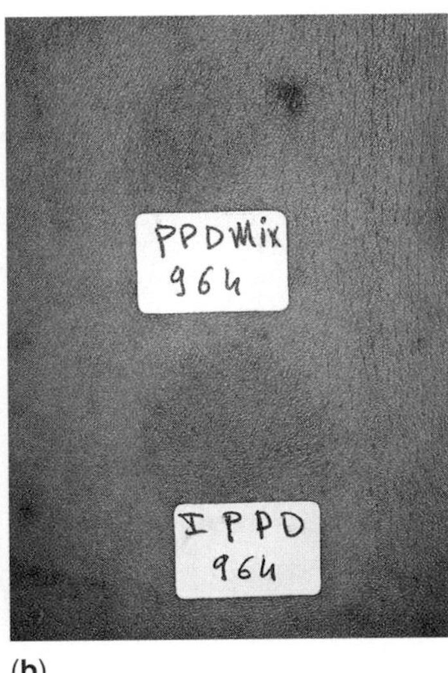

(**b**)

Figure 4.44 Allergic contact dermatitis was due to the rubber in the garter belt worn by the patient seen here. (**a**) The allergens were rubber antioxidants, which are commonly tested as a mixture formerly known as black rubber mix. (**b**) The individual components of the mix responsible for the allergy.

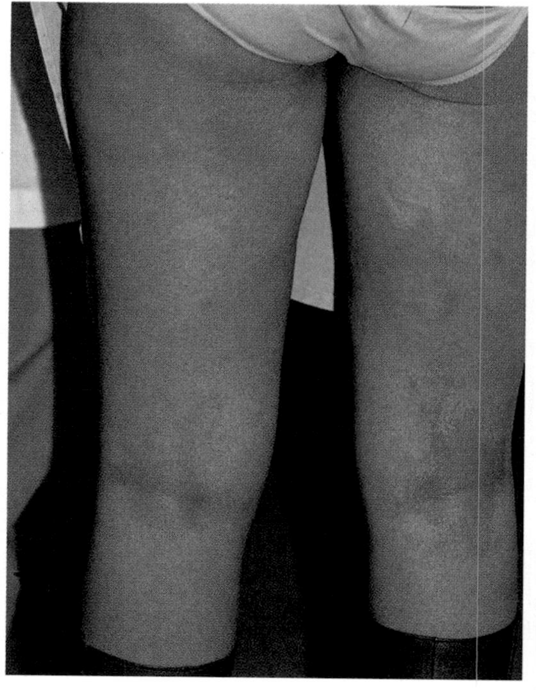

(a)

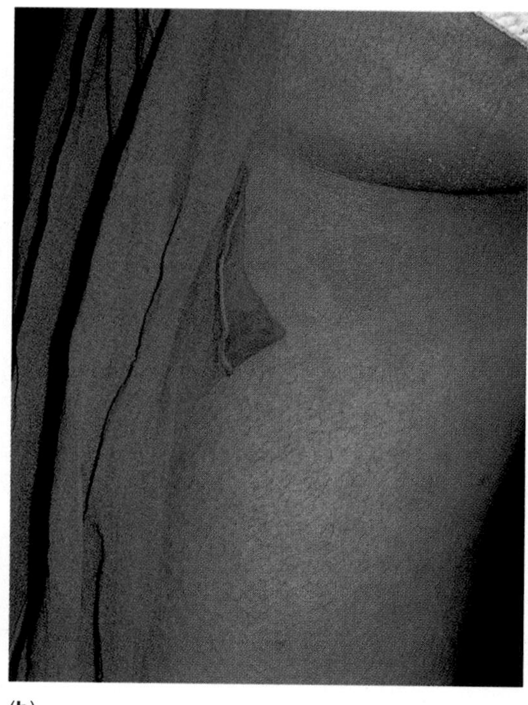

(b)

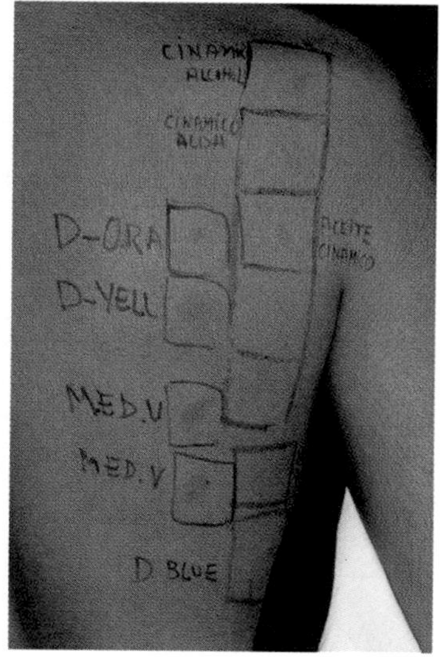

(c)

Figure 4.45 A stocking produced the dermatitis seen in (**a**) and (**b**). (**c**) The patch test reactions confirmed sensitization to disperse yellow and disperse orange. The manufacturer confirmed that both dyes were present in the stocking (Conde-Salazar et al, 1984).

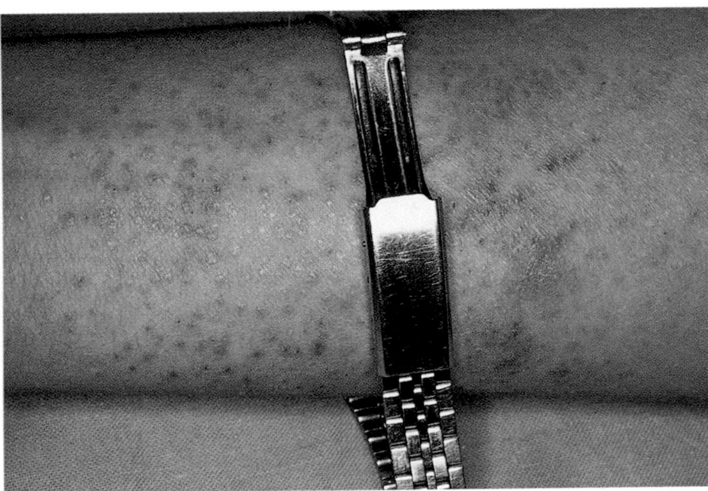

Figure 4.46 This metal watchband contained nickel, to which this patient was allergic. The papular lichenoid appearance is characteristic of nickel dermatitis.

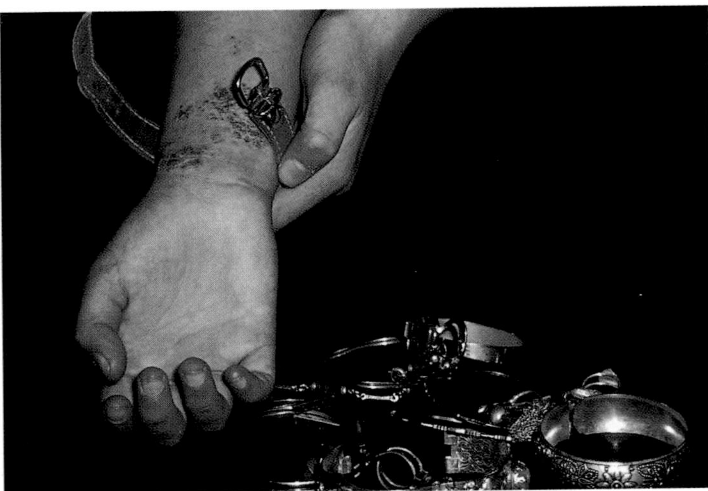

Figure 4.47 Costume jewellery frequently contains nickel: these bracelets caused this dermatitis.

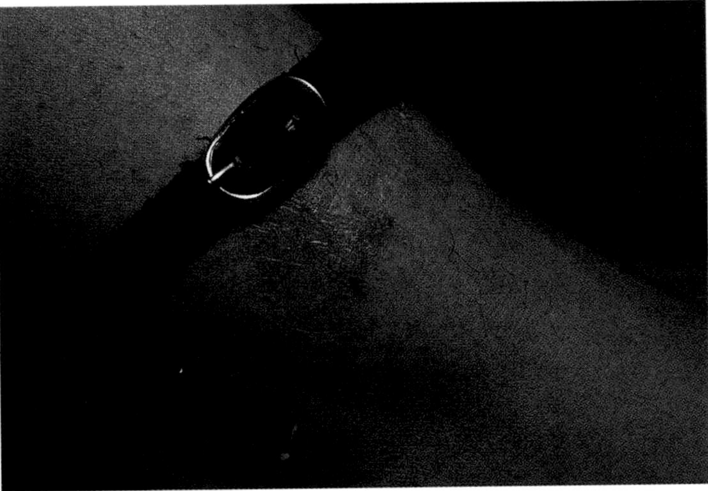

Figure 4.48 The buckle of this sandal produced a localized dermatitis near the ankle.

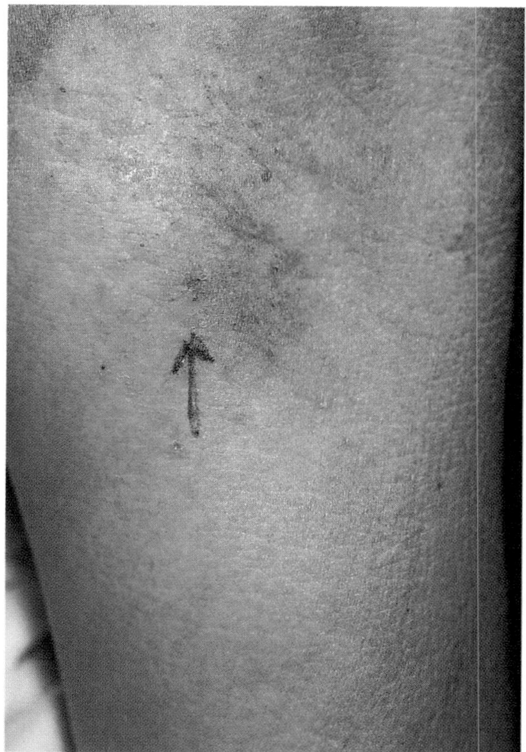

Figure 4.49 Even high-quality metal objects may contain enough nickel to cause dermatitis in a strongly allergic patient. Nickel was present in the needle used for vein puncture which led to dermatitis in this 58-year-old woman.

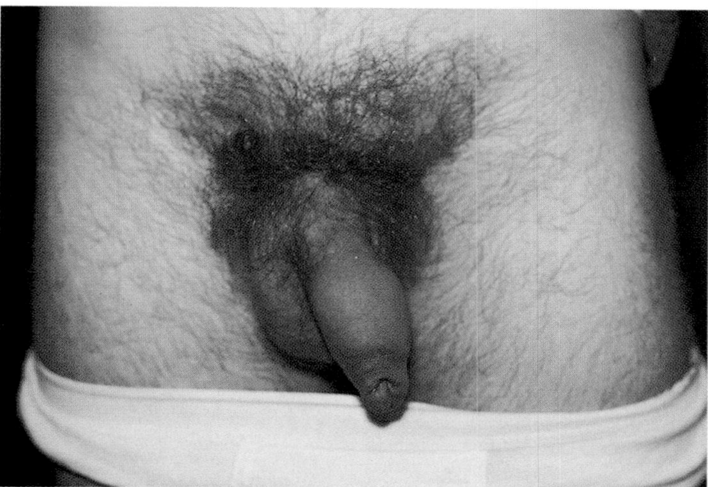

Figure 4.50 This young man had recurrent herpes simplex of the penis and treated himself with an antiviral cream containing the preservative thimerosal. He was allergic to thimerosal. Oedema is greater in the loose skin of the genitalia when allergic contact dermatitis affects this area of the body.

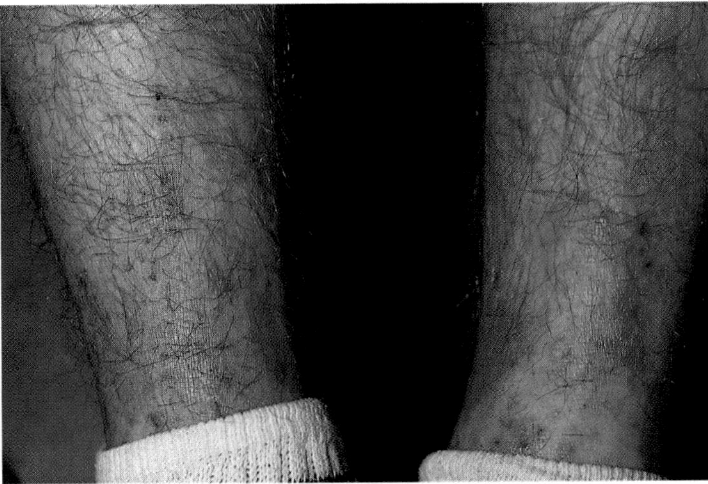

Figure 4.51 An 11-year-old boy had pruritic dermatitis on the lower legs after playing soccer. He was sensitive to mercaptobenzothiazole in the elastic in his shin protectors.

Hands

The hands interact with our environment more intensely than most other body parts do, and even though the skin in this area is thick and tough, especially on the palms, many patterns of allergic contact dermatitis can occur on the hands. Common contact allergens are given in the box. The hands may specifically manifest endogenous dermatoses that can mimic both irritant and allergic contact dermatitis. Mechanical friction can produce hyperkeratotic, fissured dermatitis (see Figures 5.21 and 5.22) that resembles psoriasis, which, in turn, is easily confused with atopic dermatitis, fungal infection, and irritant and allergic contact dermatitis.

Allergens

- Gloves
- Occupational chemicals
- Skin-care products
- Solvents
- Plants:
  - Ornamentals
  - Weeds

A diagnostic algorithm, as shown in the flow chart on the following page, may be helpful in making a specific diagnosis of dermatitis of the hands. The steps in diagnosing hand dermatitis suggested in this section are based on the flow chart.

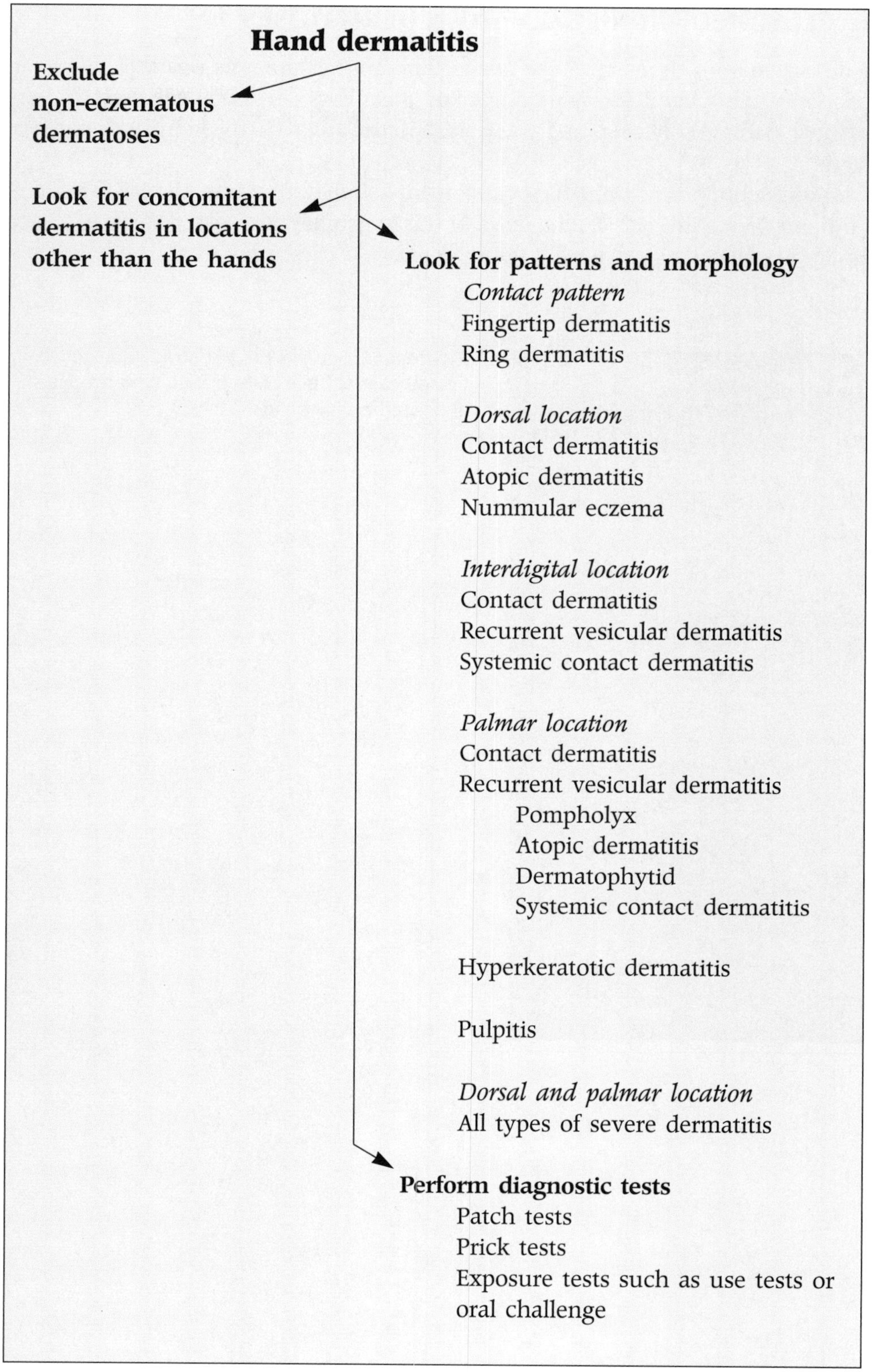

Hand dermatitis

Exclude non-eczematous dermatoses

Look for concomitant dermatitis in locations other than the hands

Look for patterns and morphology

Contact pattern
Fingertip dermatitis
Ring dermatitis

Dorsal location
Contact dermatitis
Atopic dermatitis
Nummular eczema

Interdigital location
Contact dermatitis
Recurrent vesicular dermatitis
Systemic contact dermatitis

Palmar location
Contact dermatitis
Recurrent vesicular dermatitis
- Pompholyx
- Atopic dermatitis
- Dermatophytid
- Systemic contact dermatitis

Hyperkeratotic dermatitis

Pulpitis

Dorsal and palmar location
All types of severe dermatitis

Perform diagnostic tests

Patch tests
Prick tests
Exposure tests such as use tests or oral challenge

EXCLUSION OF NON-ECZEMATOUS DERMATOSES

Non-eczematous dermatoses include guttate and plaque-type psoriasis, pustular psoriasis, acropustulosis, palmo-plantar pustulosis in non-psoriatics, lichen planus, dermatophytosis, and keratolysis exfoliativa or dyshidrosis lamellosa sicca.

At onset, bullous pemphigoid occasionally has an appearance similar to vesicular hand dermatitis, and examination of the remainder of the skin surface is necessary to make a diagnosis of bullous pemphigoid (Descamps et al, 1992).

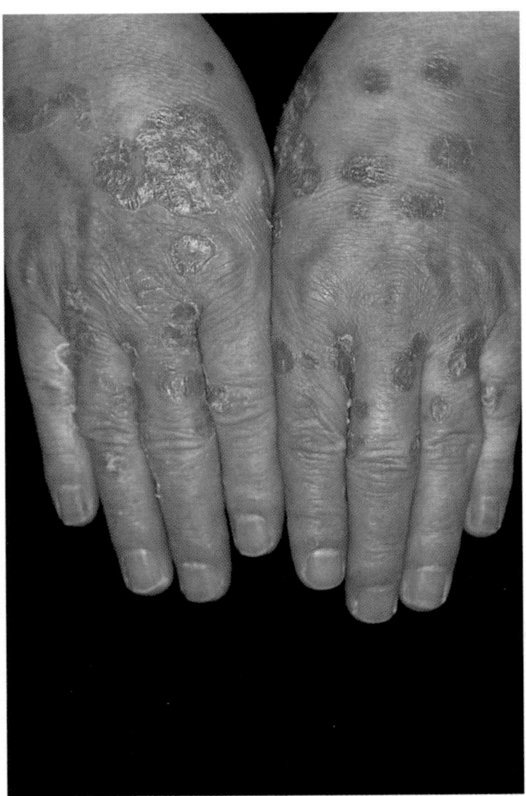

Figure 4.52 Psoriasis is the obvious diagnosis in this 46-year-old man with plaque-type psoriasis, also seen on his hands.

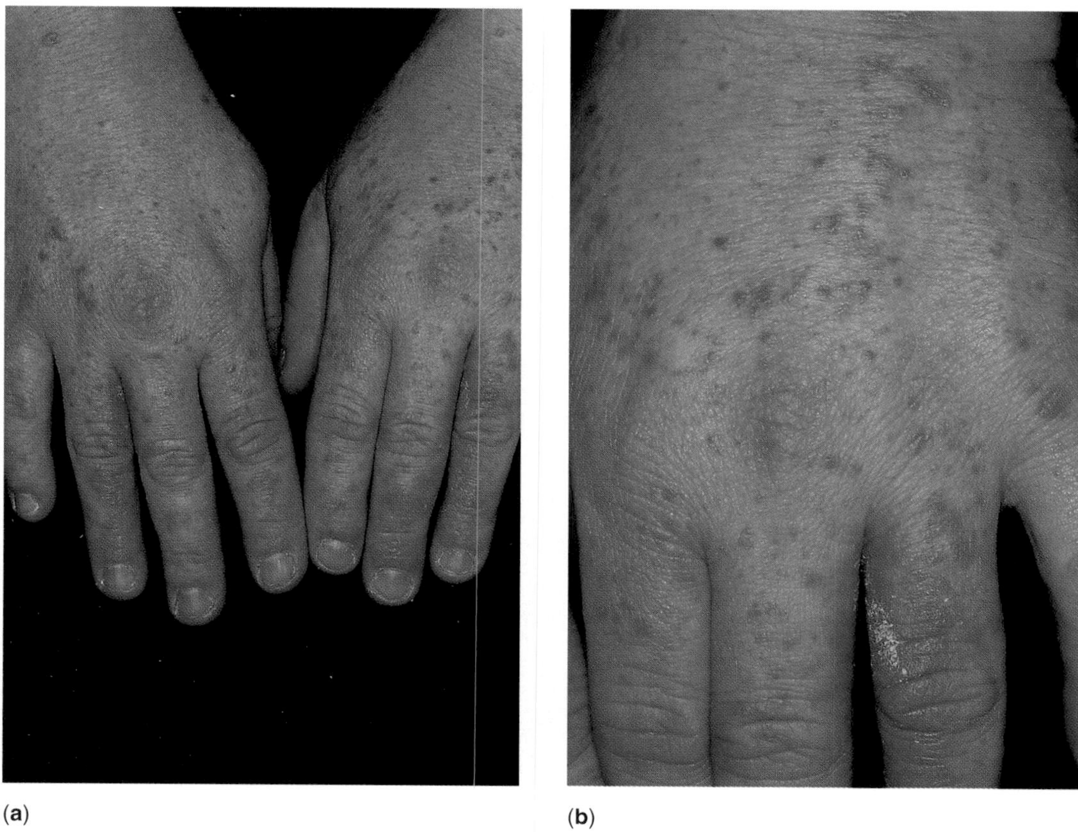

(a) (b)

Figure 4.53 (**a**) It can be difficult to make a diagnosis of psoriasis in patients with eruptive guttate psoriasis, as in this 32-year-old woman, who also has psoriasis on her hands. (**b**) Scratching the lesions reveals white psoriasiform scaling.

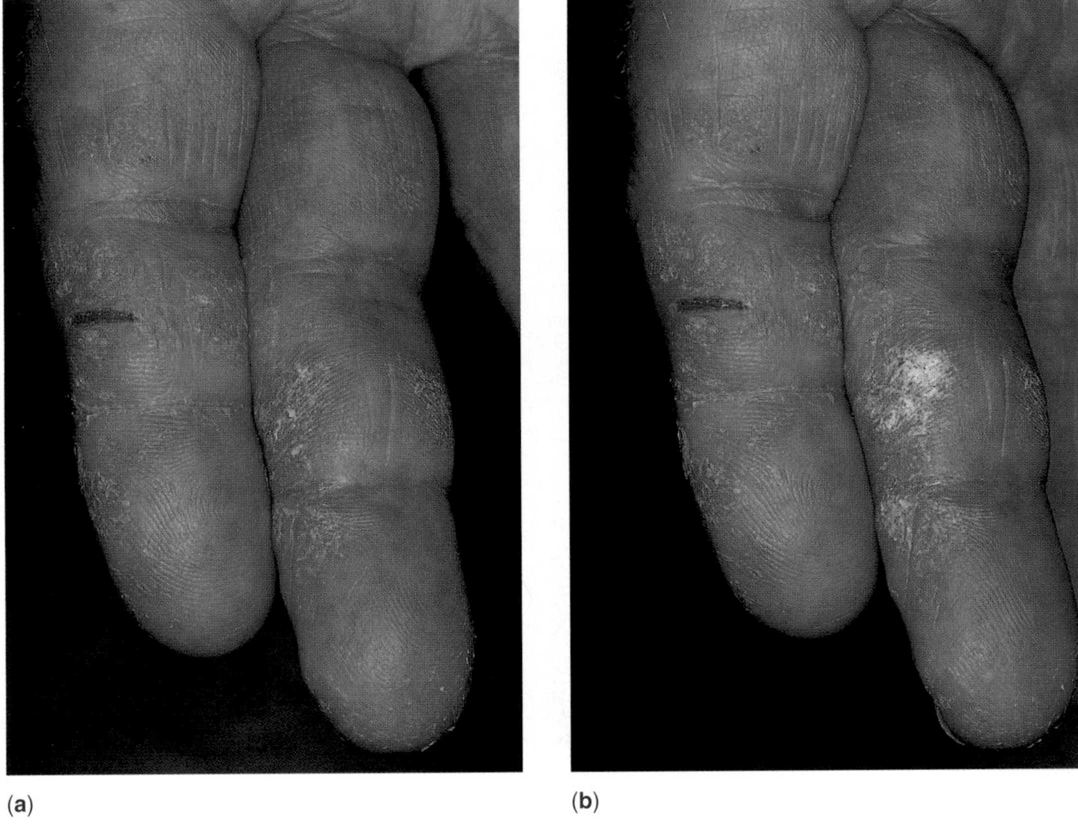

(**a**) (**b**)

Figure 4.54 (**a**) Palmar psoriasis can mimic hand dermatitis to such a degree that only the psoriasiform scaling seen in (**b**) can lead to a correct diagnosis of psoriasis. This diagnosis is also supported by a lack of pruritus and by psoriasis lesions elsewhere on the body.

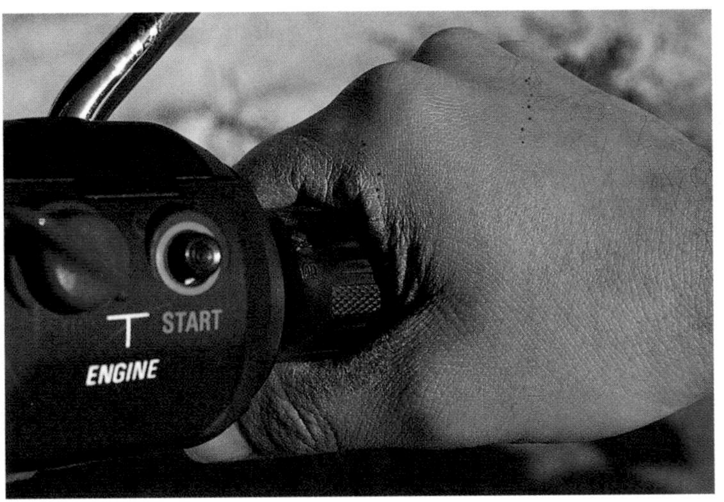

Figure 4.55 Allergic contact dermatitis caused by a hand tool. The patient was patch-test positive to the black rubber mix.

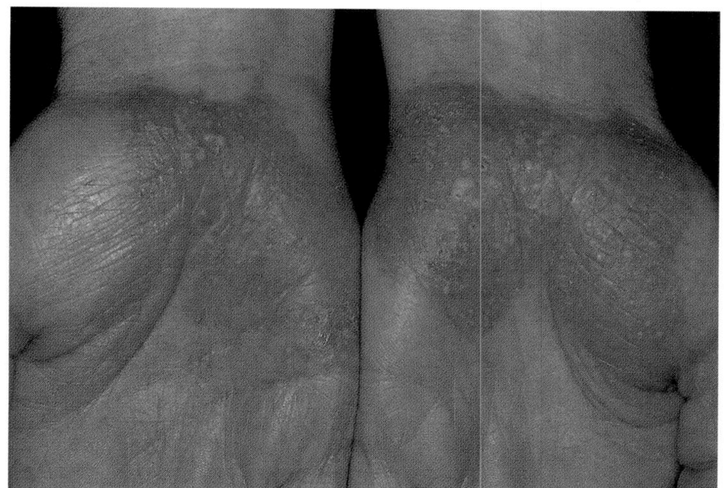
(a)

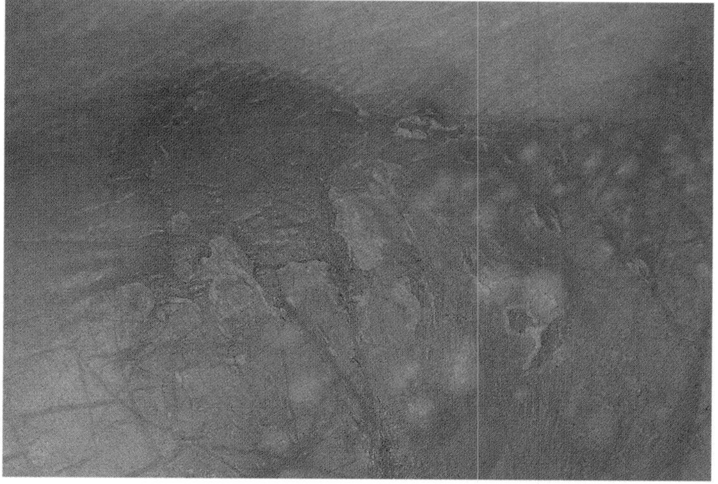
(b)

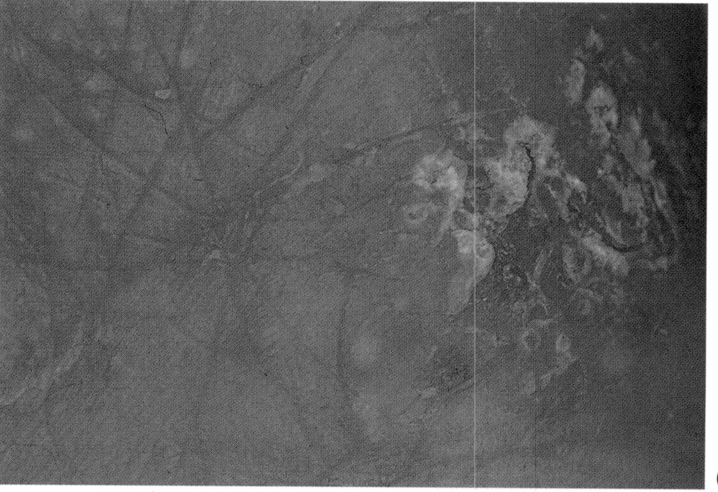
(c)

Figure 4.56 (**a**) Pustular psoriasis of the palms is often symmetrical. It may be seen simultaneously on the soles of the feet, and can be eruptive. The pustules are sterile, there is usually no pruritus, and the condition is refractory to topical treatment. (**b**) A closer view of the lesions of this 35-year-old woman shows that they are pustular from onset, as opposed to secondarily infected vesicular hand dermatitis. (**c**) The psoriasiform scaling of the lesions of the same patient.

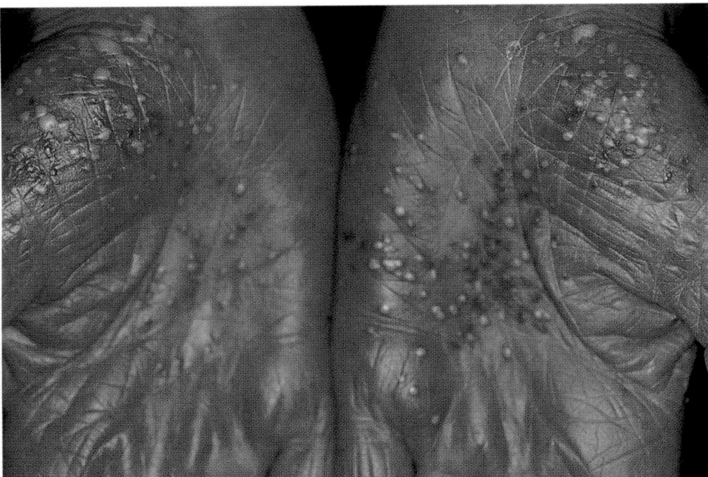

Figure 4.57 A pustular eruption known as palmoplantar pustulosis is identical to pustular psoriasis of the palms except for the lack of psoriasiform scaling. The pustules are sterile.

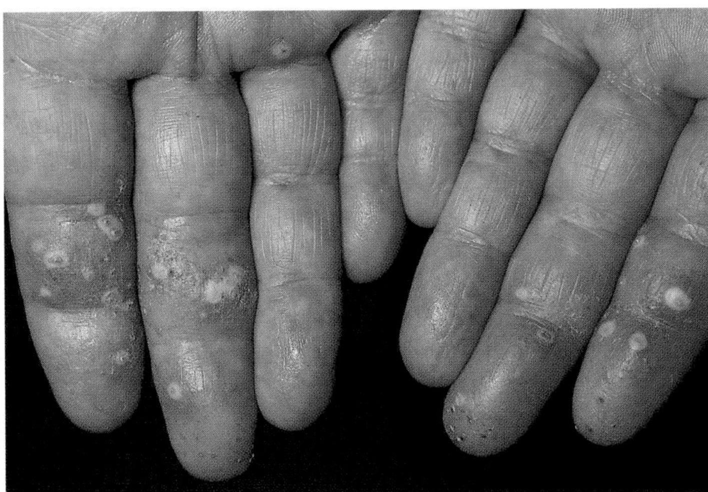

Figure 4.58 Secondarily infected hand dermatitis can easily be confused with the pustular eruptions shown in the previous figures. One clinical difference is that while the causative dermatitis is pruritic, secondarily infected dermatitis is often also painful.

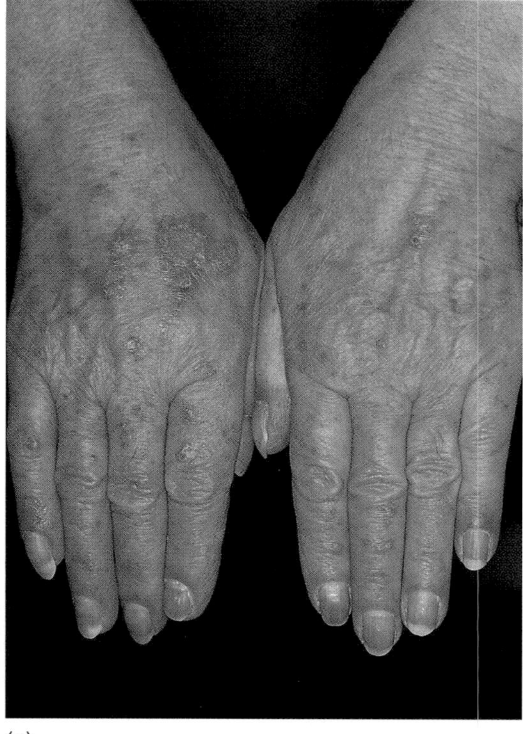

(**a**)

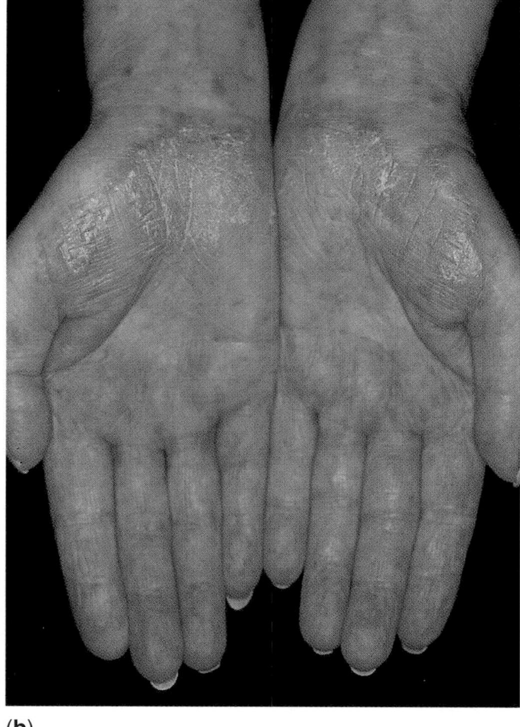

(**b**)

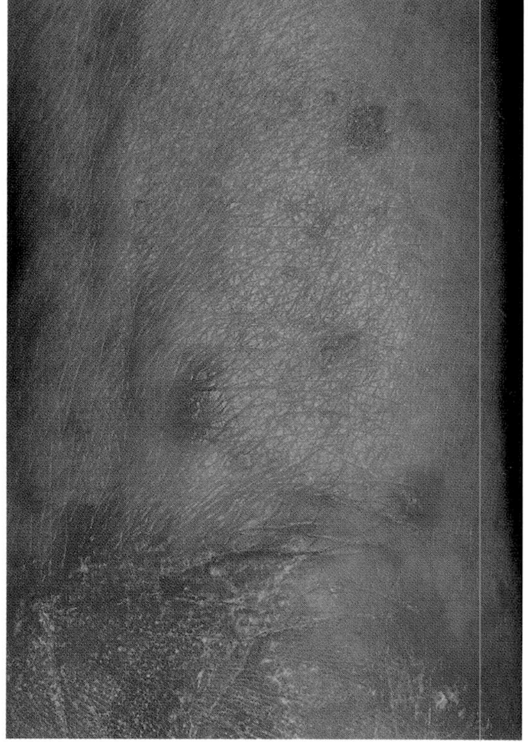

(**c**)

Figure 4.59 (**a**, **b**) Lichen planus, as seen on the hands of this 62-year-old woman, is another important differential diagnosis of hand dermatitis. There are usually lesions elsewhere on the skin surface and/or mucous membranes, and the dusky-red colour of the well-demarcated lesions, and the lichenoid lesions (**c**) commonly seen in adjacent areas, aid the diagnosis.

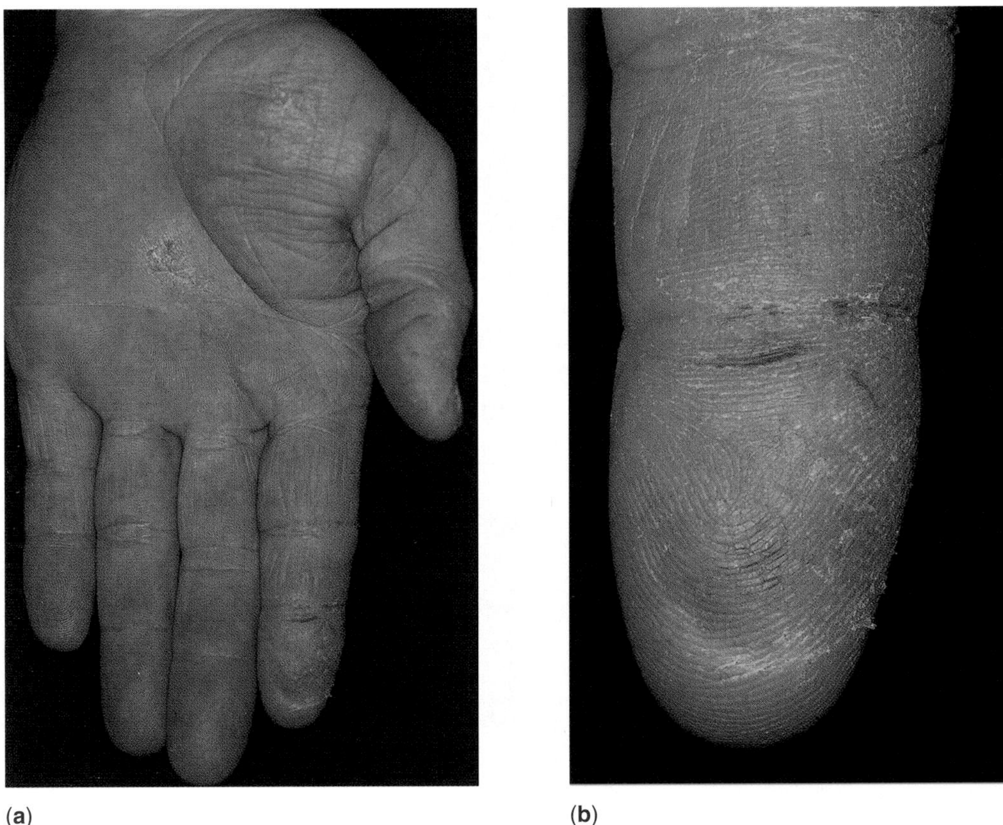

(**a**) (**b**)

Figure 4.60 (**a**) Dermatophytes – in this case *Trichophyton rubrum* – can produce lesions that mimic hand dermatitis. (**b**) A close-up of the index finger of the same patient. Dermatophytic infections of the hands are usually asymmetrical. Many patients have concomitant infections of the feet, and some have evidence of onychomycosis. It has recently been suggested that patients with dermatophytosis of the feet also acquire dermatophytosis of the dominant hand because that hand is used to scratch the feet ('one hand, two feet syndrome'). Dermatophytid has a reaction pattern that is often a 'one foot, two hands syndrome'. This is described later in this chapter in the section on 'Palmar location', p. 97.

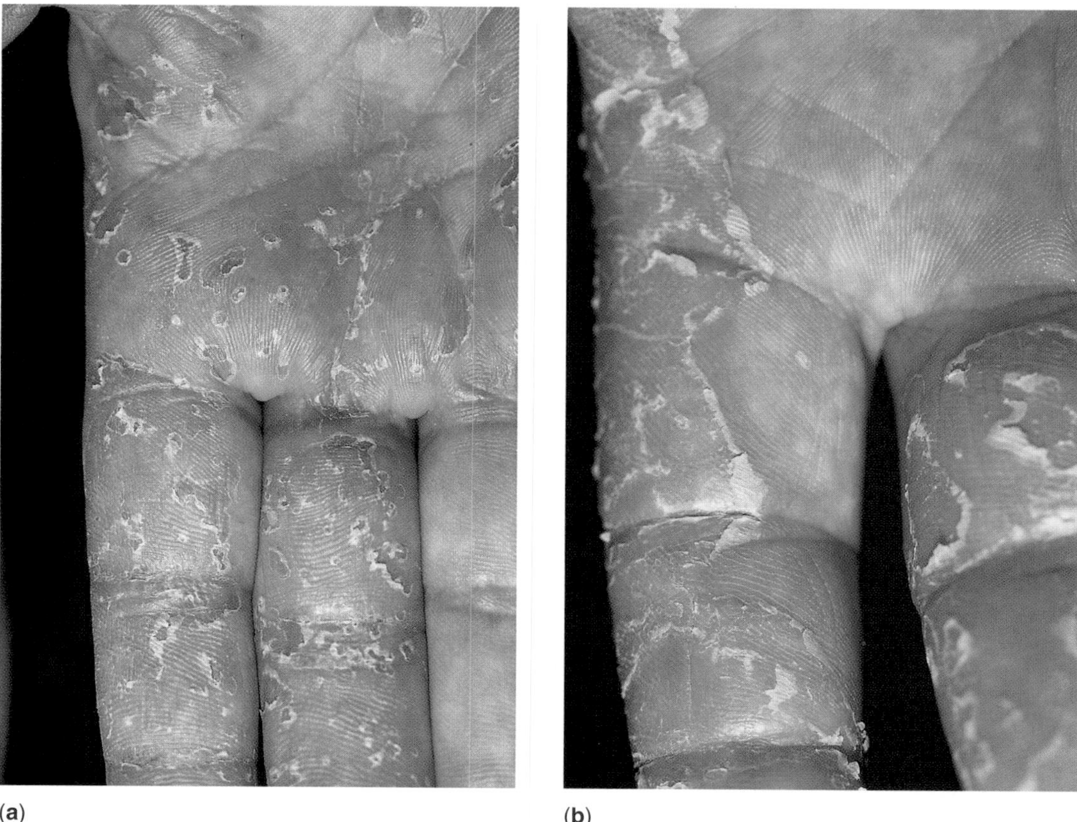

(a) (b)

Figure 4.61 The palms may periodically peel without any warning or accompanying symptoms. This condition has been given a variety of names: keratolysis exfoliativa, recurrent focal palmar peeling, lamellar dyshidrosis or dysidrosis lamellosa sicca (Lee et al, 1996). Sweat retention in the stratum corneum has been suspected by some to cause this condition. Dry scales become small dry papules, and gradually desquamate in an annular fashion. No inflammation is seen in most cases, but this 40-year-old woman has some erythema (**a**), as did this 63-year-old man with the same condition (**b**).

CONCOMITANT DERMATITIS IN LOCATIONS OTHER THAN THE HANDS

It is important to determine whether a patient with hand dermatitis has dermatitis elsewhere. Concomitant dermatitis in areas where allergic or irritant contact dermatitis is typically seen, such as at sites of contact with nickel-plated or rubber items, may suggest a diagnosis of allergic contact dermatitis.

Atopic dermatitis is a clinical diagnosis, and typical lesions at sites other than the hands may help to establish this diagnosis. White dermatographism on dermatitic skin can also point to a diagnosis of atopic dermatitis.

Seborrhoeic dermatitis may involve the hands, and is a diagnosis made clinically on the basis of scalp lesions and dermatitis in seborrhoeic and intertriginous areas.

Nummular eczema is most common on the arms and legs. When seen on the hands, it is usually on the dorsal aspects. The aetiology is unknown. Xerosis and secondary bacterial infection may play a role in the pathogenesis (Hellgren and Mobacken, 1969).

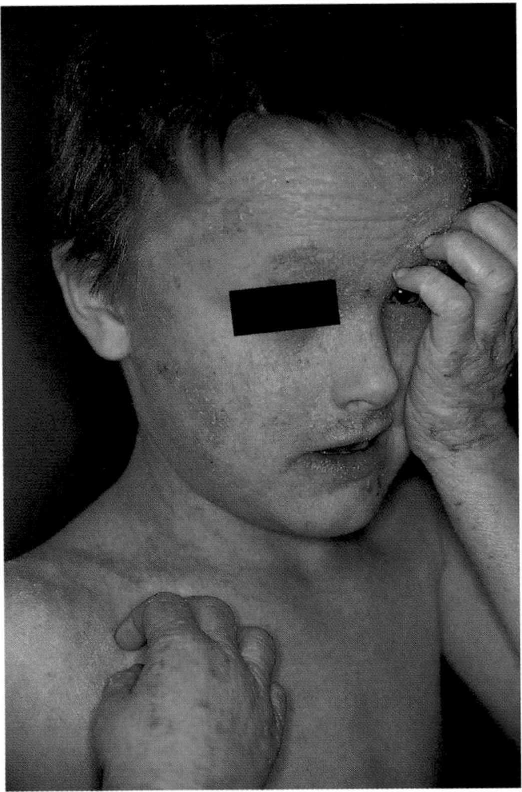

Figure 4.62 A diagnosis of atopic dermatitis of the hands was easily made for this 5-year-old boy, since he scratched constantly and had similar dermatitis in other areas of the body.

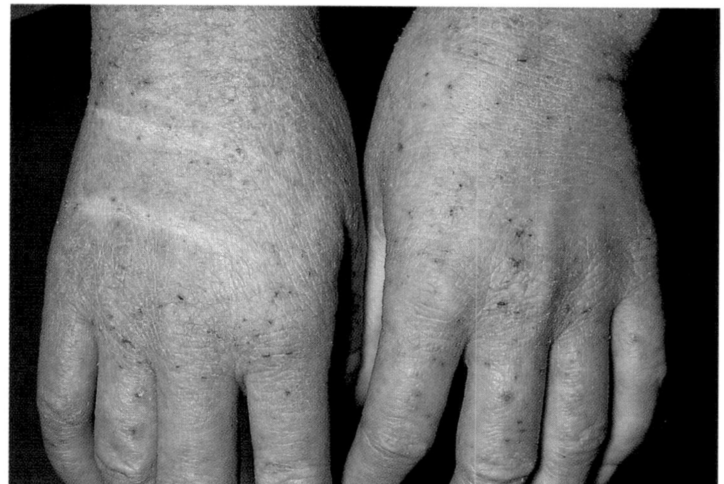

Figure 4.63 Patients with atopic dermatitis are prone to develop irritant dermatitis on the dorsal aspects of the hands. White dermatographism, as seen in this 14-year-old girl, is helpful in making the diagnosis of atopic dermatitis.

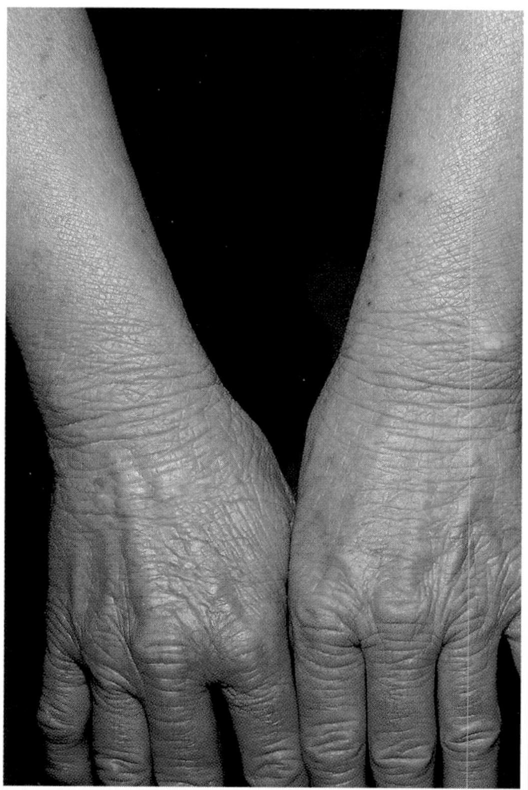

Figure 4.64 Lichenification is also an indication of atopic dermatitis.

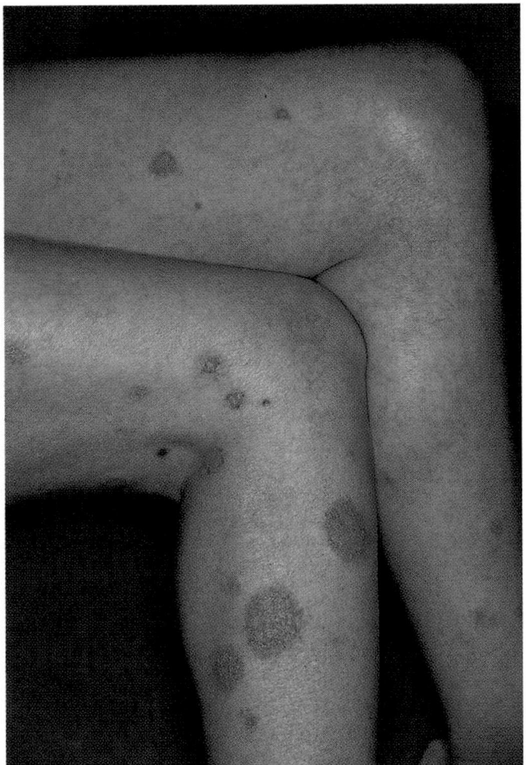

(**a**)

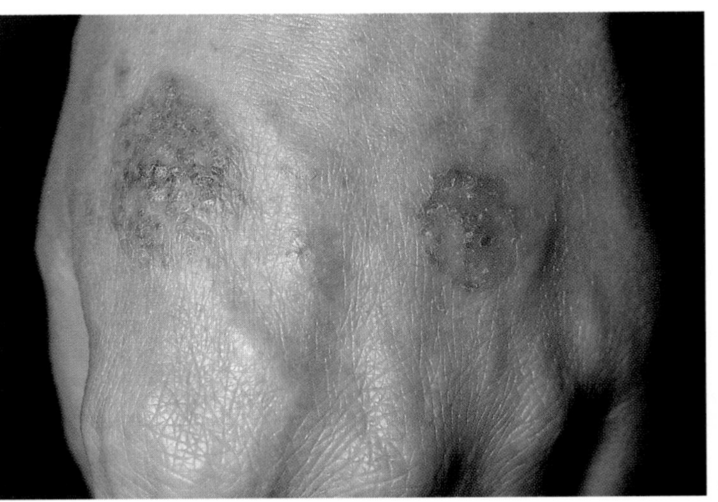

(**b**)

Figure 4.65 (**a**) This 40-year-old woman developed circumscribed areas of dermatitis with vesicles typical of nummular (coin-shaped) dermatitis. (**b**) When seen on the hands, nummular dermatitis is usually on the dorsal aspects.

PATTERNS AND MORPHOLOGY

Contact pattern

An obvious contact pattern is unusual in patients with hand dermatitis. Allergic contact dermatitis is typically asymmetrical, with the most-intense dermatitis being where the offending substance has been in contact with the skin. Both the dominant and the non-dominant hand may be involved, depending on the pattern of contact. Irritants such as detergents, soaps and cutting oils are more likely to affect both hands and cause more symmetrical dermatitis. Persons with atopic dermatitis are more prone than others to irritant contact dermatitis on the hands.

Nickel may occasionally cause dermatitis at the site of contact. Fingertip dermatitis on the first, second and third fingers of the non-dominant hand may be caused by the handling of garlic, while acrylates used in dentistry can cause similar dermatitis on the dominant hand. Allergic contact dermatitis from rubber gloves usually extends from the dorsum of the hands to the forearms, while contact urticaria from latex is usually seen only on the dorsal aspects of the hands. Protein contact dermatitis can be seen at the site of contact, with, for example, potatoes held as they are peeled, as illustrated in Figure 5.62.

Finger rings may cause a characteristic contact pattern in nickel-sensitive patients who wear inexpensive jewellery. The same pattern is occasionally also seen in gold-sensitive patients. Dermatitis under finger rings is more commonly an irritant dermatitis caused by the retention of soap, detergents and water under the rings. Ring dermatitis is most common on the dorsal aspects of the fingers but may extend to the palmar aspects and even to the same finger on the opposite hand – even if no ring is worn there.

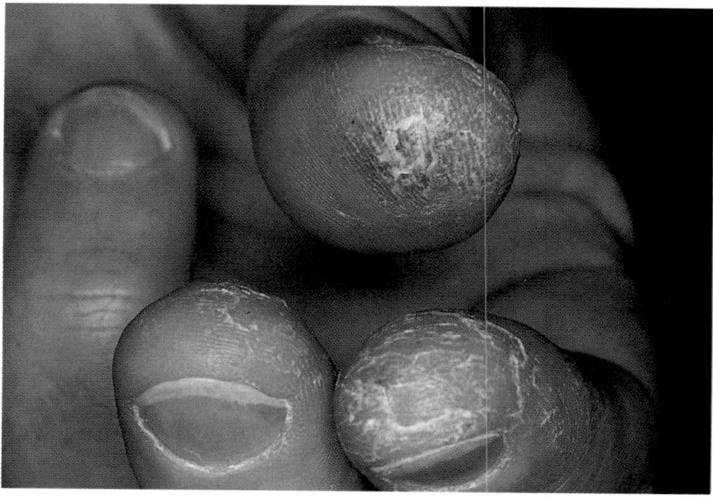

Figure 4.66 The tips of the fingers can be the exclusive site of allergic contact dermatitis, as seen in this dentist because of the nature of his exposure to acrylates. Florists may develop a nearly identical fingertip eruption from *Alstroemeria* plants (van Ketel et al, 1975). Working with tulip bulbs can likewise cause a fingertip eruption, and both garlic and onion can also produce this picture (Sinha et al, 1977). (See also Figures 7.92–7.95.)

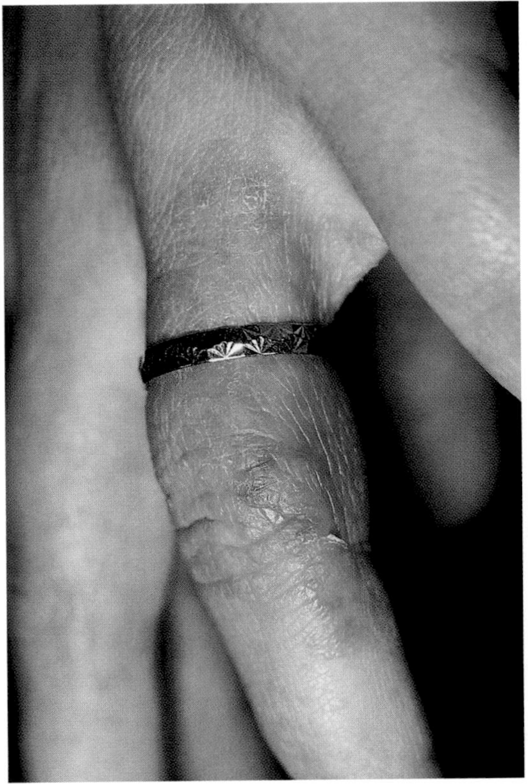

Figure 4.67 Irritant contact dermatitis may develop under rings – commonly from soap and other irritants occluded under the rings, as in this 22-year-old woman. There was no evidence of allergic contact dermatitis.

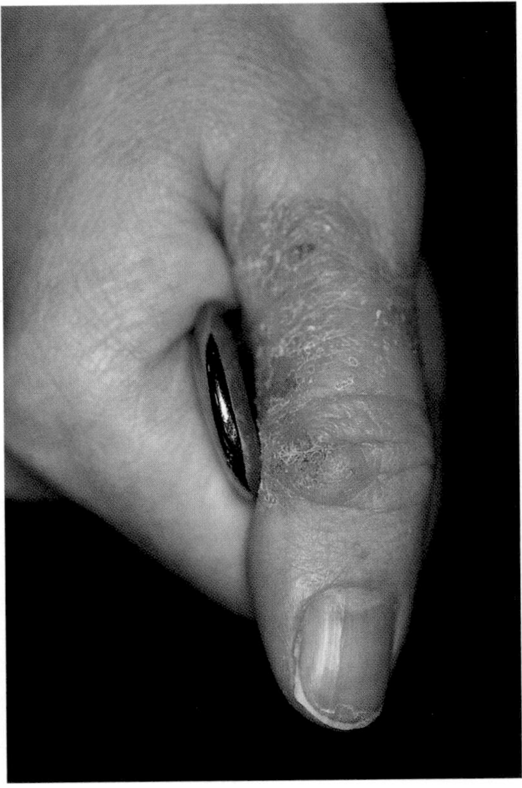

Figure 4.68 Nickel hand dermatitis as a contact pattern in a 37-year-old psychotic woman who carried her keys in her right hand all day. The dimethylglyoxime test (see Figure 6.65) showed that the key chain contained nickel.

Dorsal location

Dermatitis on the dorsal aspects of the hands is frequently associated with an external cause or atopic dermatitis. Thin dorsal skin is probably more vulnerable to irritants, and is more easily penetrated by allergens. Wet work promotes irritant contact dermatitis of the hands (Nilsson, 1986).

Interdigital location

Dermatitis at the top of the fingerwebs is usually irritant contact dermatitis, and is commonly associated with dorsal dermatitis, while vesicular, symmetrical dermatitis on the sides of the fingers may have an external cause or be systemic allergic contact dermatitis or dermatophytid. Concomitant palmar involvement is common in dermatophytid and systemic allergic contact dermatitis (Veien and Menné, 1993; Veien et al, 1994).

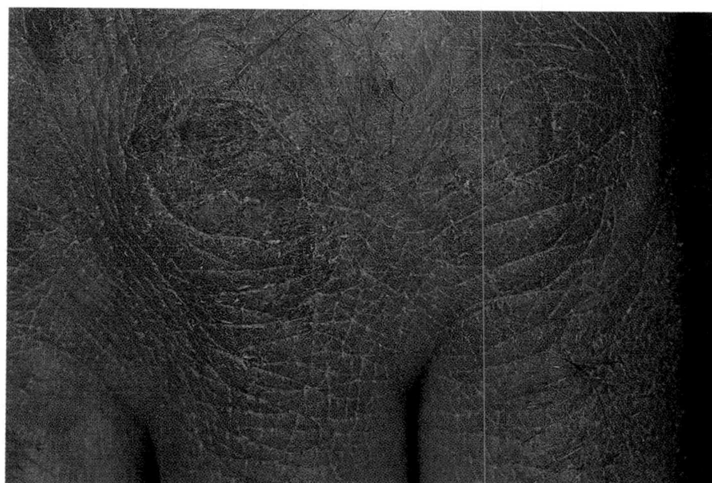

Figure 4.69 In temperate climates, chapping, especially of the knuckles in winter, is often a precursor of irritant contact hand dermatitis, as in this 26-year-old woman who worked as a cleaner.

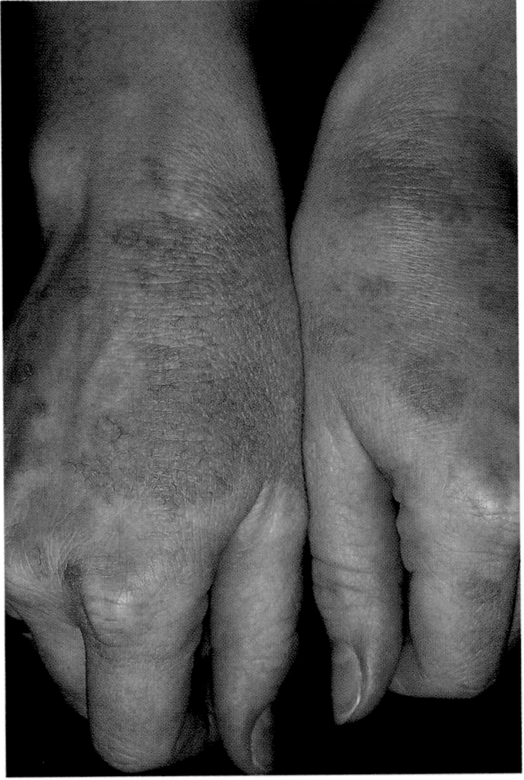

Figure 4.70 This 34-year-old woman, who worked as a cleaner, developed irritant contact dermatitis on the dorsal aspects of her hands.

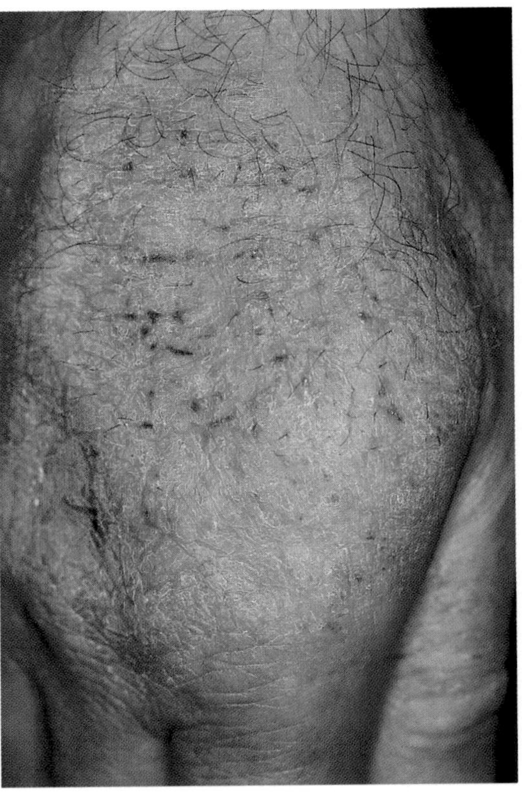

Figure 4.71 A 52-year-old male mechanic developed hand dermatitis from irritants in the oils with which he worked.

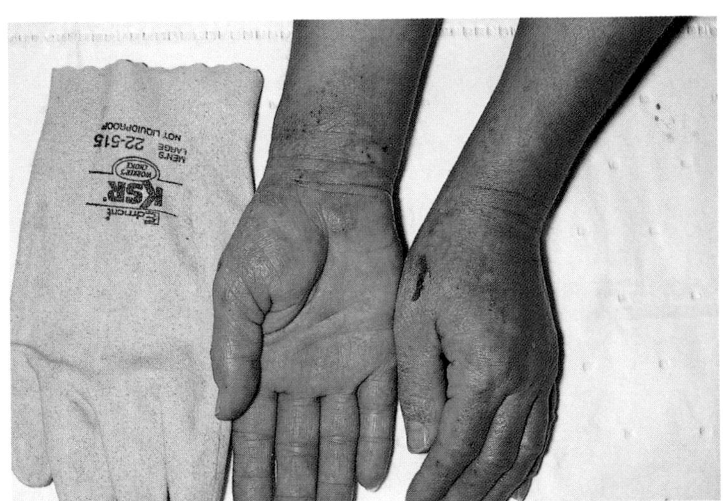

Figure 4.72 Dermatitis on the dorsal aspects of the hand extending to the distal part of the forearm is a characteristic pattern of glove dermatitis, and is usually due to rubber chemicals. This figure shows a 51-year-old woman who had a positive patch test to her glove but not to the rubber chemicals in the European Standard Patch Test Series of allergens.

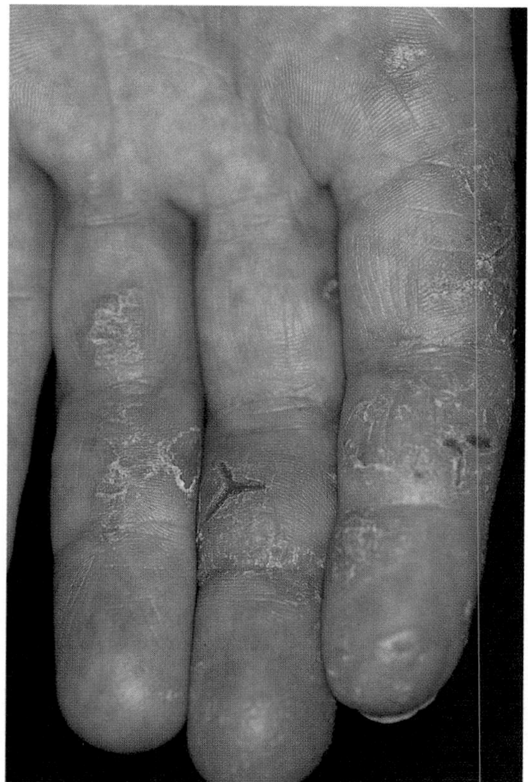

Figure 4.73 Irritant dermatitis can be superimposed on other hand disorders, as seen in this 49-year-old female cleaner with psoriasis.

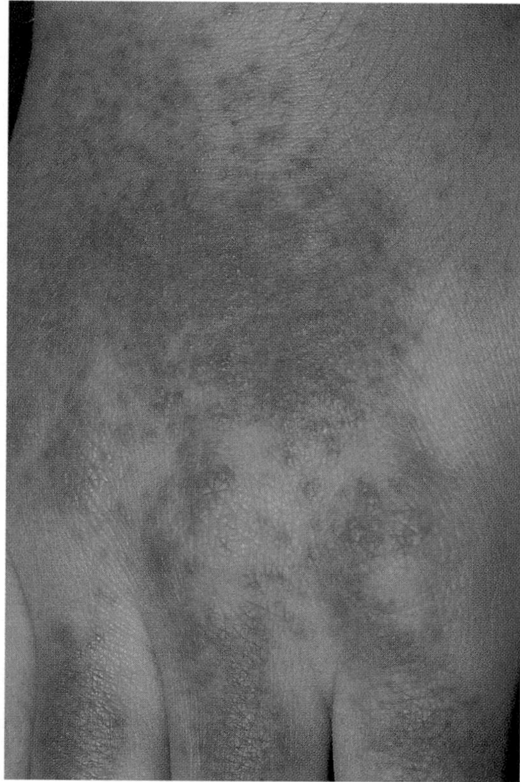

Figure 4.74 Topically applied substances can also cause dermatitis of the hands. This dermatitis on the dorsum of the hands was due to the application of an udder cream. Note the follicular morphology.

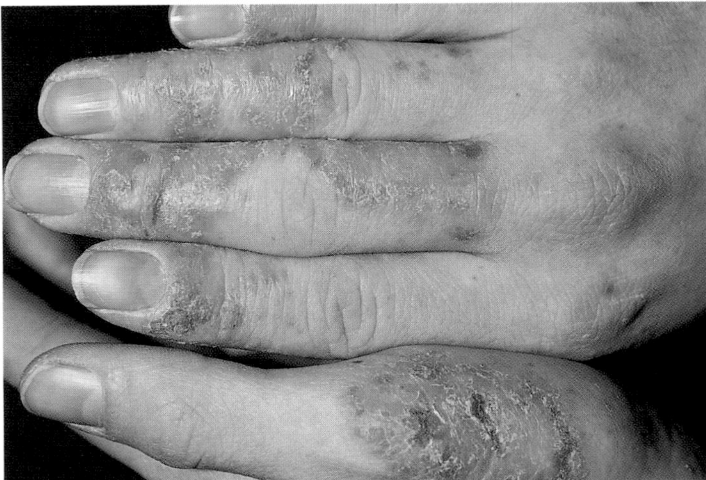

Figure 4.75 This 16-year-old boy had a positive patch test to balsam of Peru, and developed allergic contact dermatitis from contact with scented soap and shampoo.

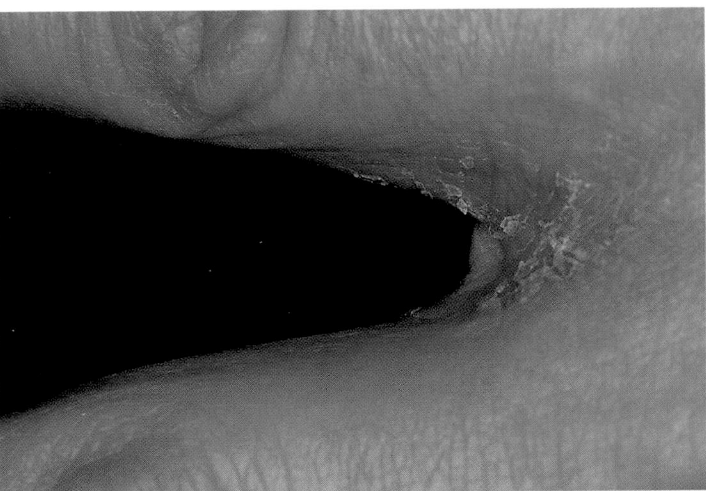

Figure 4.76 Irritant contact dermatitis in the fingerwebs of a 36-year-old woman with wet work. This dermatitis can become secondarily infected with various species of *Candida*.

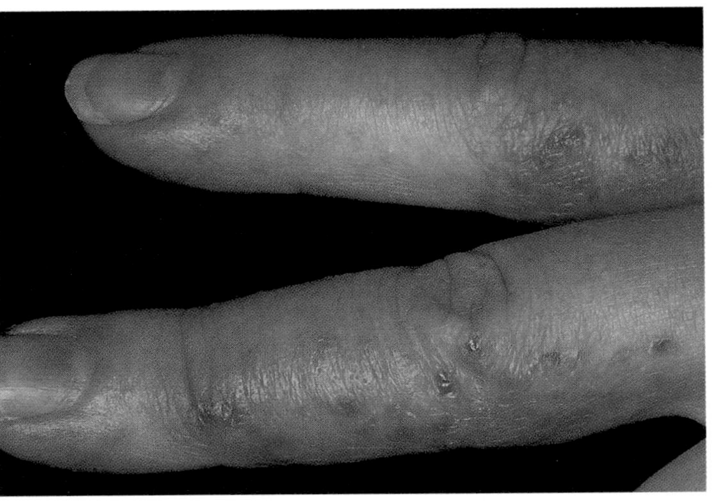

Figure 4.77 Eruptive papular and vesicular dermatitis on the sides of the fingers of a 20-year-old woman who was allergic to nickel, and who reacted to oral challenge with nickel. Her dermatitis improved after following a low-nickel diet.

Palmar location

Although, as mentioned above in the section on 'Contact pattern', dermatitis on the palms or palmar aspects of the fingers is occasionally associated with allergic contact dermatitis, it is more commonly endogenous dermatitis. There are several patterns of palmar dermatitis. One is the fairly common, usually symmetrical, recurrent, vesicular dermatitis seen on both palms. The same type of dermatitis is occasionally seen concomitantly on the soles. This dermatitis was originally described as pompholyx – a rare, eruptive dermatosis with non-inflamed vesicles, symmetrically located on both palms. The lesions heal without scarring and without progression into chronic hand dermatitis. A much more common variety is recurrent vesicular dermatitis that recurs so often that the lesions do not heal between eruptions. The resulting hand dermatitis has the appearance of chronic palmar dermatitis. The patient can describe repeated eruptions of very pruritic vesicles on the palms, around the fingernails and/or on the sides of the fingers. In many instances, this non-specific reaction pattern has no obvious cause (Veien and Menné, 1993).

Atopic dermatitis may occasionally manifest itself as a palmar vesicular eruption (Schwanitz, 1993). Some vesicular eruptions on the hands are dermatophytids – an autoimmune response to a dermatophyte infection on the foot. The diagnostic clue is that the dermatophytosis is often seen on one foot, while the immune reaction – the dermatophytid – is typically symmetrical on the hands: the 'one foot, two hands syndrome' (Menné et al, 1994). This is in contrast to chronic infection with *Trichophyton rubrum* on the hands and feet, in which case the primary infection is on the soles of the feet, and one hand (usually the dominant one that is used to scratch with) is often also infected – the 'one hand, two feet syndrome', which is non-vesicular and morphologically is dry and scaly. Another aetiology of recurrent vesicular dermatitis is systemic contact dermatitis.

Psychological stress and sweating may precipitate recurrent vesicular palmar dermatitis. There is ample evidence that the sweat ducts are not involved in the process, and thus the term 'dyshidrotic eczema' should be abandoned. The dermatitis is a spongiotic dermatitis, with vesicles as the clinical expression of the spongiosis (Veien and Menné, 1993).

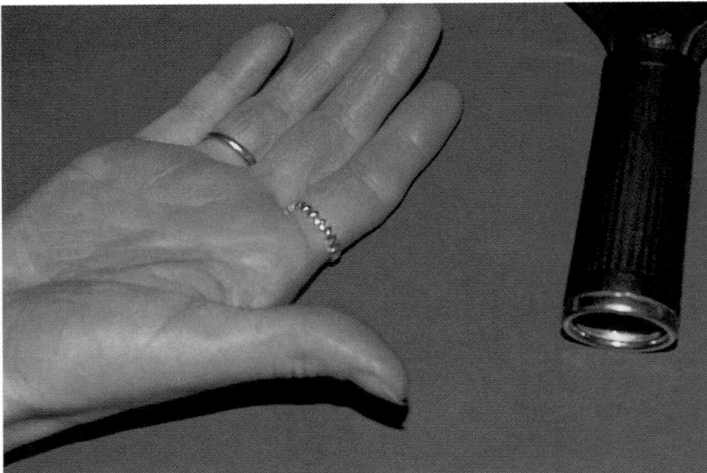

Figure 4.78 Rubber chemicals caused this palmar eruption. The localization to the palm was explained by the nature of the contact. The rubber chemical was isopropyl paraphenylenediamine, a rubber antioxidant, found in the handle of a window cleaning device.

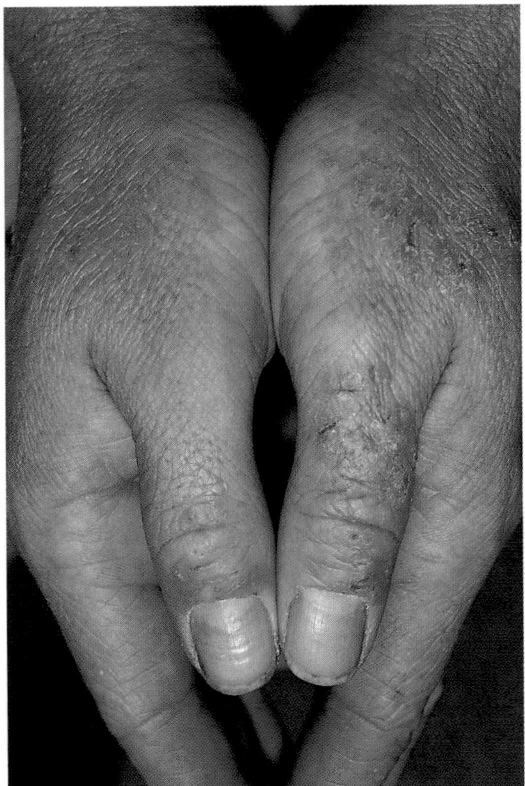

Figure 4.79 This 30-year-old man with hand dermatitis was allergic to potassium dichromate, and his hand dermatitis faded when he exchanged his leather gloves for cloth gloves.

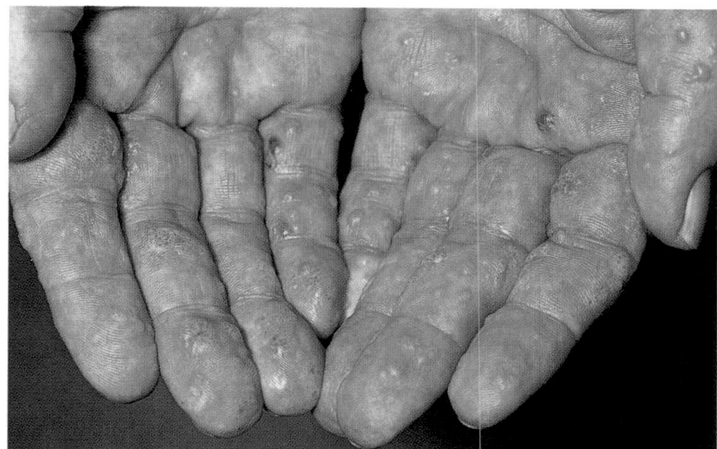

Figure 4.80 Pompholyx, as seen in this 64-year-old man, is a symmetrical eruption of pruritic vesicles in the palms and on the sides of the fingers, without any obvious explanation. The vesicles typically heal without turning into chronic hand dermatitis.

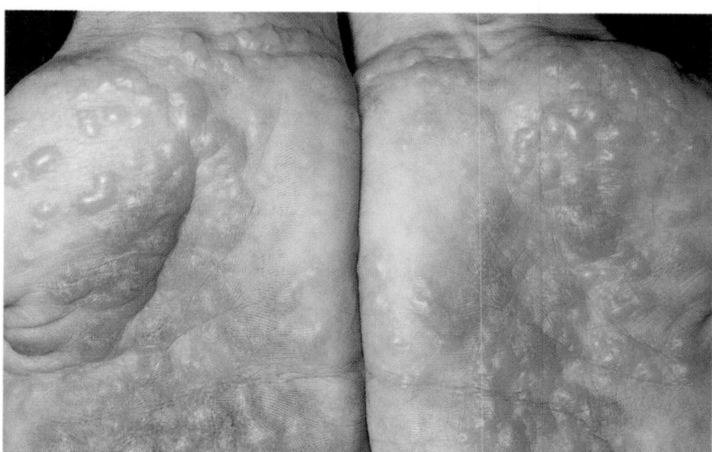

Figure 4.81 After patch testing, this 32-year-old nickel-sensitive woman developed an eruption of vesicles and bullae similar to that seen in the previous figure. Patch testing was probably carried out before her dermatitis had settled completely.

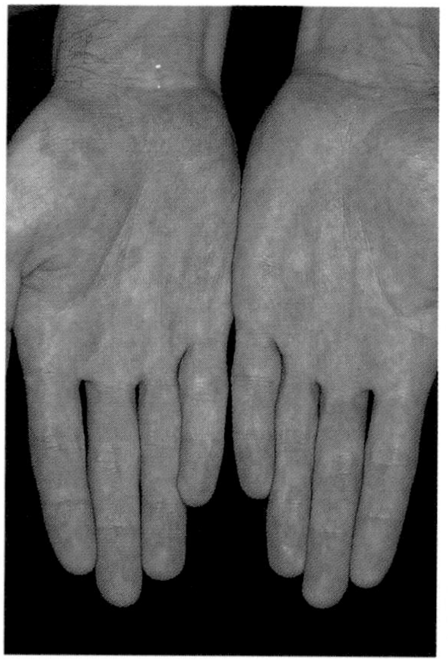

(**a**)

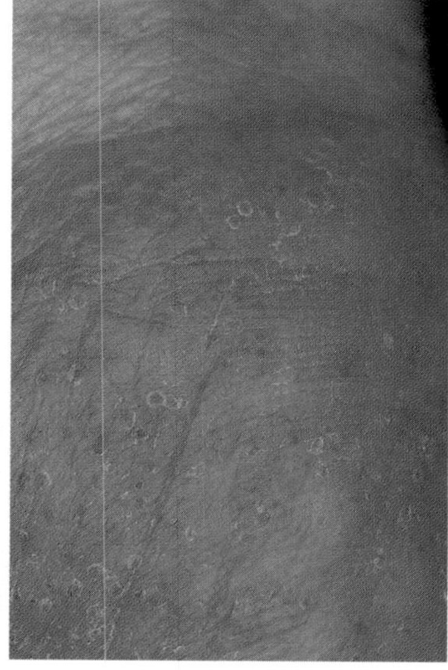

(**b**)

Figure 4.82 (**a**) A 31-year-old man had had symmetrical, pruritic vesicular eruptions of both palms for three years. A closer look (**b**) shows closely set vesicles exclusively on palmar skin, with no vesicles on the thin skin of the wrist. No cause was found, but morphologically this type of dermatitis is identical to systemic contact dermatitis caused, for example, by the metals nickel, cobalt and chromium.

Hyperkeratotic palmar dermatitis: A less common palmar dermatitis is hyperkeratotic palmar dermatitis. This is usually symmetrical and non-pruritic, there are no vesicles, and it is most common among middle-aged men (Hersle and Mobacken, 1982). It is difficult to distinguish hyperkeratotic palmar dermatitis from psoriasis. However, scratching produces white scales and Bulkley's membrane on psoriatic skin (difficult to demonstrate on thick skin). Painful fissures are common in hyperkeratotic palmar dermatitis, and may also be a feature of psoriasis. An examination of the remainder of the skin and the nails is necessary to distinguish between the two conditions.

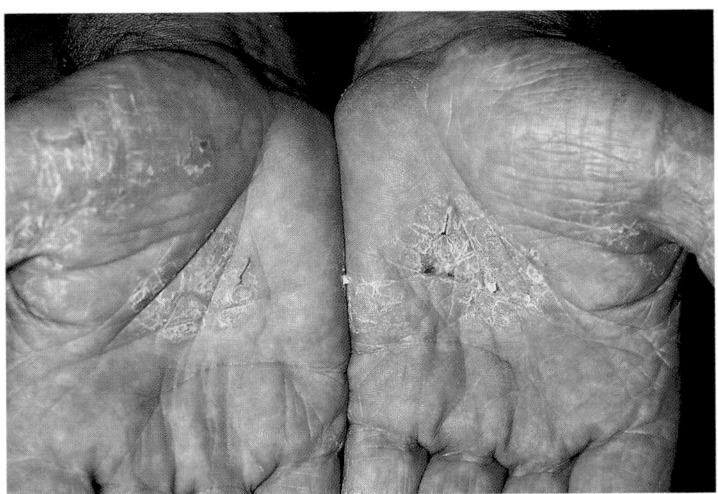

Figure 4.83 Palmar keratotic hand dermatitis is usually seen in middle-aged or older men, as in this 61-year-old man. This dermatitis is symmetrical, usually non-pruritic, and may resemble psoriasis. The cause of this condition is unknown, but it is often aggravated by mechanical friction.

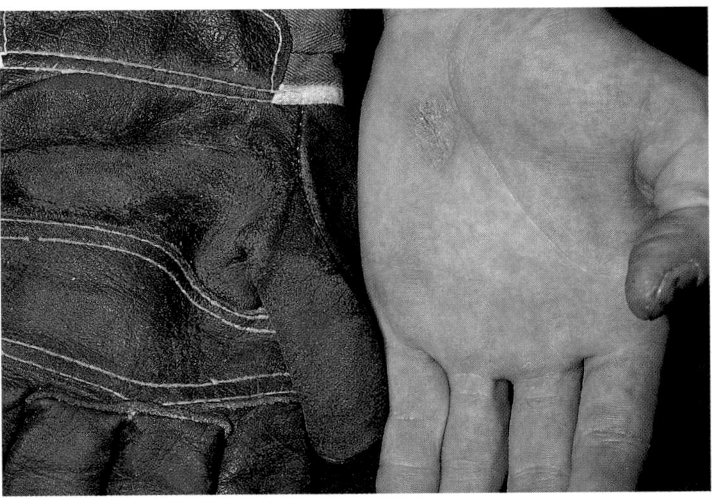

Figure 4.84 This is an example of keratotic hand dermatitis in a 25-year-old man. The role of friction was noted, since the area of greatest wear on his work glove corresponded to the area of maximum skin change. No vesicles are seen at any time in this disorder.

Pulpitis: Pulpitis is dermatitis of the fingertips. As described previously, cooks and dentists may develop allergic contact dermatitis on the fingertips that are most commonly in contact with strong allergens such as diallyl disulfide in garlic and the acrylates in dental materials. It is therefore important to note the contact pattern of these clinical manifestations of dermatitis. Most types of pulpitis other than allergic contact dermatitis are symmetrical and affect all the fingertips. Lesional skin is dry and fissured, and there are no vesicles. This suggests atopic dermatitis, mechanical irritant contact dermaitis from paper or cardboard, or irritant contact dermaitis with no obvious aetiology.

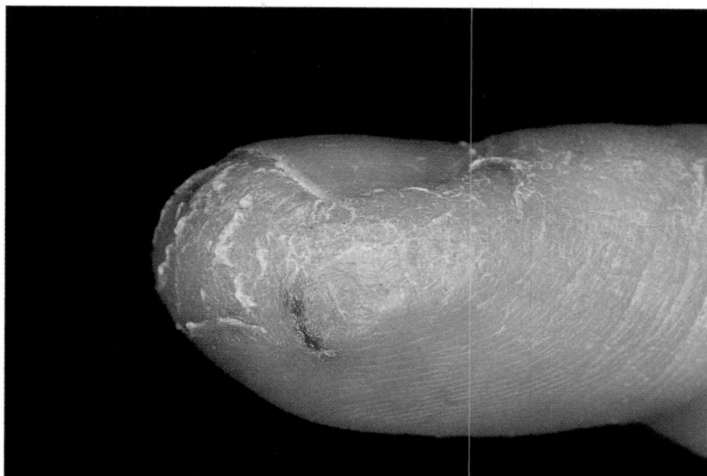

Figure 4.85 This 32-year-old woman has pulpitis. No cause could be found.

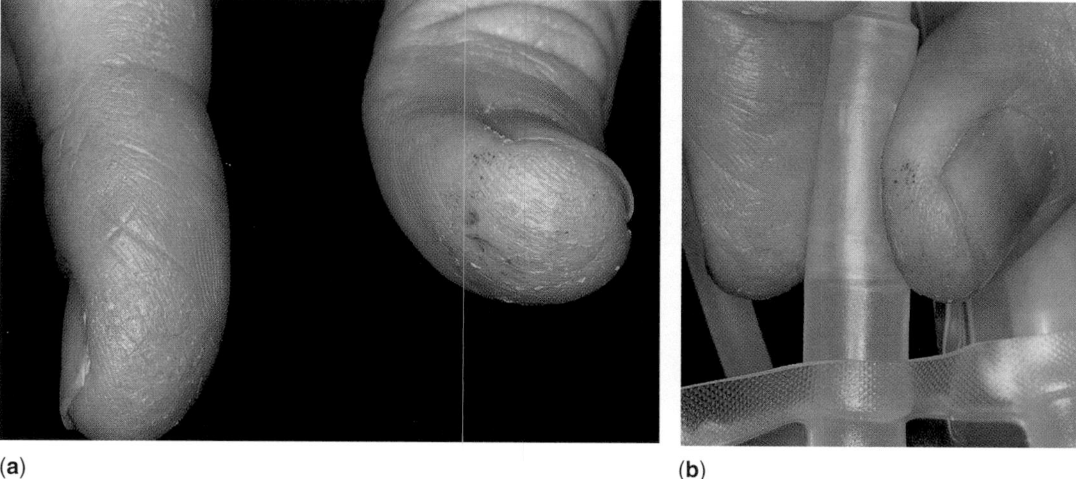

(**a**) (**b**)

Figure 4.86 (**a**) Pure mechanical friction may produce an almost-identical picture to pulpitis, as seen in this 42-year-old woman who attached and removed blood bag tubes in her job as a laboratory technician (**b**). The movements were repeated with sufficient frequency to cause mechanical dermatitis.

'Fixed' dermatitis: Systemic contact dermatitis on the hands may occur as a 'fixed' dermatitis with recurrences in one particular area and no dermatitis elsewhere. There is usually a vesicular eruption in the active phase of this dermatitis.

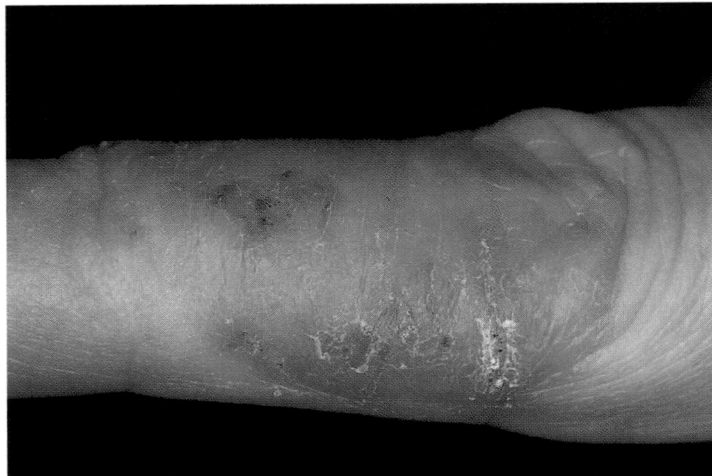

Figure 4.87 The dermatitis of this 23-year-old nickel-sensitive woman recurred in exactly the same area on her third right finger for three years. The dermatitis finally faded after she had followed a rather strict low-nickel diet for two months.

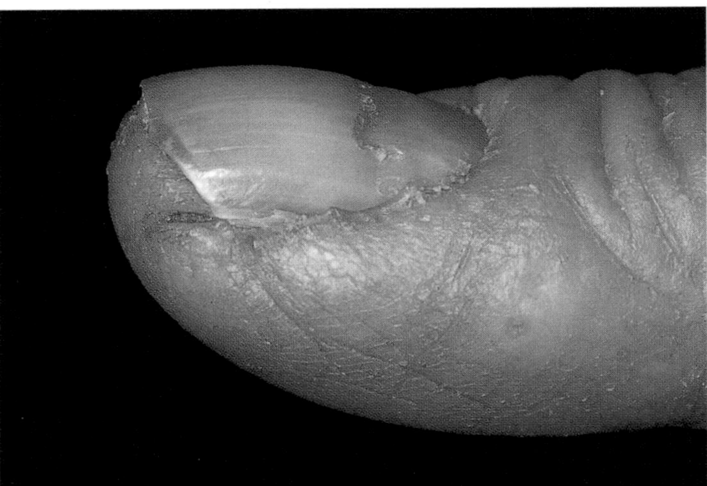

Figure 4.88 Mechanical friction can induce very painful fissures at the edges of the fingernails, as seen in this 51-year-old woman. This is a variant of fingertip dermatitis.

Dorsal and palmar location

All types of hand dermatitis can cover the entire surface of the hands, and such widespread dermatitis is common in connection with generalized dermatitis. Protein contact dermatitis caused by raw food items is a common secondary aggravating factor among housewives with extensive, chronic hand dermatitis. This is probably because the proteins can penetrate the already-damaged skin. Interestingly, even in cases of severe atopic dermatitis, the palms often remain clear.

Nails

Nail changes may occur indirectly owing to contact dermatitis of the skin surrounding the nails or owing to dermatitis developing under the nails. The nails are composed of keratin, and cannot manifest intercellular oedema or spongiotic changes, but rather reflect those changes by disorderly maturation. Dystrophic nail changes are the most common manifestation of contact dermatitis involving the proximal nail fold. Common contact allergens are given in the box.

Allergens

- Acrylates:
  - Nail varnish
  - Artificial nails
  - Screw sealants
- Ammonium thioglycolate
- Toluenesulfonamide–formaldehyde resin (tosylamide–formaldehyde resin)

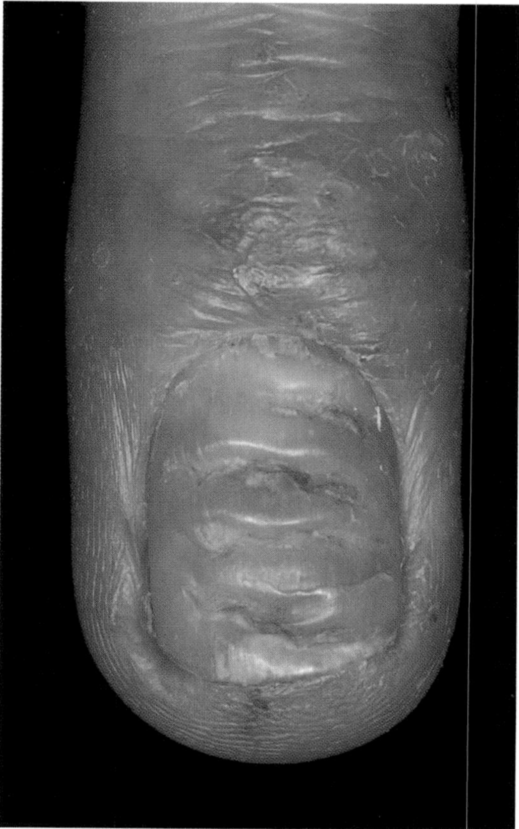

Figure 4.89 A feature of chronic or recurrent hand dermatitis is the presence of multiple Beau's lines on the fingernails of persons with hand dermatitis. The furrows are produced when dermatitis disturbs growth in the nail matrix. The nails of this 38-year-old man indicate that he has had several eruptions of hand dermatitis.

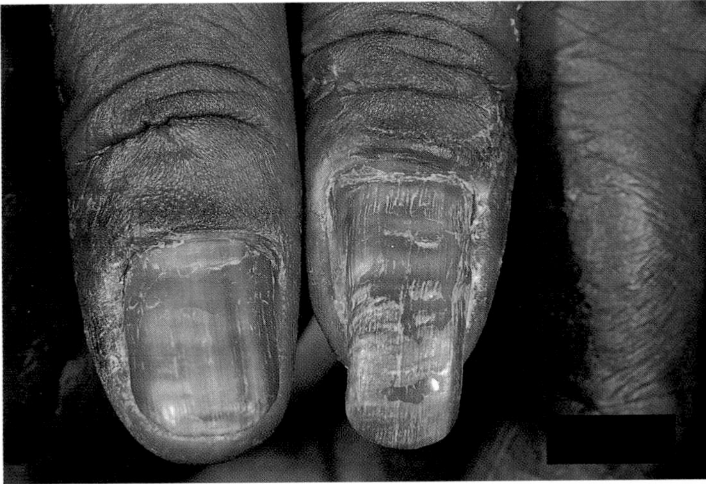

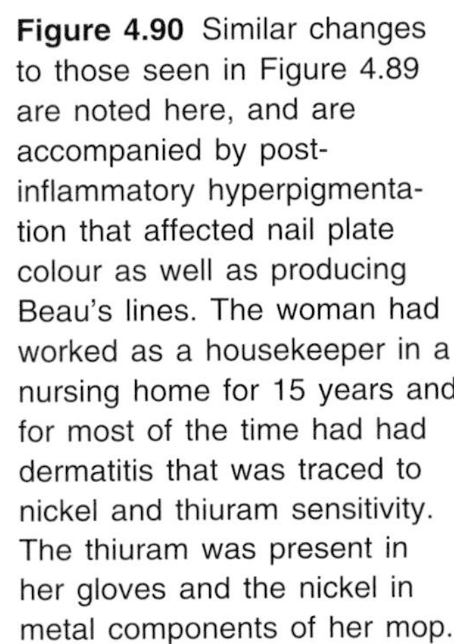

Figure 4.90 Similar changes to those seen in Figure 4.89 are noted here, and are accompanied by post-inflammatory hyperpigmentation that affected nail plate colour as well as producing Beau's lines. The woman had worked as a housekeeper in a nursing home for 15 years and for most of the time had had dermatitis that was traced to nickel and thiuram sensitivity. The thiuram was present in her gloves and the nickel in metal components of her mop.

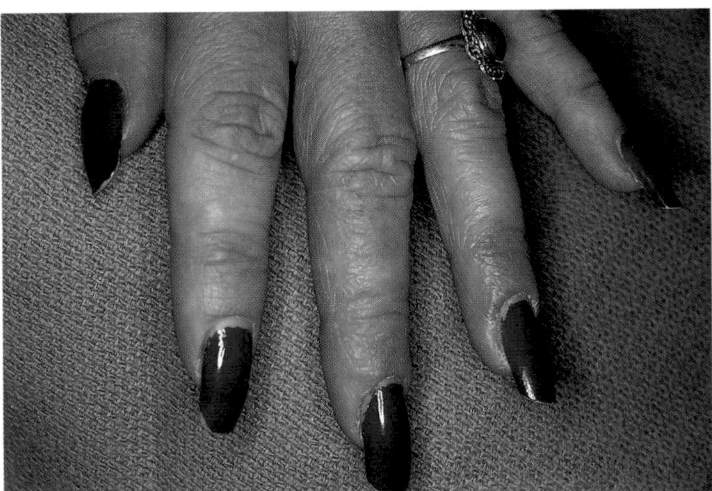

(a)

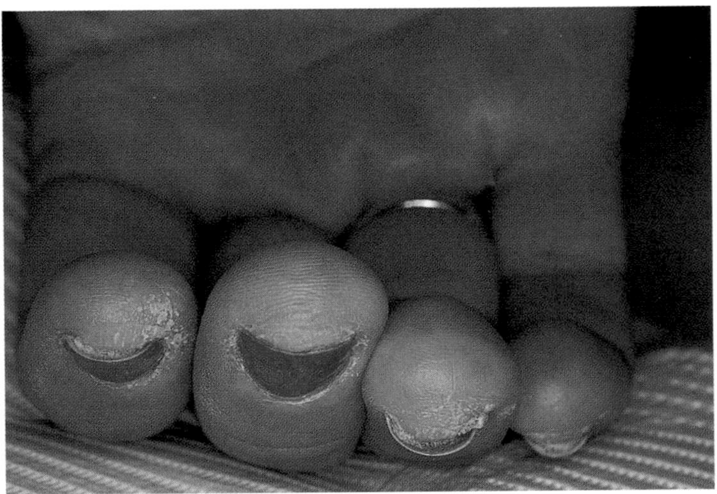

(b)

Figure 4.91 (**a**) Acrylate allergy due to artificial nails was detected as the source of periungual inflammation and (**b**) subungual keratin buildup in the onycholytic change that accompanies this type of allergic reaction (Marks et al, 1979). Methyl methacrylate was the original acrylate associated with this condition, but, as was the case in this patient, many other acrylates have been identified as contact allergens (Fisher, 1980; Hemmer et al, 1996). This reaction can sometimes lead to permanent loss of nails (Fisher, 1989).

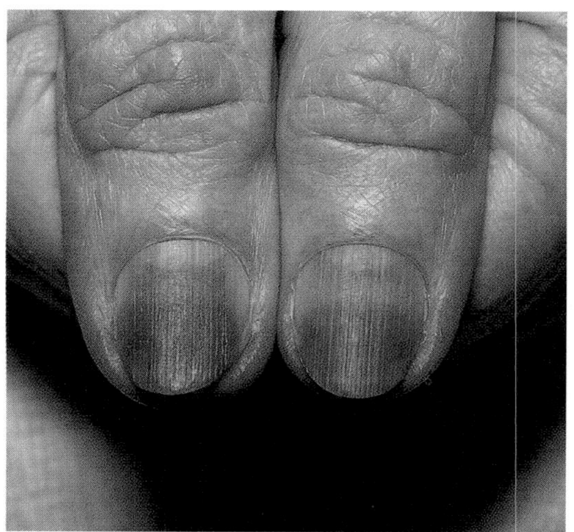

Figure 4.92 At times, topically applied agents can stain the nail, as seen in this woman who applied a hydroquinone-containing cream to her hands to treat melanoses. Hydroquinone, which is used to bleach hyperpigmentation, can, paradoxically, hyperpigment the nails (Garcia et al, 1978).

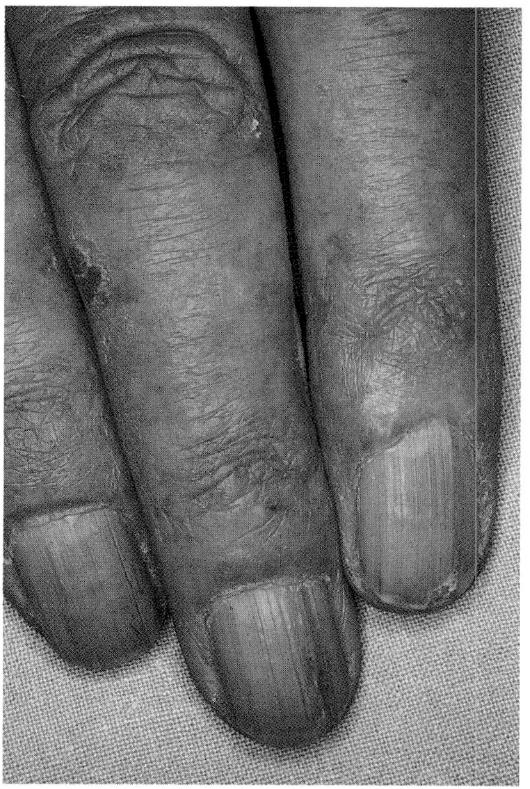

Figure 4.93 A change of nail colouring, and the appearance of streaks, in a radiologist suffering from chronic radiodermatitis (Conde-Salazar et al, 1987).

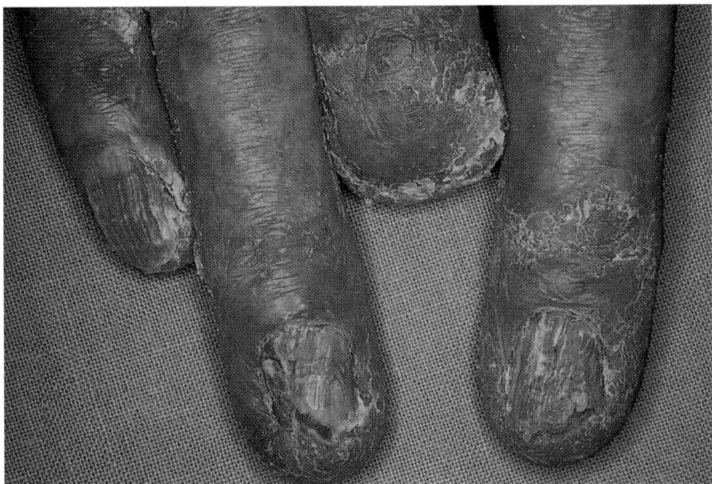

Figure 4.94 Total destruction of the nails with the appearance of pre-malignant lesions on the back of the fingers of a radiologist suffering from chronic radiodermatitis. The distal third of a finger was amputated due to the presence of squamous cell carcinoma (Conde-Salazar et al, 1987).

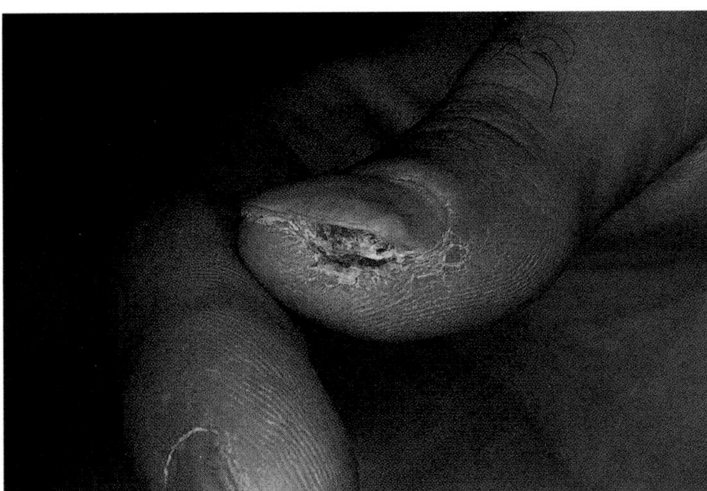

Figure 4.95 Pre-malignant lesion in the subungal region of a patient with occupational radiodermatitis produced by iridium-192 (Conde-Salazar et al, 1986).

Feet

Exogenous dermatitis of the feet is commonly caused by components of footware. The allergens present in shoes include chromate found in leather, rubber components and rubber cements used to bind the components together, and dyes (Saha et al, 1993; Freeman, 1997). If socks are worn with the footware, the allergens must traverse the sock before becoming available to the skin for absorption and subsequent dermatitis. Allergens may be retained in socks even after washing and boiling (Rietschel, 1984). In some cases, the allergens in footware remain unidentified even after careful patch testing. The use of pieces of specific shoes and socks can be of assistance as patch test devices in such cases. Common contact allergens are given in the box below.

Allergens

Medications
Socks

Shoes:
- Leather
- Glues
- Rubber components

ALLERGEN ALTERNATIVES

If the dermatitis is on the dorsum of the foot and there is no allergy to leather (chromate) then a hand-sewn leather upper shoe can be selected if it is unlined. Glues are the most common allergens in this setting, and can also be avoided with a plain canvas-topped shoe. In the USA, the penny loafer known as the Bass Weejun is available in an unlined leather upper style.

Several canvas shoes are available, such as the Docksider by Sperry for men and Keds for women. The least-expensive versions of these shoes are sewn together, and do not have multilayer construction that requires glues.

If the dermatitis is on the soles then a protective insole is required. Neoprene insoles are acceptable if the patient is allergic to thiuram, mercaptobenzothiazole or carbamates. However, if the patient is allergic to thioureas, neoprene should be avoided and an activated charcoal insole can be used as a temporary measure. Plastizote can be moulded to form an insole for any shoe, and is available at orthopaedic brace and limb shops. It is a suitable alternative even if the patient's allergen is unknown and the dermatitis is confined to the sole.

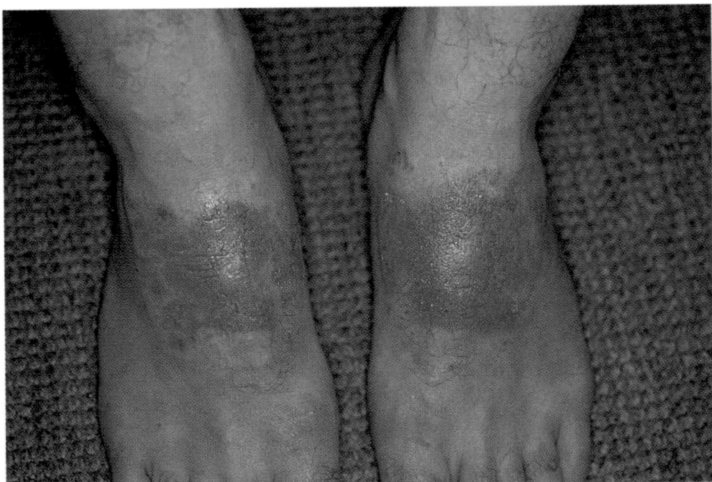

Figure 4.96 Symmetrical dermatitis of the feet can be a clue that shoe components are responsible for the dermatitis.

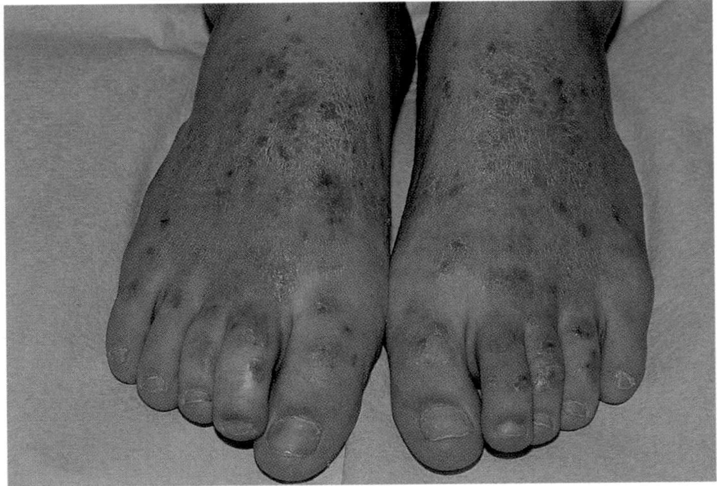

Figure 4.97 This shoe dermatitis is easily distinguished from dermatophyte infections of the feet, since the interdigital areas are spared because they are not in contact with the components of the shoes containing the allergen. Tinea pedis usually begins between the toes and spreads from that site. Here the interdigital areas were clearly spared.

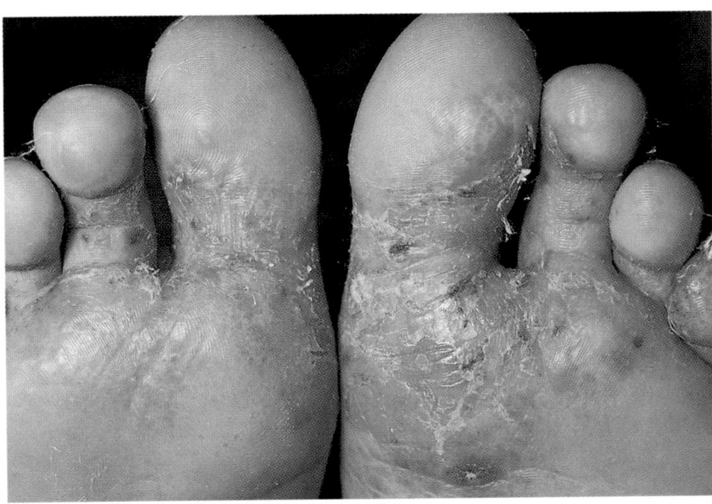

Figure 4.98 Children with pruritic, plantar forefoot dermatitis with vesicles should be suspected of having allergic contact dermatitis as seen in this 10-year-old boy. He had a positive patch test to the rubber vulcanizer, mercaptobenzothiazole, and the dermatitis was caused by rubber in his shoes.

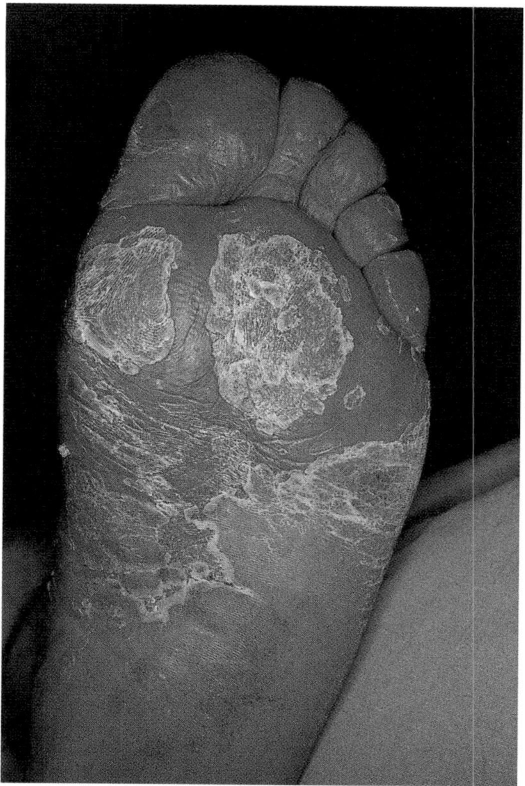

Figure 4.99 The rubber insole of the black rubber boots worn by a construction worker was responsible for this plantar dermatitis. The allergens proved to be the antioxidants added to the insole: *N*-isopropyl-*N'*-phenyl-*p*-phenylene-diamine (IPPD) and cyclohexyl-phenyl-paraphenylenediamine (CPPD).

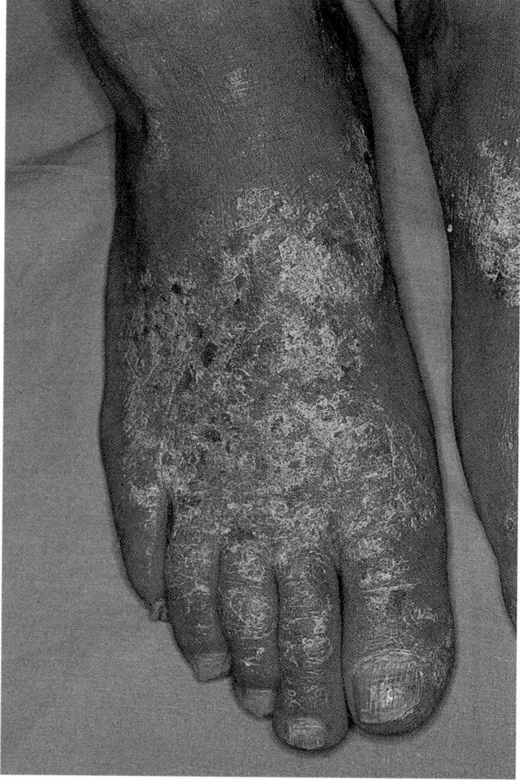

Figure 4.100 This chronic dermatitis on the dorsum of the foot was caused by chromate contained in the leather of Spanish-manufactured footware.

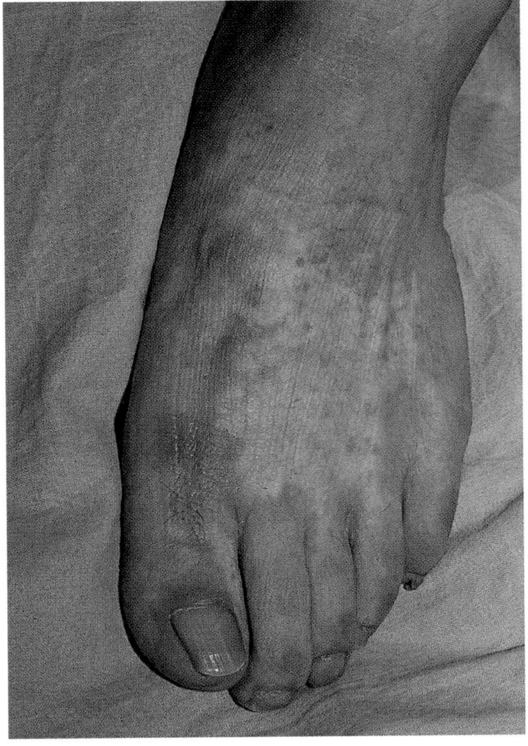

(**a**)

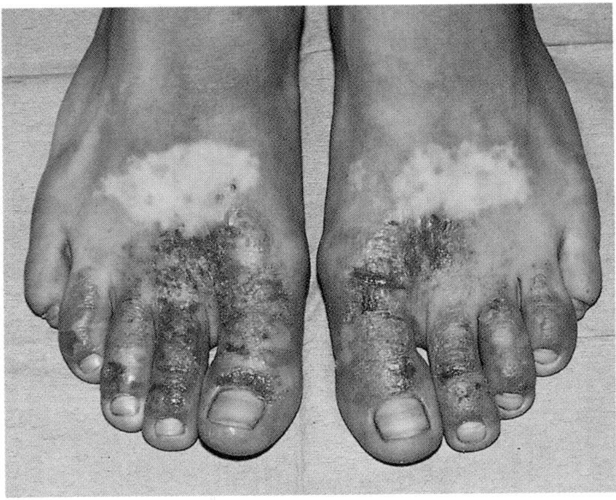

(**b**)

Figure 4.101 (**a**) The cause of the loss of pigment on the dorsum of the foot was an adhesive that contained *p-tert*-butylphenol–formaldehyde resin. The depigmentation was not post-inflammatory. This type of depigmentation does not require antecedent dermatitis, and is seen in industrial exposures to this same class of compounds (Rietschel and Fowler, 1995, p.770). (**b**) An example of post-inflammatory depigmentation.

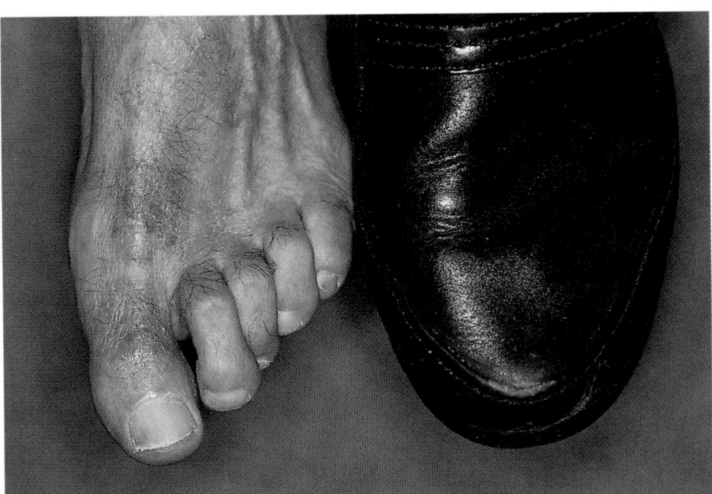

Figure 4.102 Shoe contact dermatitis is most commonly seen on the dorsal aspects of the feet, as in this 69-year-old man. He did not have positive patch tests to the standard series or his own shoes, but the dermatitis faded when he stopped wearing the shoes he himself suspected as being the cause of the dermatitis.

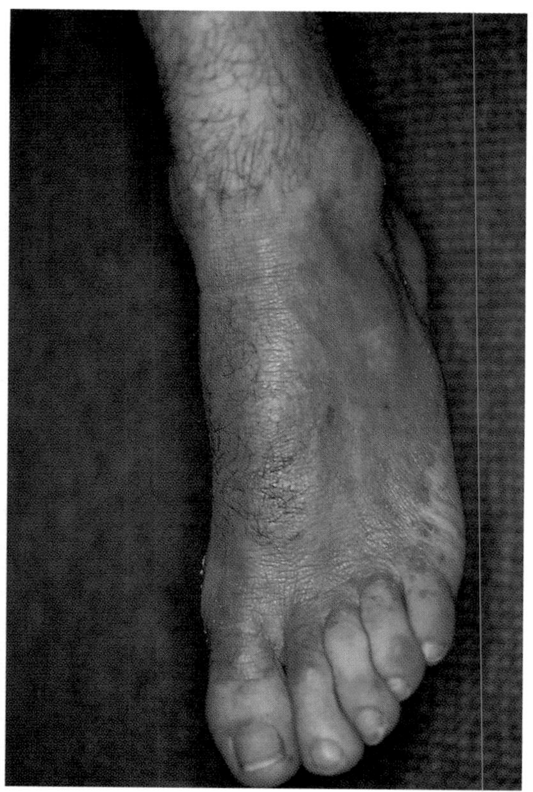

Figure 4.103 This welder was allergic to chromate, which is found in welding flux. He began to react to his leather work shoes, and had to switch to a vinyl work boot (Mathias and Maibach, 1979).

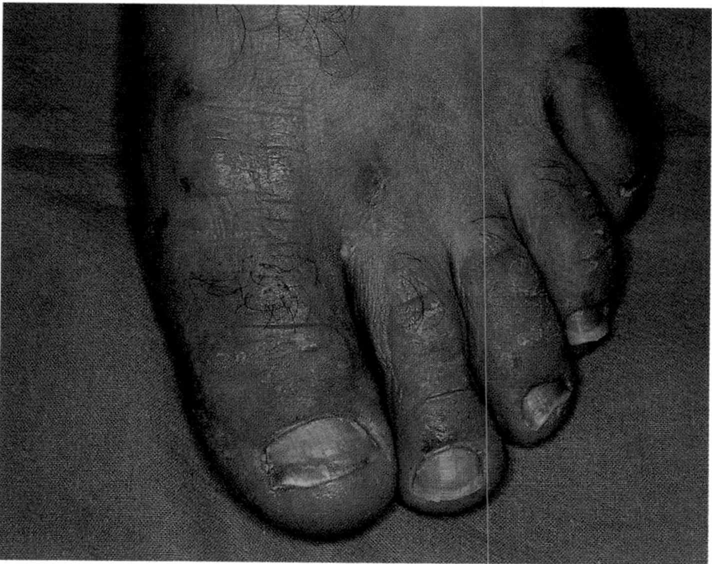

Figure 4.104 The dermatitis on this foot was caused by an azo dye found in the patient's nylon inner stocking.

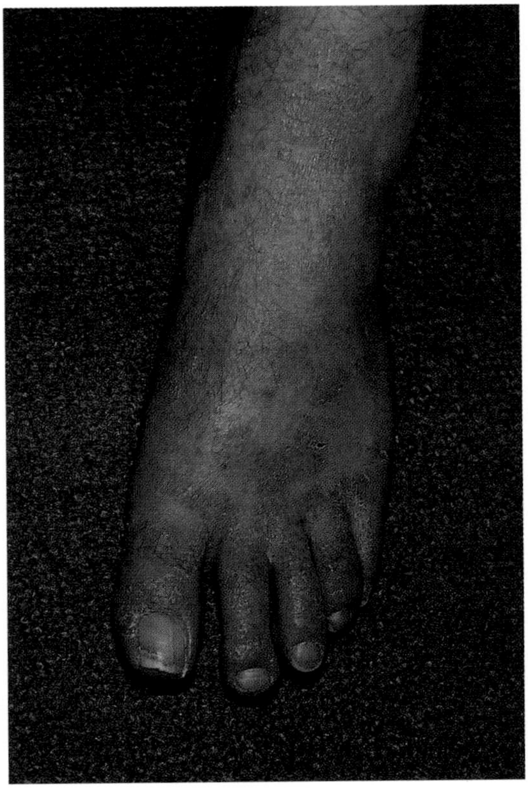

(a) 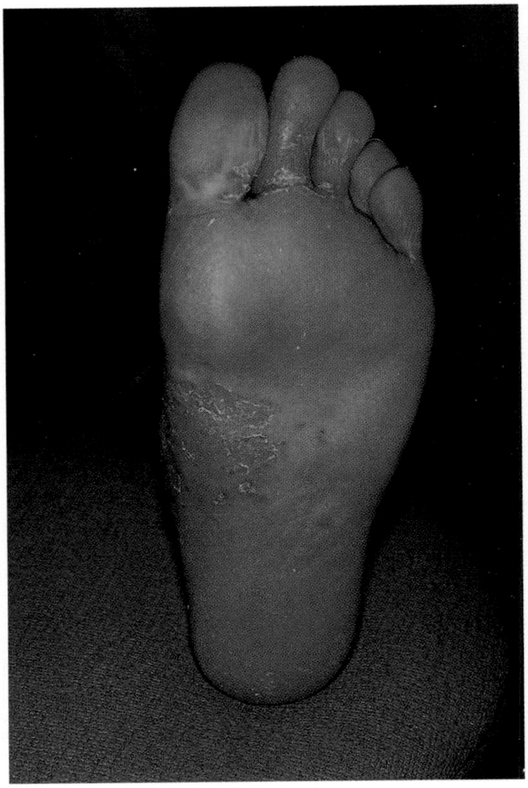 (b)

Figure 4.105 Sometimes foot dermatitis is multifactorial, as was the case in this patient who was patch-test positive to tixocortol pivalate, which indicates hydrocortisone allergy. He had been using hydrocortisone to treat his foot problem, which proved to be psoriasis. A papulosquamous dermatitis was present over the dorsum (**a**) of his foot, and vesicular dermatitis was seen on the instep (**b**).

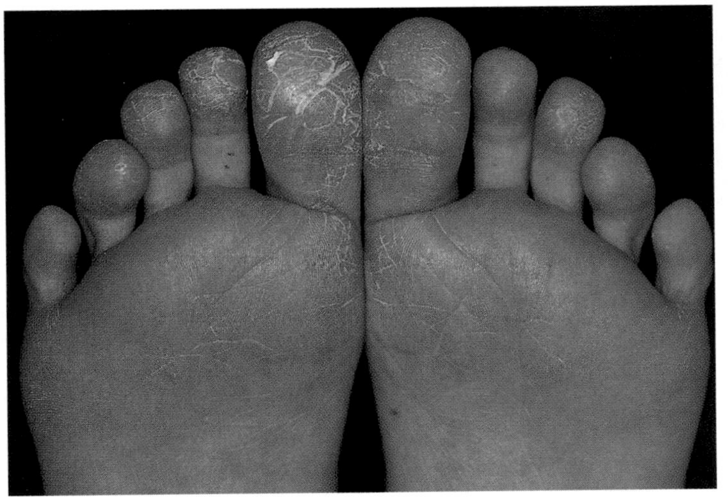

Figure 4.106 Dry, fissured dermatitis of the pressure areas of the plantar aspects of the forefoot with little pruritus is likely to be dermatitis plantaris sicca, a mechanical dermatitis, most commonly seen in patients with atopic dermatitis (Svensson, 1988).

REFERENCES

Ancona Alayon A, Escobar-Marques R, Gonzalez-Mendoza A et al (1976) Occupational pigmented contact dermatitis from Naphthol AS. *Contact Dermatitis* **2**:129–34.

Calnan CD (1975) Resorcinol monobenzoate. *Contact Dermatitis* **1**:59.

Conde-Salazar L, Guimaraens D, Romero L, Harto A (1984) Dermatitis de contacto por colorantes azoicos. *Medicina y Seguridad del Trabajo* **124**:29–34.

Conde-Salazar L, Guimaraens D, Romero L (1986) Occupational radiodermatitis from Ir-192 exposure. *Contact Dermatitis* **15**:202–4.

Conde-Salazar L, Gonzalez MA, Guimaraens D, Romero L (1987) Radiodermatitis profesional. *Medicina y Seguridad del Trabajo* **134**:26–9.

Descamps V, Flageul B, Vignon-Pennamen D et al (1992) Dyshidrosiform pemphigoid: report of three cases. *J Am Acad Dermatol* **26**:651–2.

Dooms-Goossens A (1993) The red face: contact and photocontact dermatitis. *Clin Dermatol* **11**:289–95.

Dooms-Goossens A, Debusschere K, Gevers D et al (1986) Contact dermatitis caused by airborne agents. *J Am Acad Dermatol* **15**:1–10.

Edman B (1985) Sites of contact dermatitis in relationship to particular allergens. *Contact Dermatitis* **13**:129–35.

Fisher AA (1976) Epoxy resin dermatitis. *Cutis* **17**:1027.

Fisher AA (1980) Cross reactions between methyl methacrylate monomer and acrylic monomers presently used in acrylic nail preparations. *Contact Dermatitis* **6**:345.

Fisher AA (1989) Permanent loss of fingernails due to allergic reaction to an acrylic nail preparation. *Cutis* **43**:404.

Fowler JF Jr, Skinner SM, Belsito DV (1992) Allergic contact dermatitis from formaldehyde resins in permanent press clothing: an underdiagnosed cause of generalized dermatitis. *J Am Acad Dermatol* **27**:962–8.

Freeman S (1997) Shoe dermatitis. *Contact Dermatitis* **36**:247–51.

Garcia RL, White JW Jr, Willis WF (1978) Hydroquinone nail pigmentation. *Arch Dermatol* **114**:1402–3.

Goh CL (1989) Eczema of the face, scalp and neck: an epidemiological comparison by site. *J Dermatol* **16**:223–6.

Hatch KL, Maibach HI (1985) Textile fiber dermatitis. *Contact Dermatitis* **12**:1–11.

Hatch KL, Maibach HI (1986) Textile chemical finish dermatitis. *Contact Dermatitis* **14**:1–13.

Hellgren L, Mobacken H (1969) Nummular eczema – clinical and statistical data. *Acta Derm Venereol (Stockh)* **49**:189–96.

Hemmer W, Focke M, Wantke F et al (1996) Allergic contact dermatitis to artificial fingernails prepared from UV light-cured acrylates. *J Am Acad Dermatol* **35**:377–80.

Hersle K, Mobacken H (1982) Hyperkeratotic dermatitis of the palms. *Br J Dermatol* **107**:195–201.

Jenni C, Zala L (1980) Das Unterschenkelekzem – klinische, allergologische und differentialdiagnostische Aspekte. *Schweiz Med Wochenschr* **110**:124–8.

Jordan WP Jr, Bourlas MC (1975) Allergic contact dermatitis to underwear elastic chemically transformed by laundry bleach. *Arch Dermatol* **111**:593–5.

Jordan WP Jr, Dahl MV (1972) Contact dermatitis from cellulose ester plastics. *Arch Dermatol* **105**:880.

Lee YC, Rycroft RJ, White IR, McFadden JP (1996) Recurrent focal palmar peeling. *Australas J Dermatol* **37**:143–4.

Liden C, Berg M, Farm G et al (1993) Nail varnish allergy with far-reaching consequences. *Br J Dermatol* **128**:57–62.

McDonagh AJ, Wright AL, Cork MJ et al (1992) Nickel sensitivity: the influence of ear piercing and atopy. *Br J Dermatol* **126**:16.

McKenna KE, McMillan C (1992) Facial contact dermatitis due to black rubber. *Contact Dermatitis* **26**:270.

Marks JG, Bishop ME, Willis WP (1979) Allergic contact dermatitis to sculptured nails. *Arch Dermatol* **115**:100.

Mathias CGT, Maibach HI (1979) Polyvinyl chloride work boots in the management of shoe dermatitis in industrial workers. *Contact Dermatitis* **5**:249–50.

Menné T, Veien NK, Sjølin K-E, Maibach HI (1994) Systemic contact dermatitis. *Am J Contact Derm* **5**:1–12.

Nethercott JR, Nield G, Holness DL (1989) A review of 79 cases of eyelid dermatitis. *J Am Acad Dermatol* **21**:223–30.

Nilsson E (1986) Individual and environmental risk factors for hand eczema in hospital workers. *Acta Derm Venereol (Stockh)* Suppl 128:1–62.

Ophaswongse S, Maibach HI (1995) Allergic contact cheilitis. *Contact Dermatitis* **33**:365–70.

Patruno C, Auricchio L, Mozzillo R et al (1990) Allergic contact dermatitis to tromantadine hydrochloride. *Contact Dermatitis* **22**:187.

Pegum JS (1966) Contact dermatitis from plastics containing tri-aryl phosphates. *Br J Dermatol* **78**:626.

Rietschel RL (1984) Role of socks in shoe dermatitis. *Arch Dermatol* **120**:398.

Rietschel RL, Fowler JF Jr (1995) *Fishers' Contact Dermatitis.* Baltimore, MD: Williams and Wilkins.

Roed-Petersen J, Batsberg W, Larsen E (1990) Contact dermatitis from Naphthol AS. *Contact Dermatitis* **22**:161–3.

Saha M, Srinivas CR, Shenoy SD et al (1993) Footwear dermatitis. *Contact Dermatitis* **28**:260–4.

Schwanitz H (1993) Palmar eczema in atopics. In: *Hand Eczema* (Menné T, Maibach HI, eds). Boca Raton, FL: CRC Press: 49–55.

Sinha SM, Pasricha JS, Sharma R et al (1977) Vegetables responsible for contact dermatitis of the hands. *Arch Dermatol* **113**:776–9.

Svensson A (1988) Prognosis and atopic background of juvenile plantar dermatosis and gluteofemoral eczema. *Acta Derm Venereol (Stockh)* **68**:336–40.

Valsecchi R, Iberti G, Martino D et al (1992) Eyelid dermatitis: an evaluation of 150 patients. *Contact Dermatitis* **27**:143–7.

Van Ketel WG, Mijnssen GAWV, Nerring H (1975) Contact eczema from *Alstroemeria. Contact Dermatitis* **1**:323.

Veien NK (1995) Clinical features. In: *Textbook of Contact Dermatitis,* 2nd edn (Rycroft RJG, Menné T, Frosch PJ, eds). Berlin: Springer-Verlag: 153–204.

Veien NK, Menné T (1993) Acute and recurrent vesicular hand dermatitis (pompholyx). In: *Hand Eczema* (Menné T, Maibach HI, eds). Boca Raton, FL: CRC Press: 57–73.

Veien NK, Hattel T, Laurberg G (1994) Plantar *Trichophyton rubrum* infections may cause dermatophytids on the hands. *Acta Derm Venereol (Stockh)* **74**:403–4.

5

Patterns of Contact Dermatitis

Systemic Contact Dermatitis

The traditional route of exposure to contact allergens is epicutaneous. The nature of some allergens is such that ingestion can be anticipated and may lead to a systemic reaction of limited or generalized nature. Typical clinical reaction patterns of systemic contact dermatitis include symmetrical recurrent vesicular palmar and/or interdigital dermatitis, dermatitis in skin folds, such as the antecubital fossae, axillae and anogenital area, or more widespread dermatitis. Repeated oral ingestion of allergens can also result in a lower level of reactivity to the allergen or tolerance (Lowney, 1974). The distribution of systemic contact dermatitis is illustrated below. Common causes of systemic contact dermatitis are given in the box on the following page.

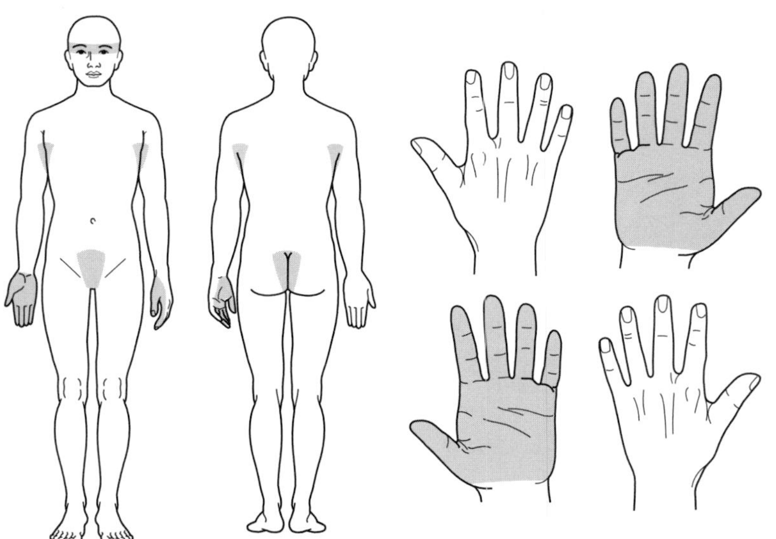

Typical distribution of systemic contact dermatitis

Allergens	
Flavouring agents	Metals:
Medications	Nickel
Sesquiterpene lactones	Cobalt
	Potassium dichromate

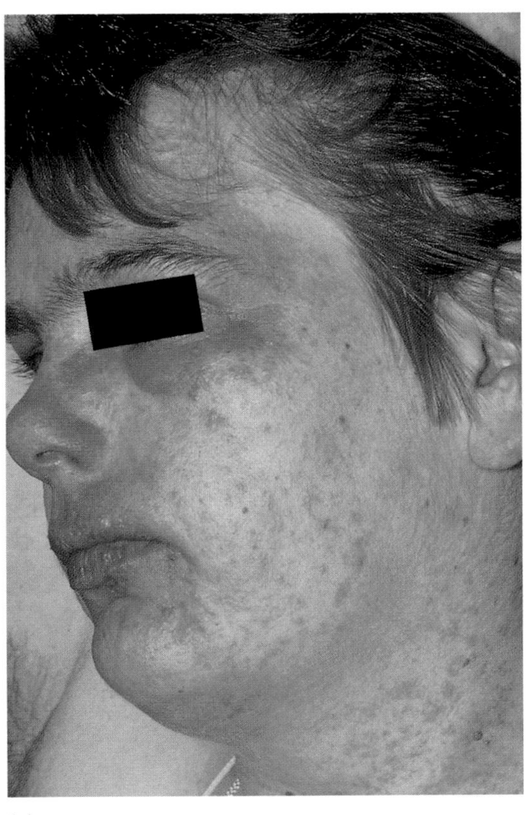

(**a**)

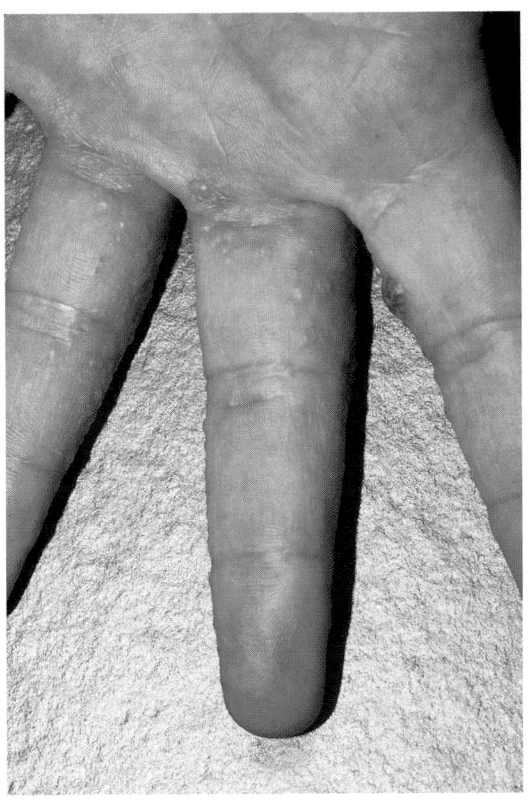

(**b**)

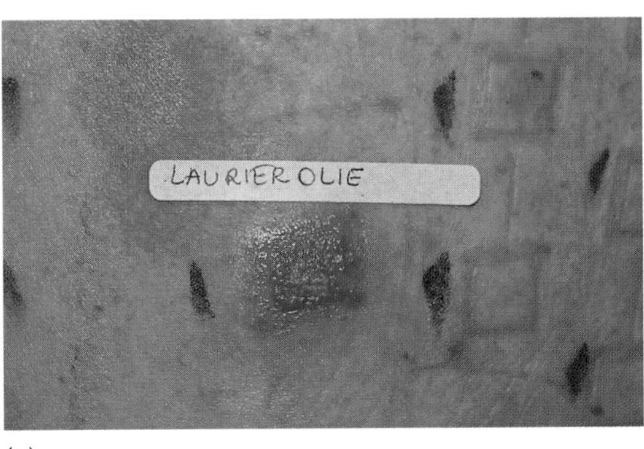

(**c**)

Figure 5.1 (**a**) Dermatitis of the face due to systemic exposure to sesquiterpene lactones in the form of bay leaf or laurel. (**b**) The bay leaf exposure also caused vesicular lesions of the hands. (**c**) This positive patch test was due to laurel oil.

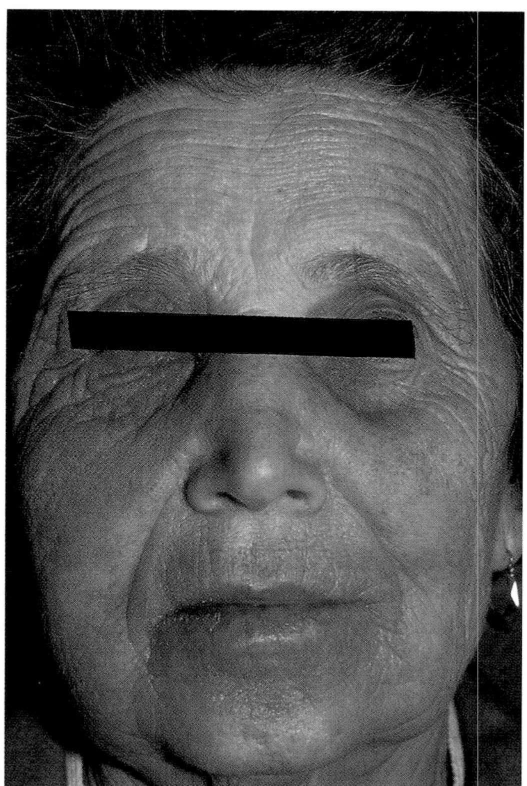

Figure 5.2 This individual was sensitive to thimerosal and received a vaccine that was preserved with thimerosal, resulting in a systemic reaction confined to the face.

Figure 5.3 (*below*) Ethylenediamine-sensitive patients can experience generalized reactions if they receive intravenous aminophylline. Aminophylline contains theophylline and ethylenediamine to solubilize the theophylline (Petrozzi and Shore, 1976). (**a**) Systemic contact dermatitis presenting as generalized pustular erythroderma was induced by intravenous administration of aminophylline in an ethylenediamine-sensitive patient. (**b**) Close-up view.

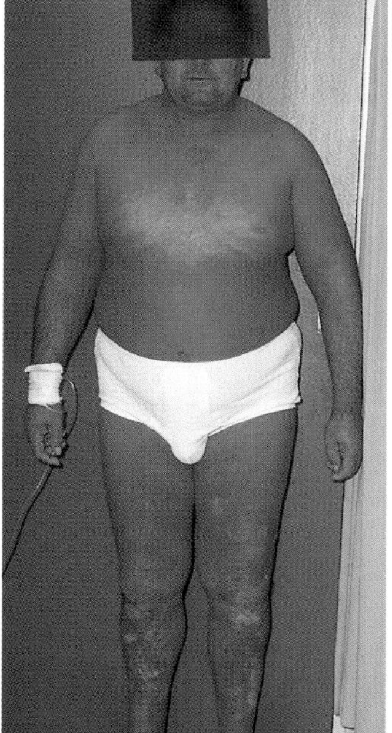

(**a**)

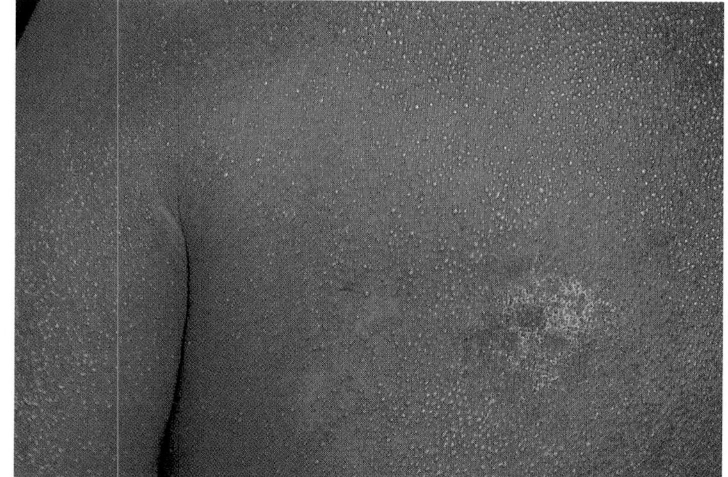

(**b**)

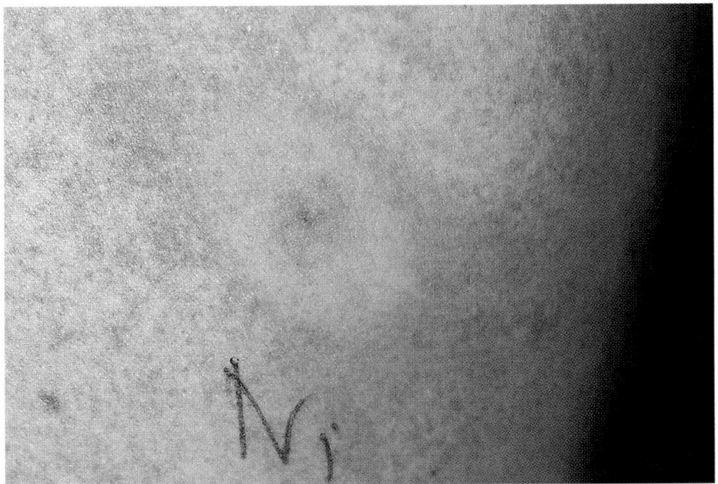

(a)

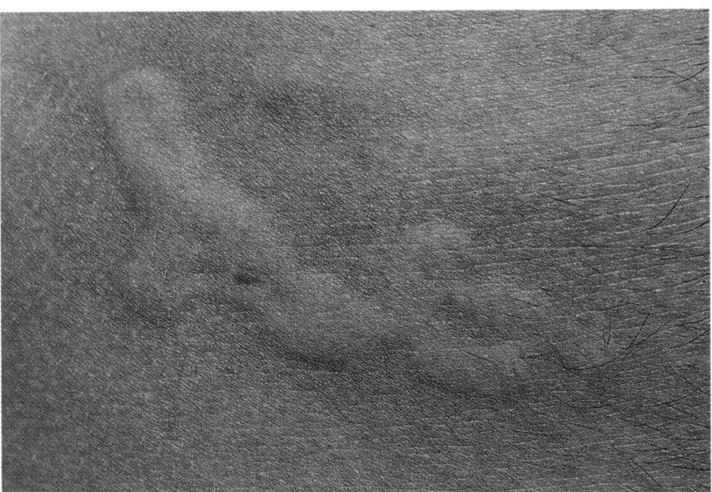

(b)

Figure 5.4 Placebo-controlled oral challenge with the hapten can provide valuable information about the clinical features of systemic contact dermatitis. A dose of 2.5 mg of nickel, given as 11.2 mg nickel sulfate ($NiSO_4.6H_2O$), to a nickel-sensitive patient resulted in a flare of oedema and pruritus at a recent nickel patch test site within 12 hours (Veien, 1989). (**b**) A similar exceptional urticarial contact reaction can be seen following contact with nickel-plated items.

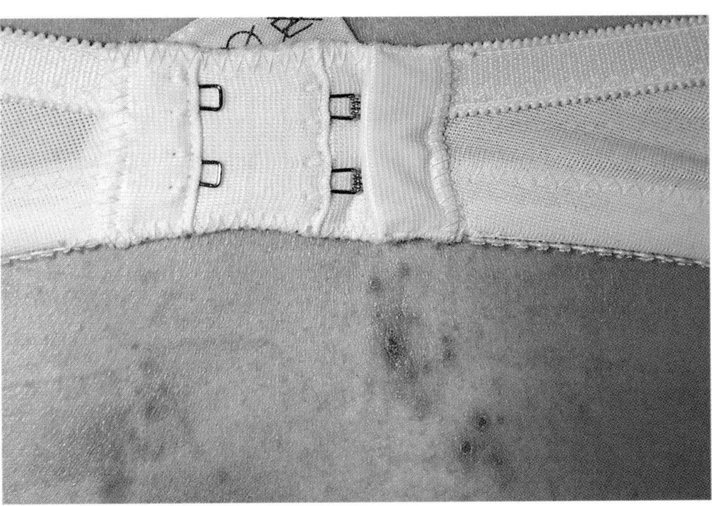

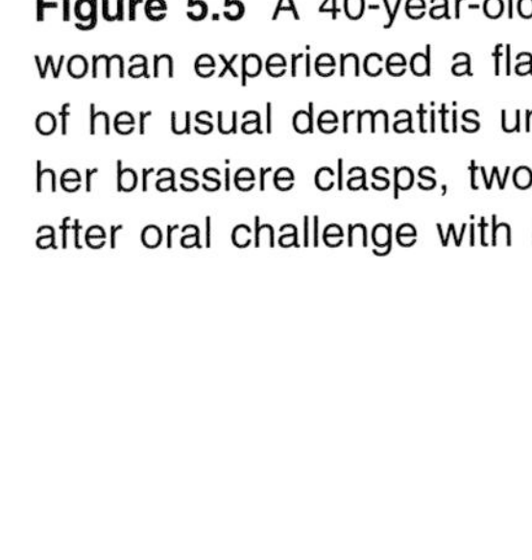

Figure 5.5 A 40-year-old woman experienced a flare-up of her usual dermatitis under her brassiere clasps, two days after oral challenge with nickel.

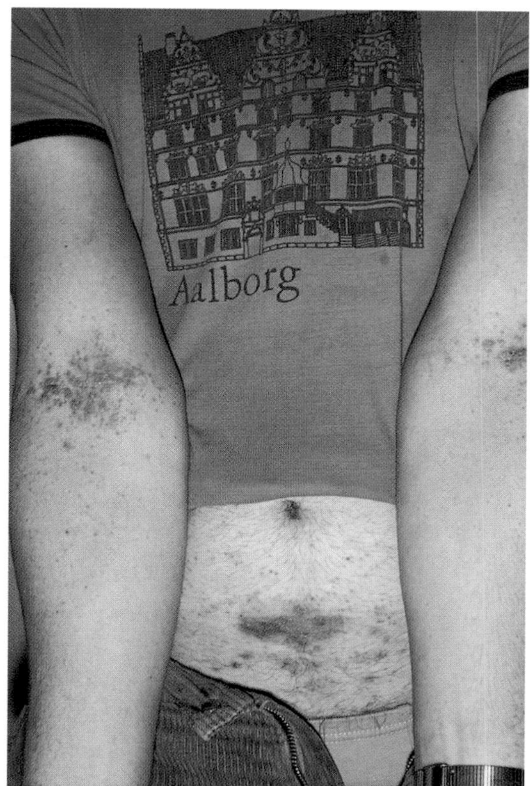

Figure 5.6 Persistent exposure to an allergen may increase the degree of sensitivity and cause dermatitis beyond the area of direct contact. This phenomenon is seen in nickel-sensitive patients who do not remove nickel-plated items that are in direct contact with the skin, with a resultant flexural dermatitis, as seen in this 19-year-old man.

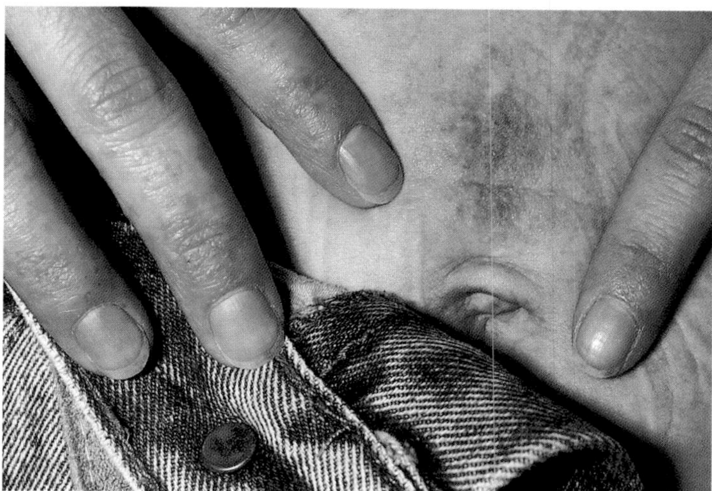

Figure 5.7 The hands may also be an area of distant dermatitis, as seen in this 28-year-old woman who had persistent nickel exposure from the button of her jeans, and developed symmetrical vesicular dermatitis on her fingers.

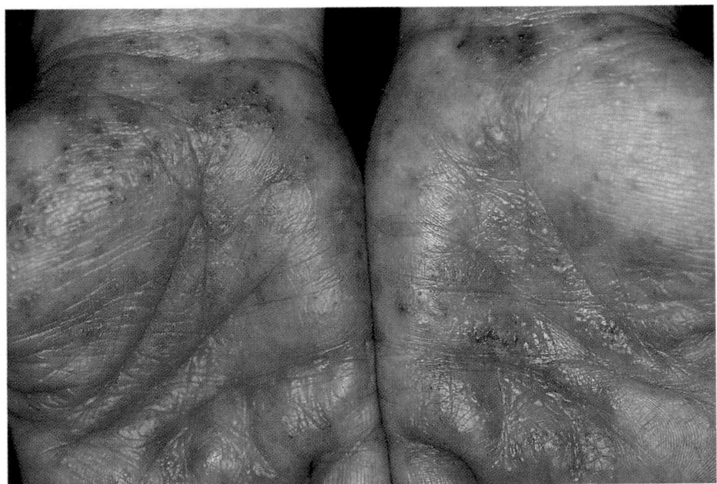

(a)

Figure 5.8 Recurrent vesicular hand dermatitis is the most common clinical disease among nickel-sensitive patients with systemic contact dermatitis (Veien, 1989). (**a**) A 46-year-old woman presented with severe recurrent, vesicular palmar dermatitis, as seen here. She had a positive patch test to nickel, and had a flare of her vesicular palmar dermatitis after placebo-controlled oral challenge with 2.5 mg nickel. (**b**) Close-up view of one finger. (**c**) Similar dermatitis may be seen on the sides of the fingers.

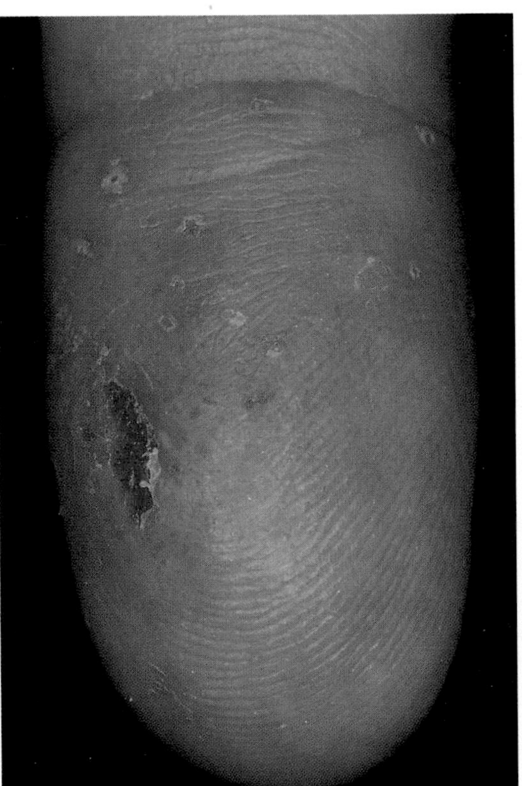

(b)

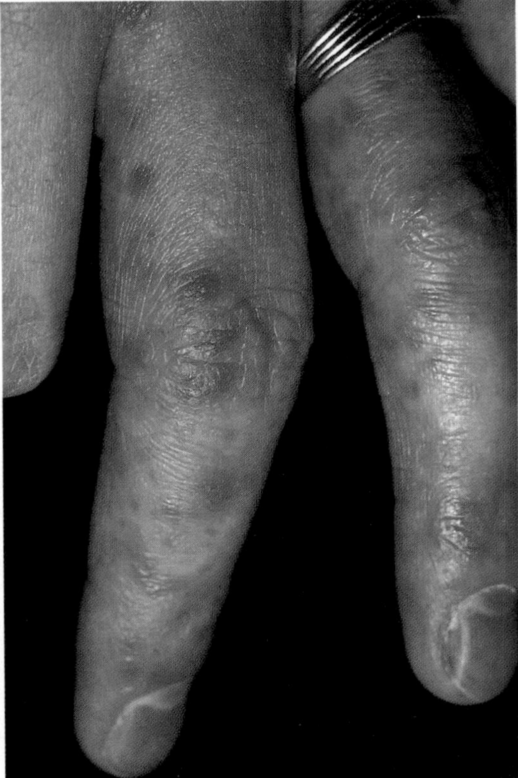

(c)

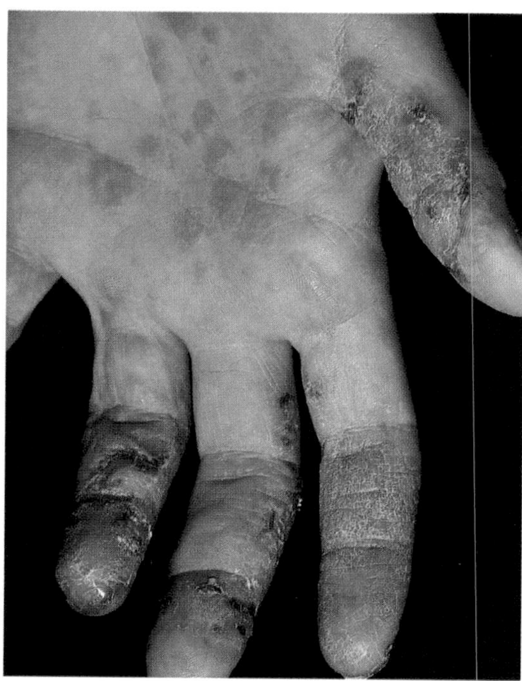

Figure 5.9 After one to two weeks on a weight-reducing diet, severe vesicular palmar dermatitis was seen in this 26-year-old nickel-sensitive woman. A close look at the diet showed that most of the foods on it were high in nickel content (Veien et al, 1993).

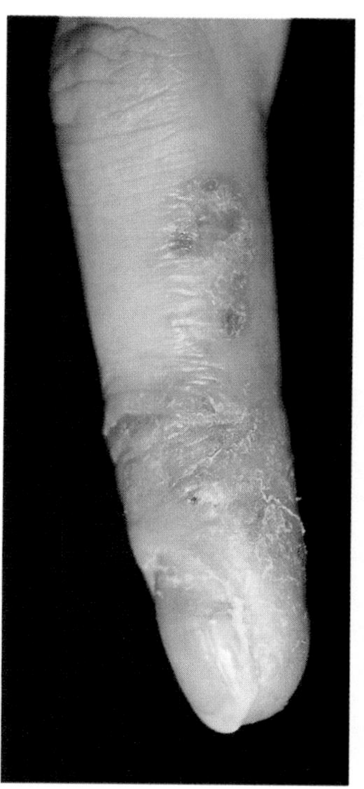

(**a**)

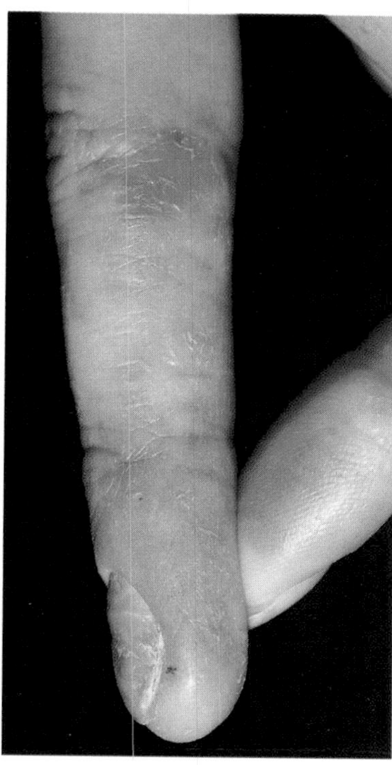

(**b**)

Figure 5.10 The benefit of a low-nickel diet is seen in these before-diet (**a**) and after-diet (**b**) photographs.

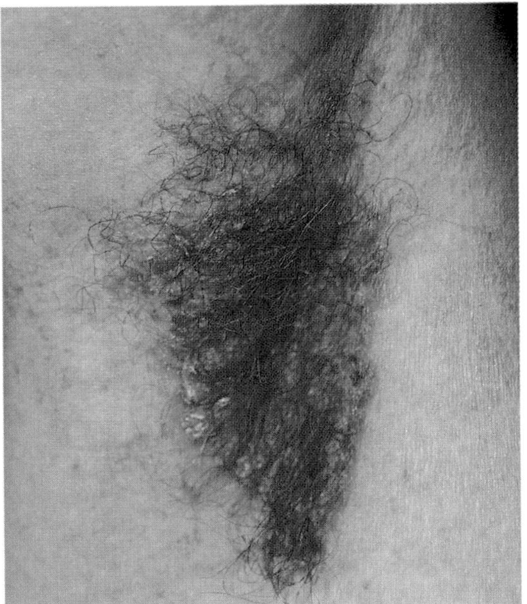

(**a**)

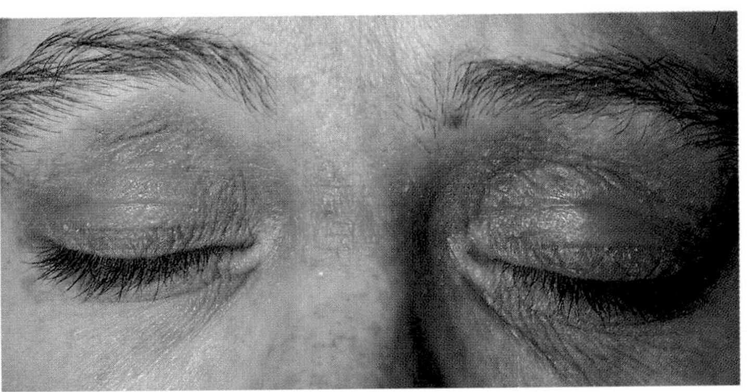

(**b**)

Figure 5.11 Systemic contact dermatitis can preferentially affect body folds, such as the axilla (**a**) or be seen as symmetrical eyelid dermatitis (**b**).

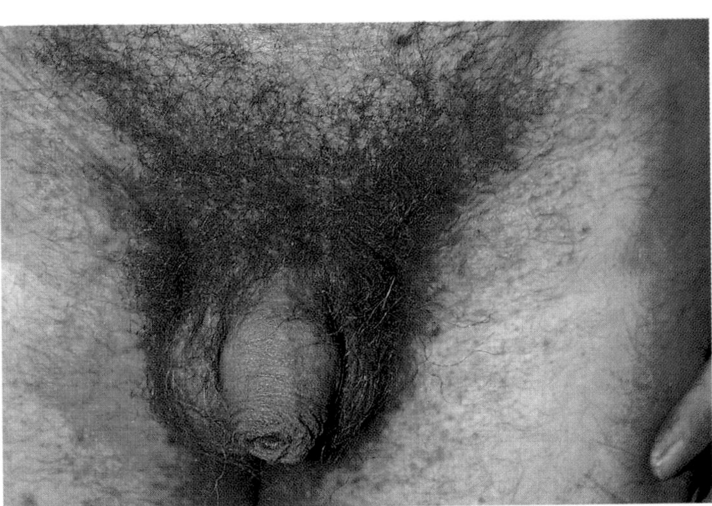

Figure 5.12 Brisk erythema of the buttocks and/or genital skin has been reported after systemic exposure to contact allergens – it is called the 'baboon syndrome' (Andersen et al, 1984); see also Figure 6.33.

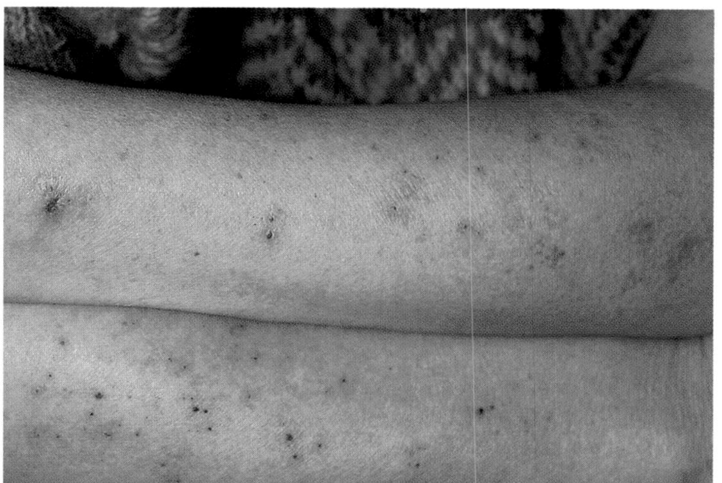

(a)

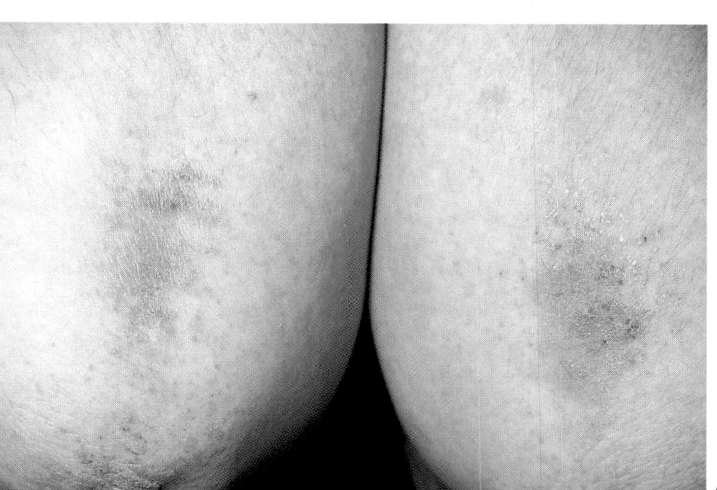

(b)

Figure 5.13 (**a**) Nickel-sensitive patients may also experience vasculitis-like eruptions. (**b**) This reaction may commonly be seen on the elbows.

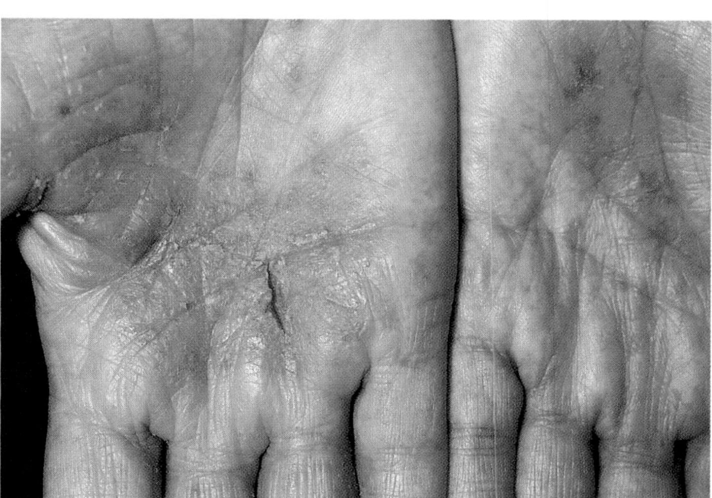

Figure 5.14 Systemic contact dermatitis may be caused by balsams as well as by nickel (Dooms-Goossens et al, 1990). A 72-year-old woman developed vesicular and fissured palmar dermatitis after placebo-controlled oral challenge with 1 g balsam of Peru.

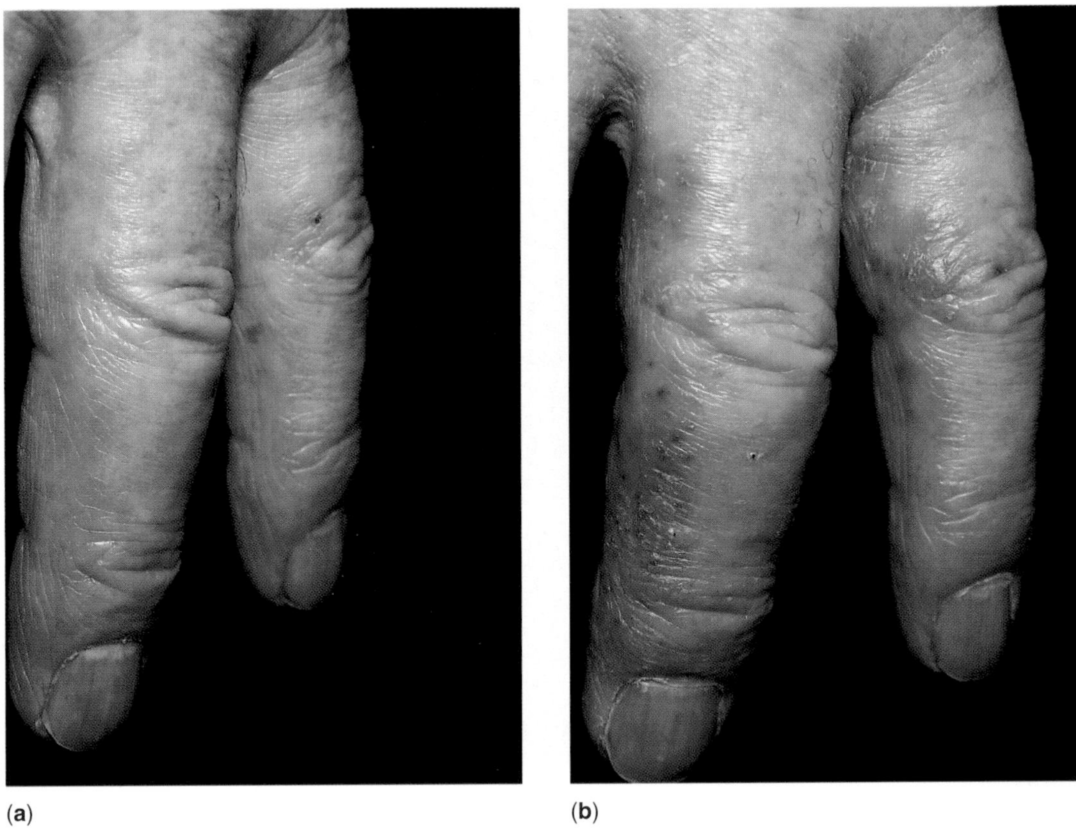

(**a**) (**b**)

Figure 5.15 (**a**) A potassium dichromate-sensitive patient with vesicular, interdigital dermatitis reacted with interdigital vesicles (**b**) after oral challenge with 2.5 mg chromium, given as potassium dichromate (Veien et al, 1994).

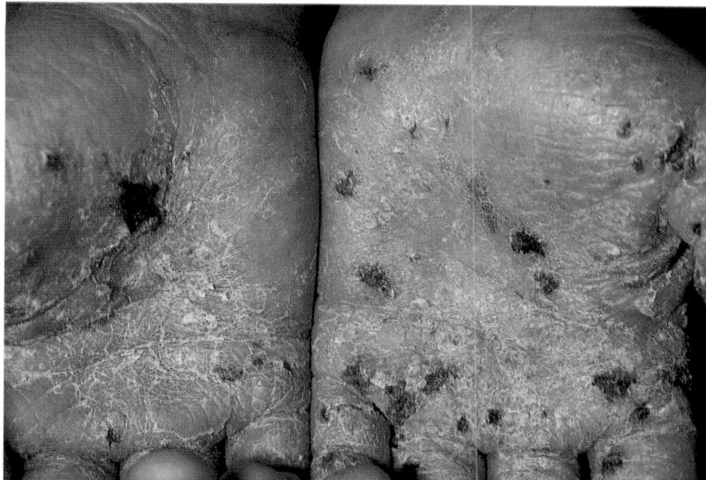

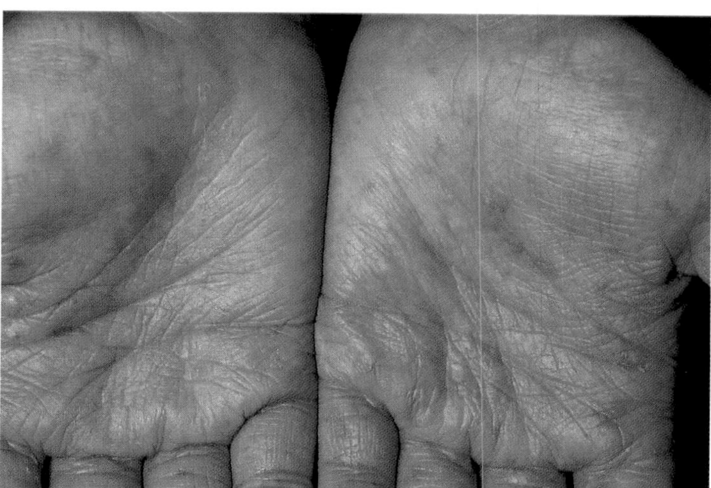

Figure 5.16 A 17-year-old girl with atopic dermatitis and a positive patch test to the paraben mixture was challenged orally with a mixture of parabens. (**a**) She experienced a severe flare-up of palmar dermatitis, which faded after she followed a diet low in preservatives (**b**) (Veien et al, 1996).

Non-Eczematous Contact Dermatitis

The classic presentation of contact dermatitis is an inflammatory reaction accompanied by spongiosis histologically and manifesting as vesiculation macroscopically. There are less common patterns such as erythema multiforme-like eruptions, purpuric reactions, pigmented patterns, lichen planus-like eruptions, pustular eruptions, granulomas, and frictional or hyperkeratotic patterns (Rietschel and Fowler, 1995, pp.92–113).

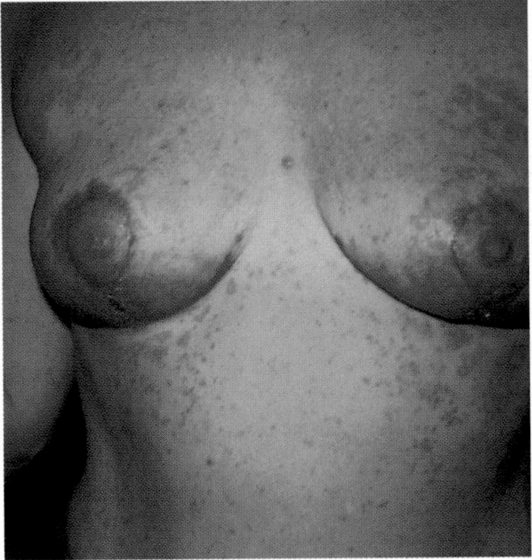

Figure 5.17 Erythema multiforme patterns are most commonly associated with exotic woods and vegetation. This patient had persistent fixed areas of erythema and oedema that were somewhat urticarial in quality. She had undergone reduction mammoplasty and was applying vitamin E from several sources to her scars in hopes of improving the cosmetic appearance of her operation. Patch tests were positive to vitamin E, with an eczematous patch test morphology, but the clinical pattern did not demonstrate vesiculation (Saperstein et al, 1984).

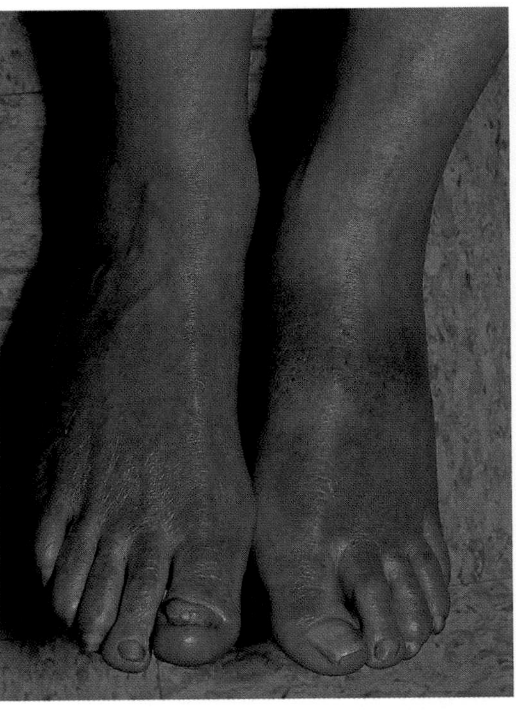

Figure 5.18 Purpuric patterns are frequently associated with clothing. Wool, fabric finishes of formaldehyde–urea, optical whiteners in laundry detergent, and rubber components of garments are most frequently incriminated. Schamberg's disease-like patterns may occur. Wool socks were blamed for this eruption.

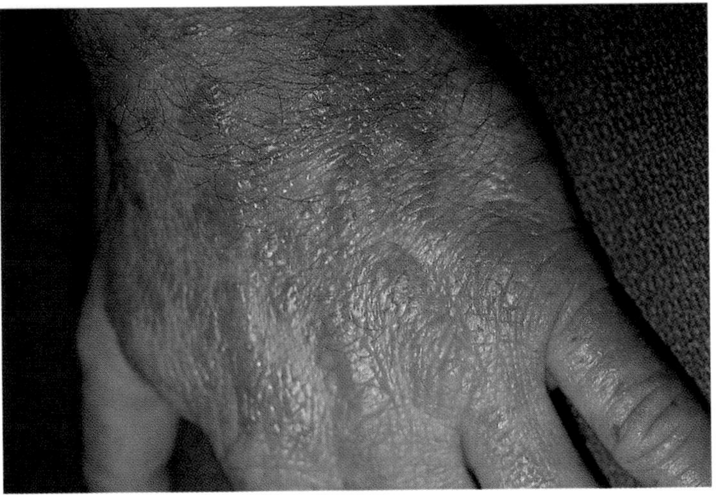

Figure 5.19 This eruption was biopsied and interpreted as classic lichen planus. The eruption was due to a chromate primer applied to aircraft, and the patient was sensitive to both chromate and one other proprietary component of the primer. Avoidance of further contact was curative.

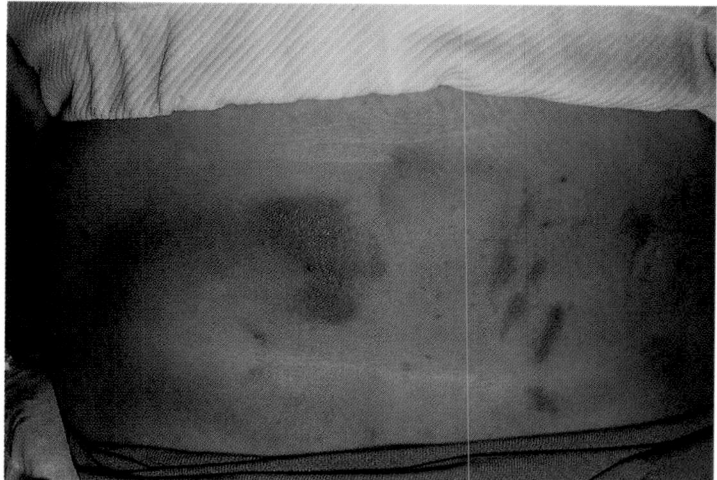

Figure 5.20 Hyperpigmentation is a common component of phototoxic reactions. This subject will be covered more extensively in the following section. In this example, lime juice splashed onto the abdomen of this woman while she was mixing drinks outdoors. She was wearing a two-piece bathing suit, which allowed the lime peel to spray onto the skin of the abdomen and combine with sunlight to produce this pigmented photocontact dermatitis. The peel of limes contains psoralens, which are responsible for the phototoxicity.

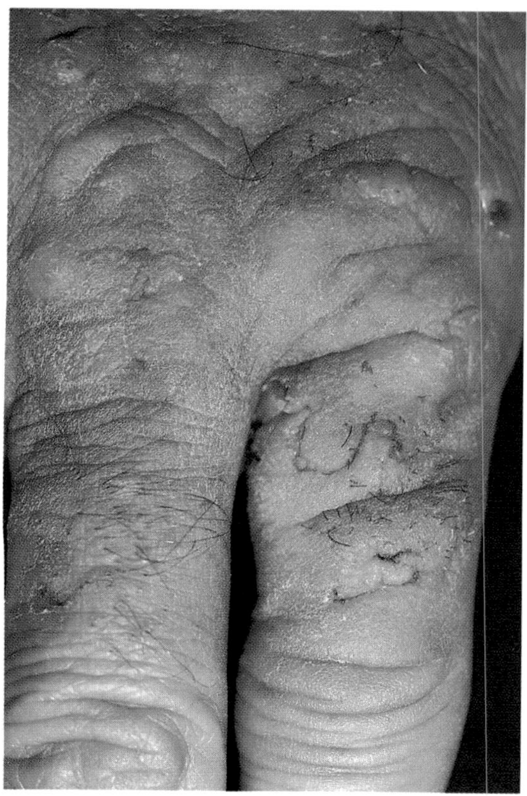

Figure 5.21 Friction can cause a variety of dermatoses. This 86-year-old man rubbed his right hand on the ulnar aspect of his left hand and developed a course, keratotic change of the skin on the first two fingers of the left hand. Note the broken hairs in the involved area, which is a sign of intense rubbing.

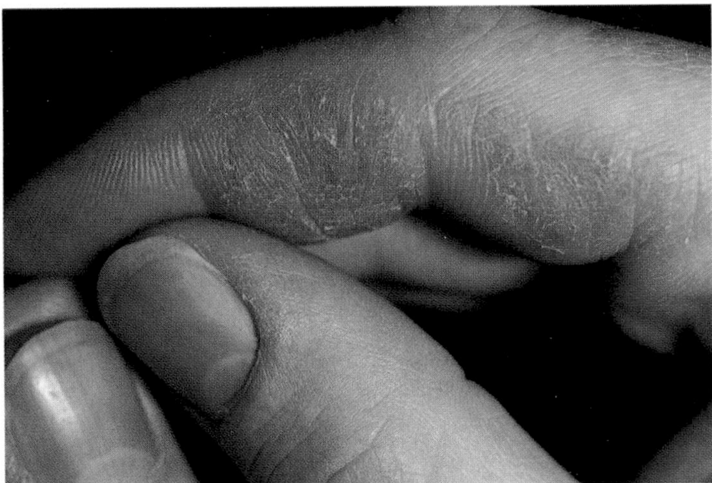

Figure 5.22 A 25-year-old man had keratotic dermatitis on the palmar aspects of both second fingers after tic-like rubbing of his thumb against these areas.

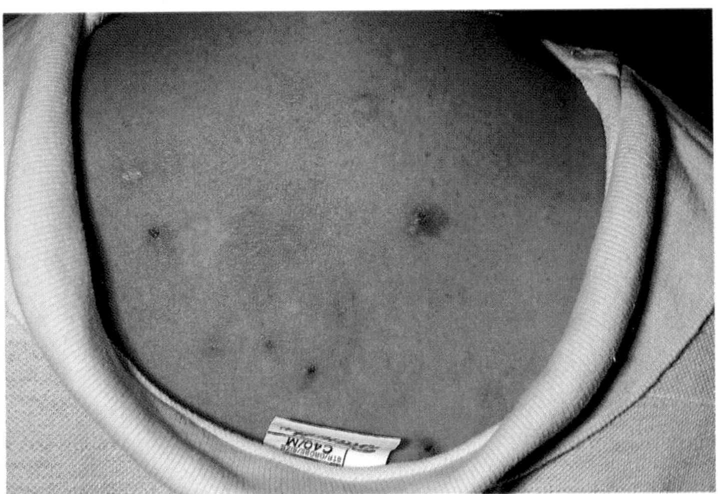

Figure 5.23 A 62-year-old woman presented with pruritic, excoriated dermatitis on her neck. She had had atopic dermatitis and now had mechanical dermatitis caused by the coarse fibres in the labels in her clothing. The condition had persisted for several years, and, in addition to the mechanical 'label dermatitis', she had self-induced 'creeping neurotic excoriations' on the neck, as illustrated by the linear scars above the label.

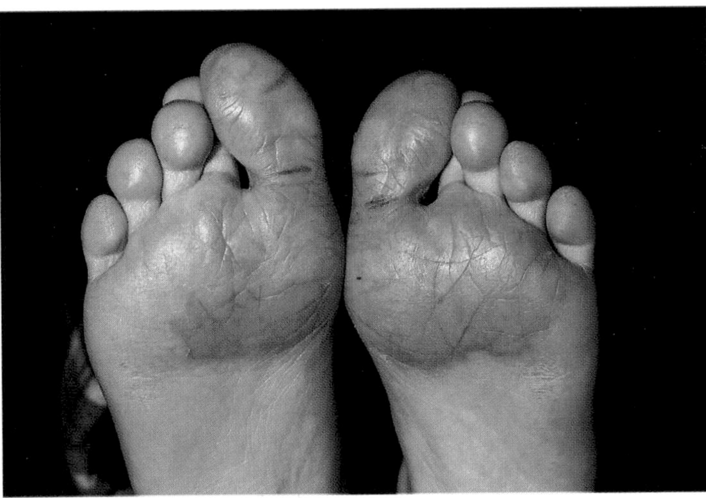

Figure 5.24 This 10-year-old boy was diagnosed as having juvenile plantar dermatitis. The cause of this condition is unknown, but a relationship to atopic dermatitis is common. Friction appeared to be a dominant factor in this case. The condition is seen in the prepubertal years (Verbov, 1989).

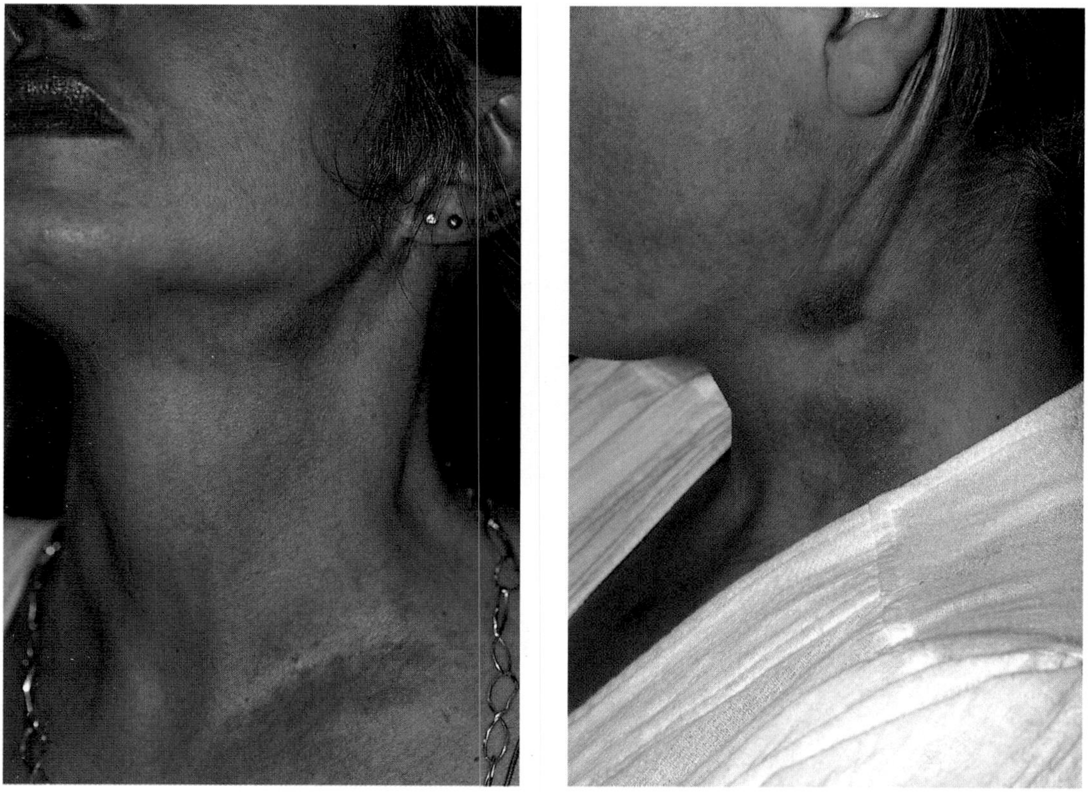

(a) (b)

Figure 5.25 (**a**) This 55-year-old amateur violinist suffered from 'fiddler's neck' – frictional contact dermatitis of the mandibular and clavicular areas where the violin is supported while being played. (**b**) This woman has a combination of 'fiddler's neck' and nickel dermatitis, the latter being caused by the nickel in the chin rest.

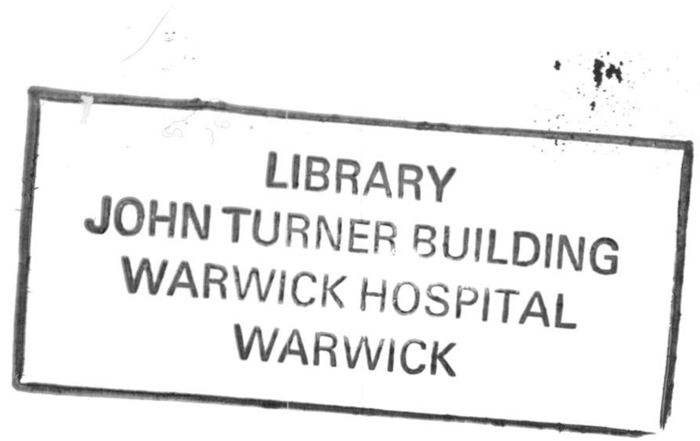

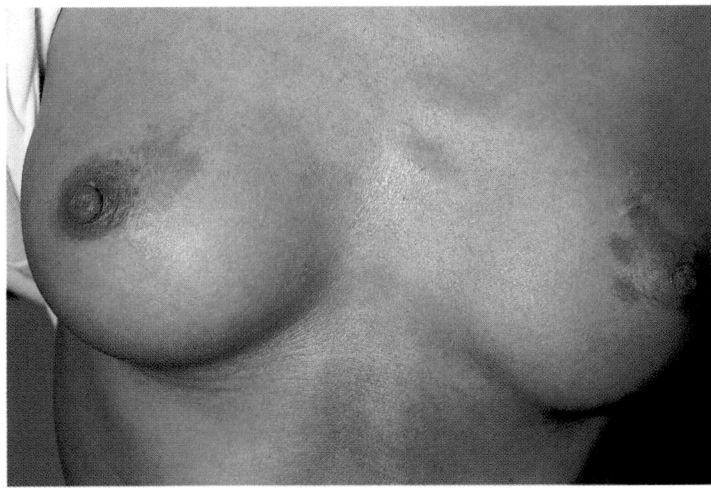

(**a**)

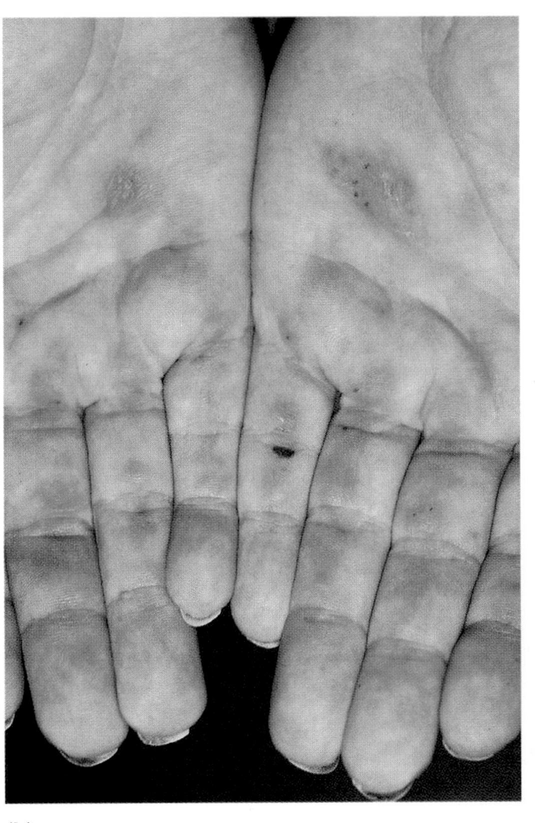

(**b**)

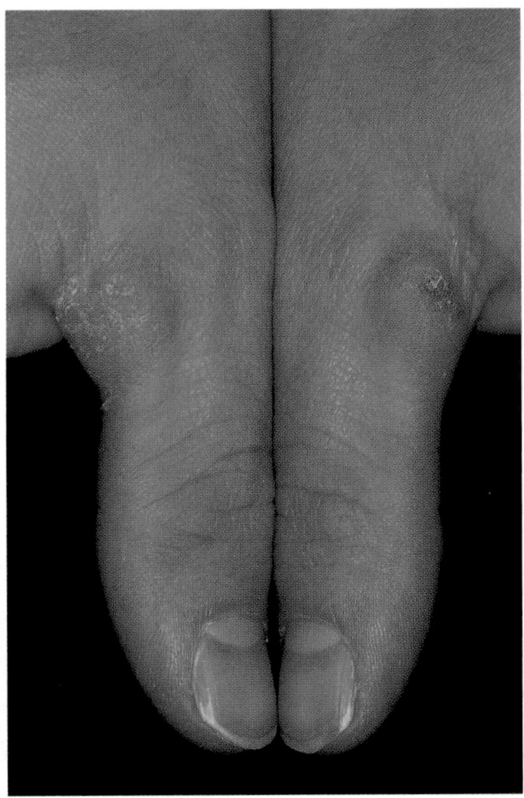

(**c**)

Figure 5.26 Various sports are associated with mechanical contact dermatitis caused by friction and pressure on the skin. Typical examples include jogger's nipples (**a**), striped palmar dermatitis in weightlifters (**b**), and keratotic papules on the hands of kayak rowers (**c**).

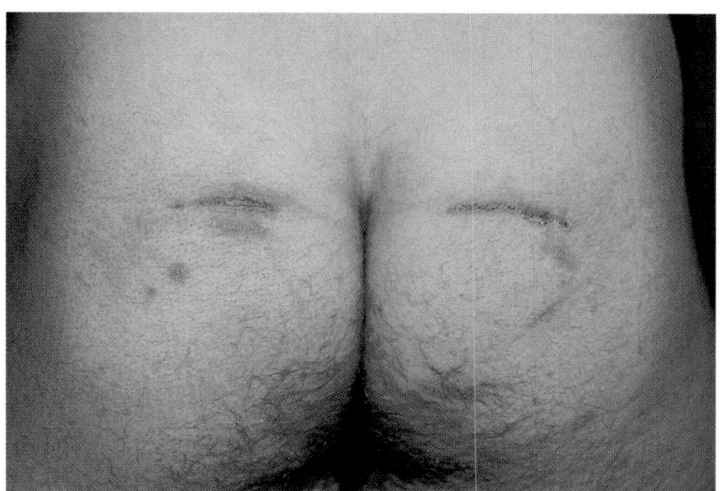
(a)

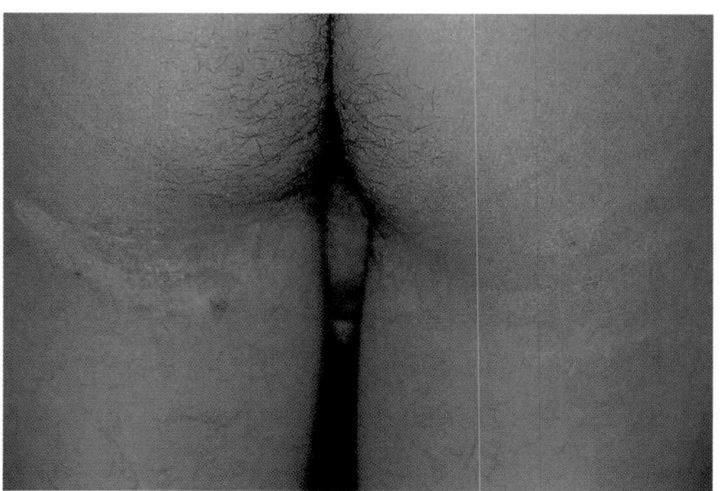
(b)

Figure 5.27 (**a**) Rower's rump. (**b**) Cyclist's bottom.

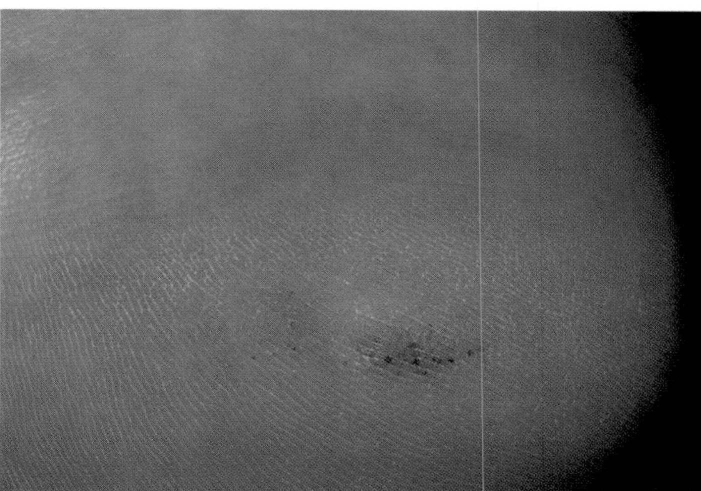

Figure 5.28 'Black heel' – purpura caused by friction, typically seen on the medial aspects of the heel in those engaged in sports that involve rapid accelerations and sudden stops, such as badminton.

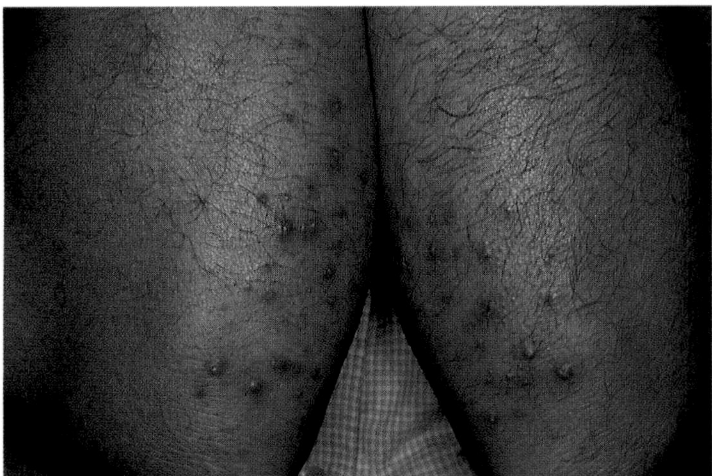

Figure 5.29 Oil boils on a worker exposed to machinery oils and lubricants (Alomar et al, 1985).

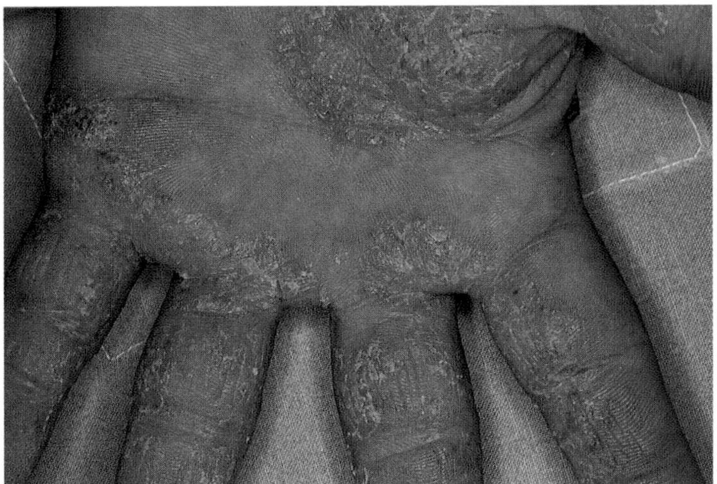

Figure 5.30 Tinea on the hands (*Trichophyton mentagrophytes*) in an agricultural worker who handled many agrochemical products. This should be considered in the differential diagnosis of allergic contact dermatitis.

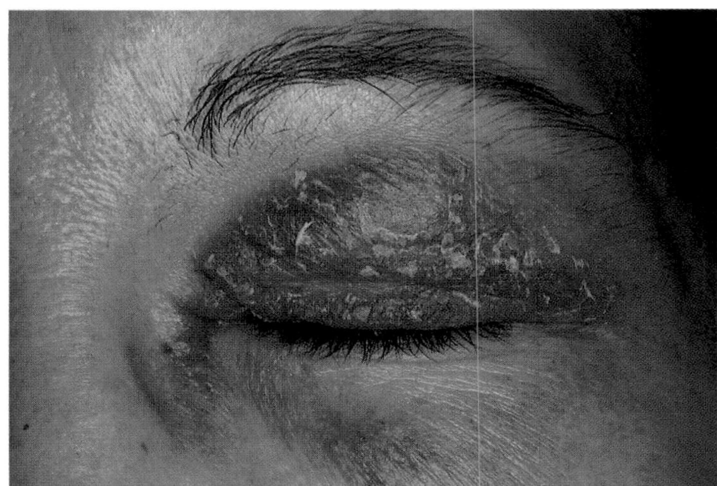
(a)

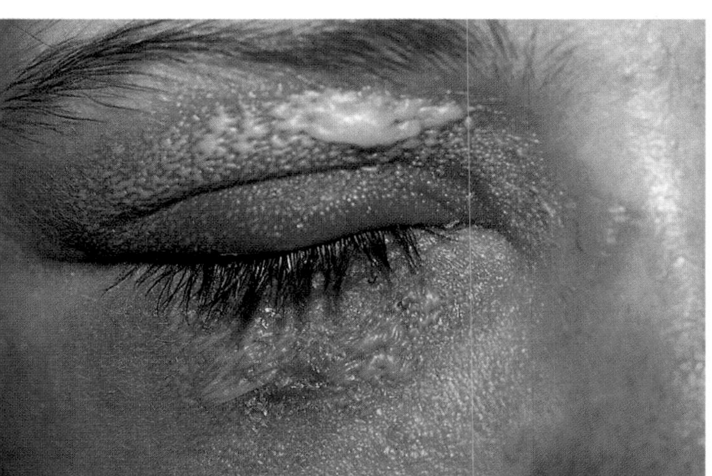
(b)

Figure 5.31 (**a**) Factitious dermatitis in a woman who worked in the chemical industry. The lesion occurred in only one eye, and trauma and petechiae were observed. The lesions were self-inflicted, the reason being that she wanted to change her job. Standard allergy tests with the products she handled gave negative results. (**b**) Artefact dermatitis caused by rubbing with the sap of a cactus.

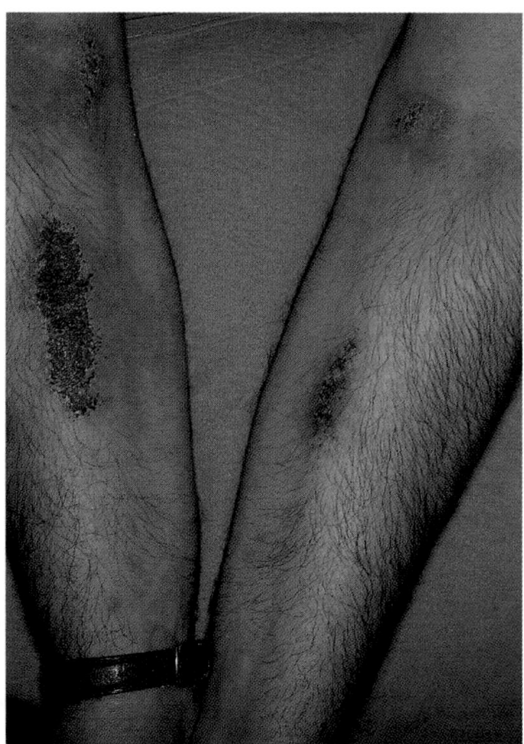

Figure 5.32 Factitious dermatitis in a tobacco worker, who stated that contact with tobacco powder caused intense stinging, and that lesions appeared when he was at home. The patient had not worked for six months for this reason, and was requesting a life-long pension.

Phototoxic and Photoallergic Reactions

Phototoxic reactions usually resemble sunburn and recur in exposed areas. The typical distribution is illustrated on the facing page. The time required to produce a phototoxic reaction is usually much less than that required to produce a similar degree of erythema in the absence of the phototoxic material. Potentially anyone may develop phototoxic reactions if a sufficient amount of chemical penetrates the skin and if this is then exposed to sufficient light energy. The amount of chemical and the amount of light energy required can vary widely among individuals, as is the case for irritant contact dermatitis.

Photoallergic reactions require the participation of the immune system, with specific sensitization to a photoproduct that is the result of the interaction of ultraviolet light and a sensitizing chemical. Most photoallergic reactions involve ultraviolet light in the UV-A range of 320–400 nm. Phototoxic reactions can result from either UV-B or UV-A. Common phytophototoxic substances and photoallergens are given in the box.

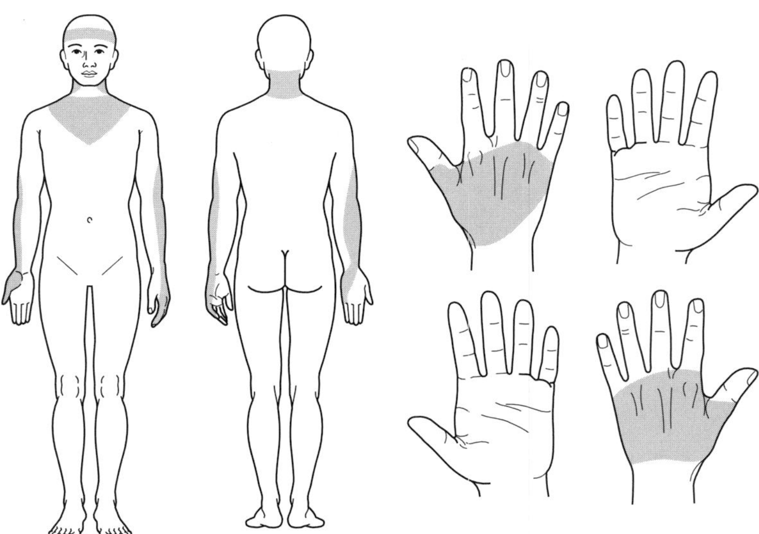

Typical distribution of phototoxic and photoallergic dermatitis

Phytophototoxic substances	Photoallergens
Furocoumarins (psoralens) in Umbilliferae and other plants such as: Giant hogweed Parsley Celery Parsnip Fig plant Citrus fruits such as lime, lemon	Antimicrobials: Triclosan Salicylanilides Chlorhexidine Fragrances: Oak moss Musk ambrette Sunscreens: Benzophenone Methoxycinnamates *p*-Aminobenzoic acid Other types: Sulfanilamide Coal tar

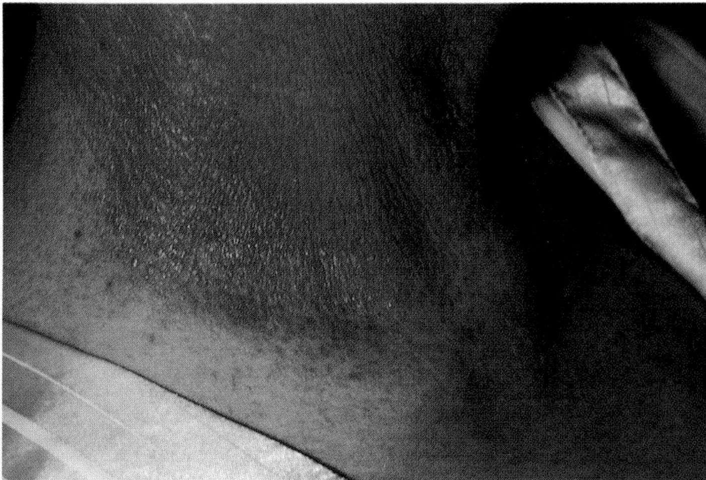

Figure 5.33 Photodermatoses are usually sharply demarcated on the neck, as in this 71-year-old woman, as opposed to dermatitis caused by dust, which commonly extends to the area under the collar.

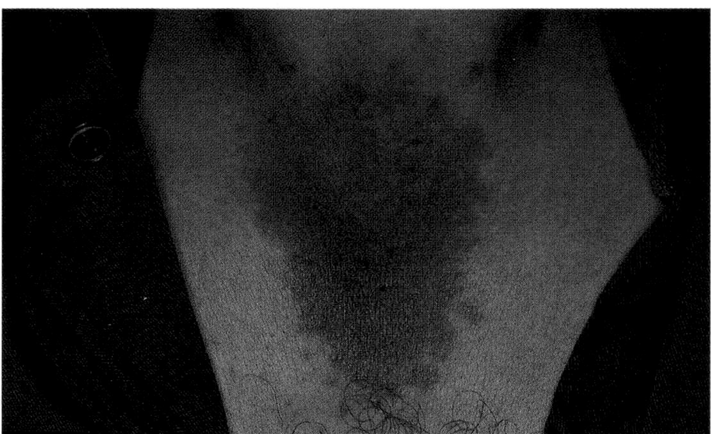

Figure 5.34 Sharply demarcated dermatitis in the jugular region is also characteristic of photodermatitis.

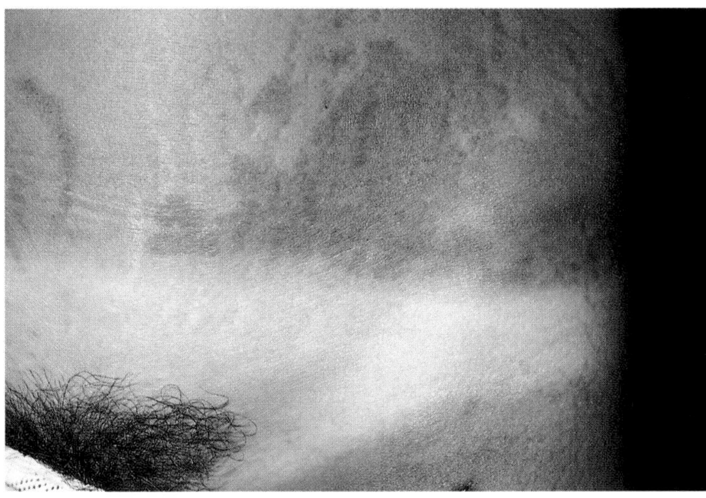

Figure 5.35 If a photodistribution, such as that seen in this 34-year-old woman, is presented in combination with a striped pattern, phytophotodermatitis is a common cause.

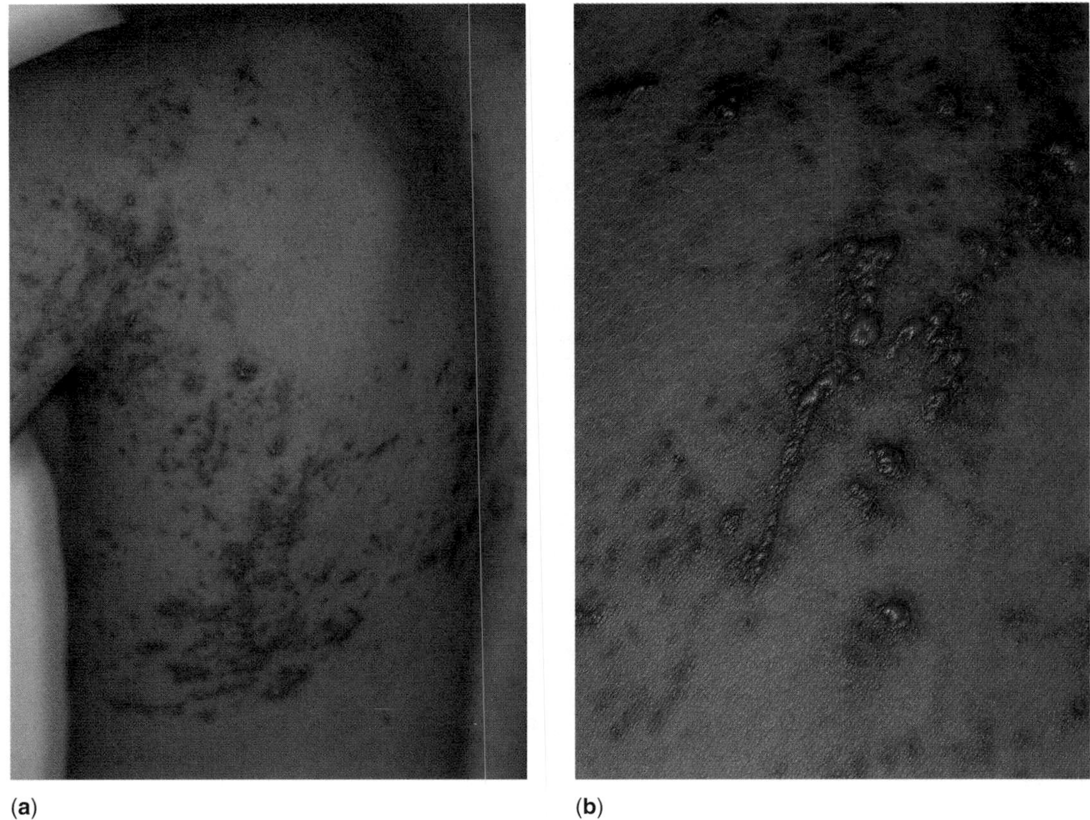

(a) (b)

Figure 5.36 (**a**) A striped pattern in combination with acute bullous dermatitis is a characteristic pattern of plant exposure. (**b**) Close-up view. If the plant contains phototoxic materials, and there is sufficient exposure to the sun, photodermatitis may occur. Some of the plants commonly associated with phytophotodermatitis are Umbilliferae (see box above) (Rietschel and Fowler, 1995, p.495).

SPECIFIC PLANT-INDUCED PHOTOREACTIONS

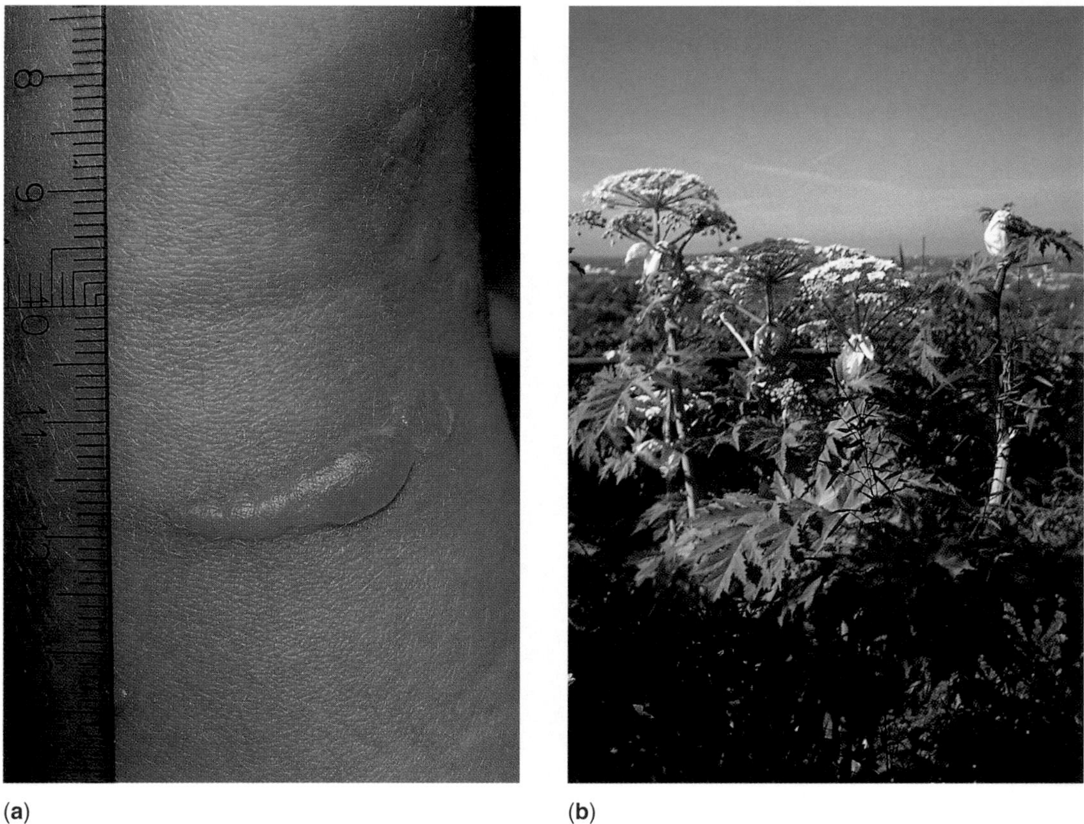

(a) (b)

Figure 5.37 (**a**) A 9-year-old boy with acute, striped, bullous, phototoxic contact dermatitis caused by giant hogweed. (**b**) Giant hogweed (*Heracleum mantegazzianum*). These particular plants were 3m tall.

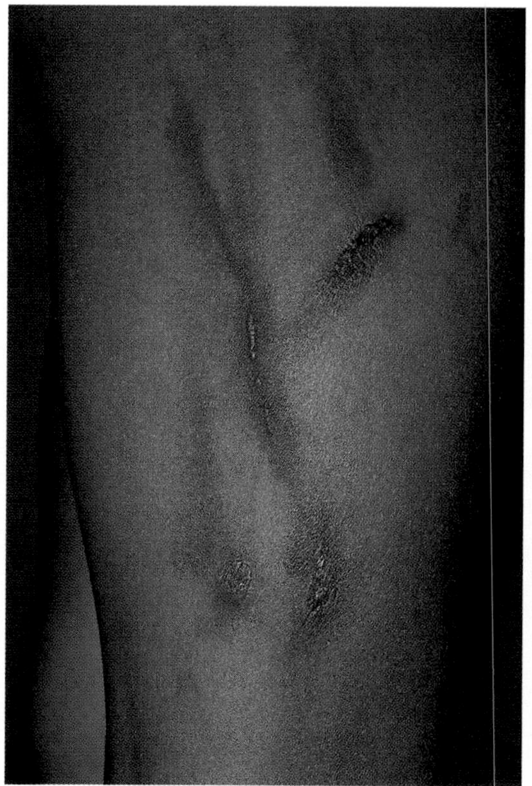

Figure 5.38 A 10-year-old girl with a striped pattern of dermatitis and hyperpigmentation following phototoxic contact dermatitis from giant hogweed.

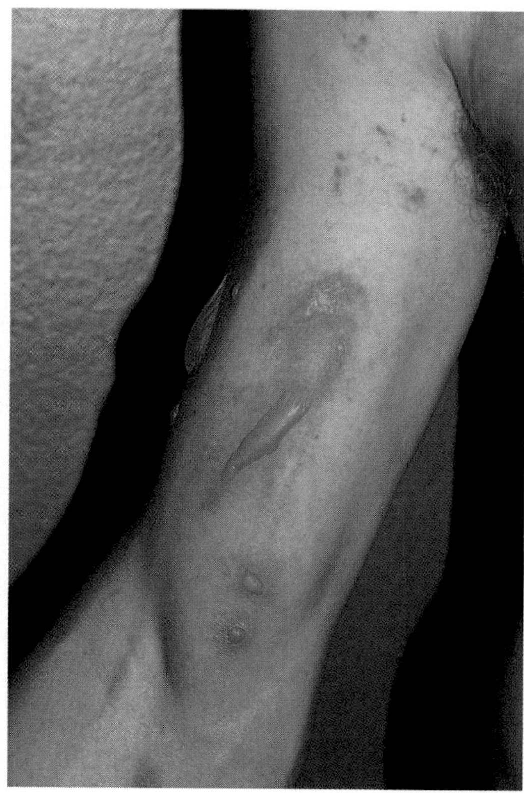

Figure 5.39 The bullous and linear lesions seen on the arm are typical of photocontact dermatitis. This phototoxic reaction was caused by contact with giant hogweed.

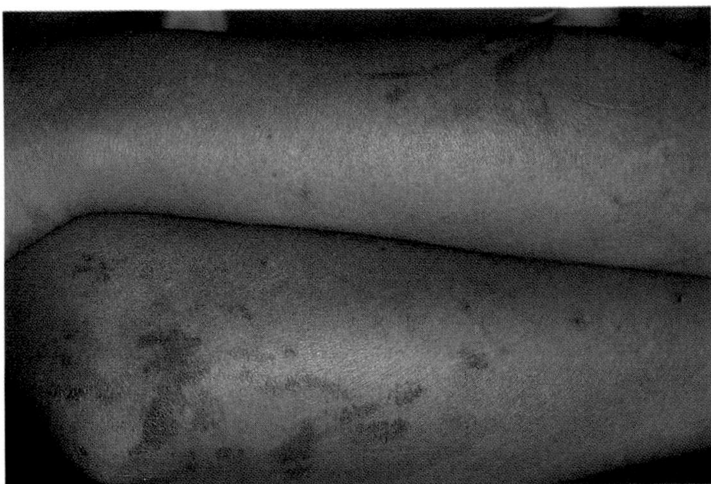

Figure 5.40 A 46-year-old woman with striped hyperpigmentation as a sequela of working with parsley plants in sunshine.

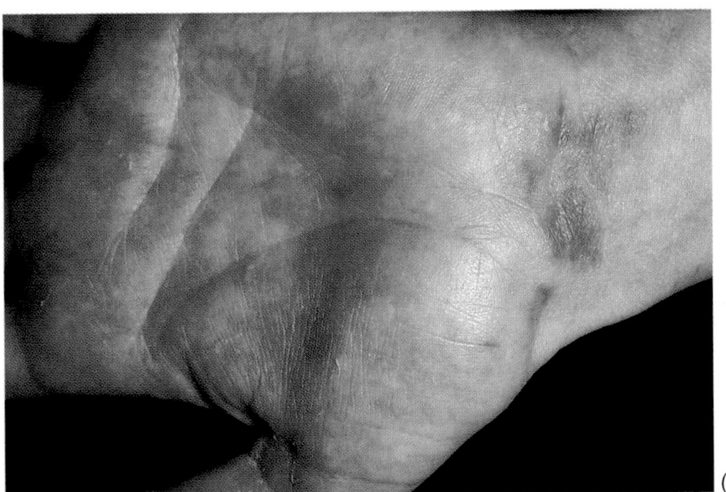

(a)

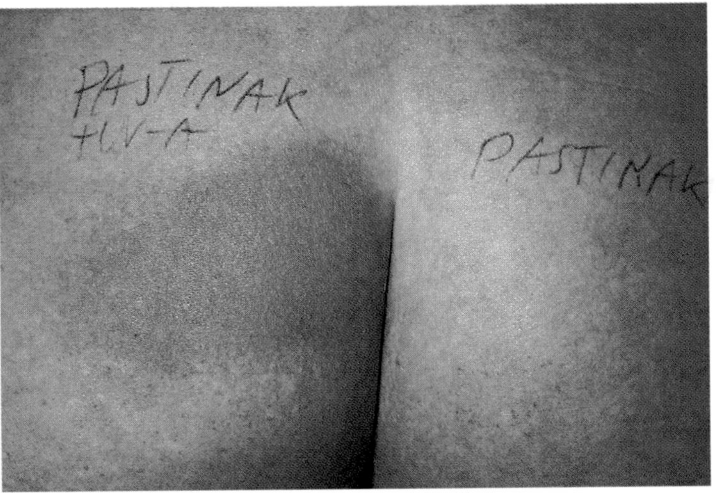

(b)

Figure 5.41 (**a**) A 32-year-old woman who had prepared parsnip and was then exposed to UV-A on a tanning bed developed this reaction. (**b**) A photo test with parsnip juice applied to both buttocks, followed by UV-A exposure on the left buttock, was positive. No reaction was seen on the right buttock, which was not exposed to UV-A.

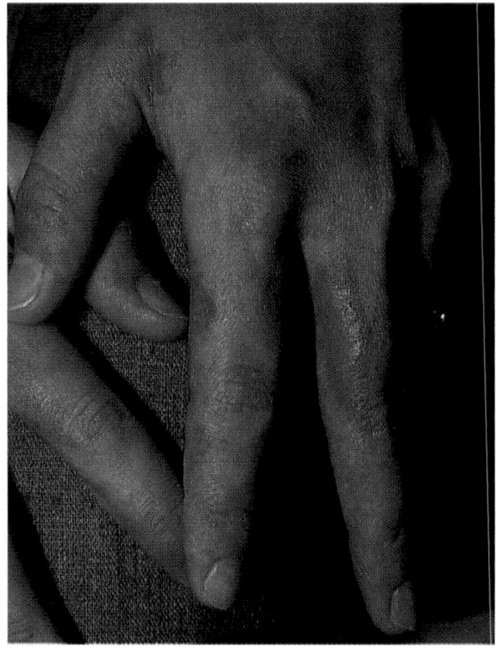

Figure 5.42 Squeezing limes outdoors led to hyperpigmented dermatitis of the fingers.

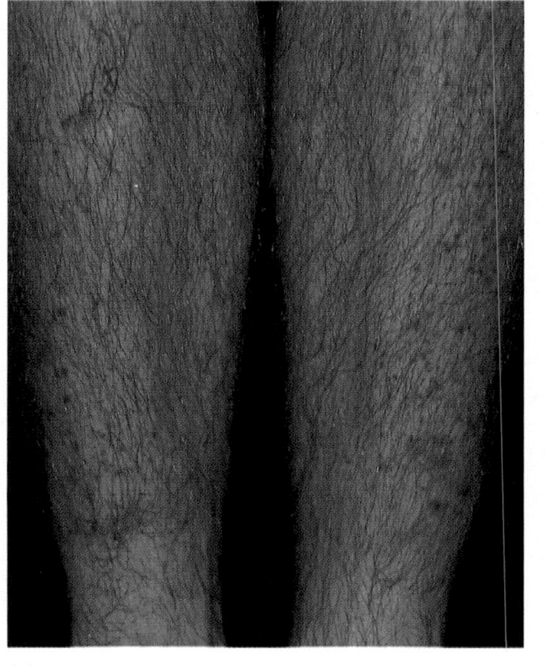

(**a**)

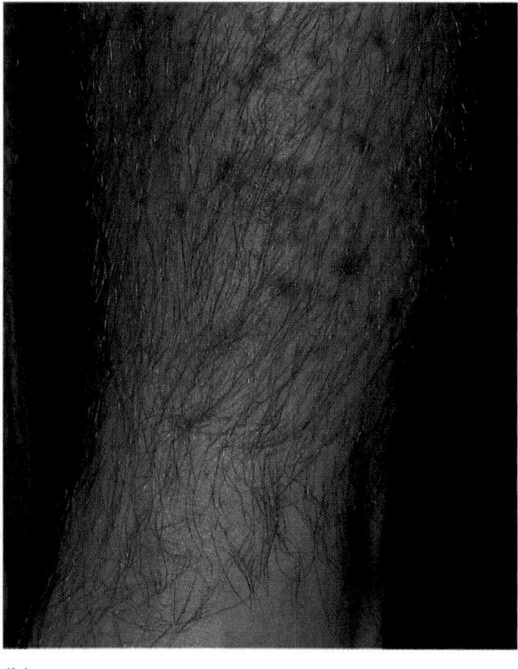

(**b**)

Figure 5.43 (**a**) A 24-year-old man with 'weed eater' or 'strimmer's dermatitis' is seen with scattered areas on the lower extremities affected by cutting weeds with a string trimmer. The weeds contained psoralen, and resulted in this phytophotodermatitis. (**b**) This close-up shows the eruption, which resembles purpura and was caused by drops of plant juice on the skin, which were then exposed to the sun.

OTHER CAUSES OF PHOTODERMATITIS

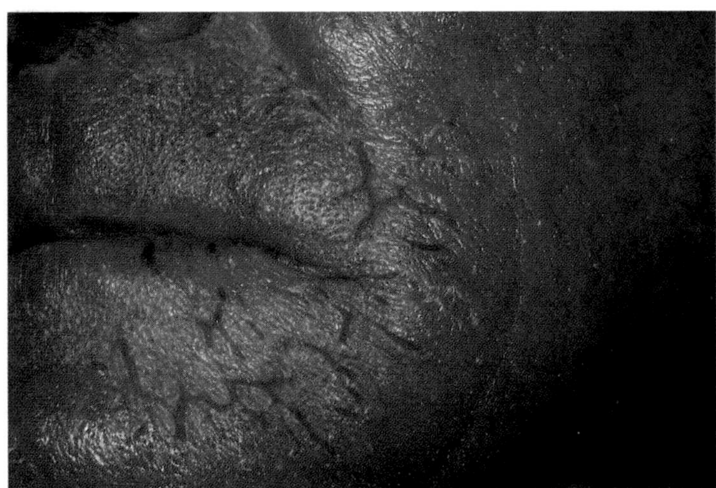

Figure 5.44 Photoallergic contact dermatitis of the beard area due to musk ambrette in an aftershave lotion (Gonçalo et al, 1991). Persistent photosensitivity has been reported after the development of this photoallergic state (Lan et al, 1994).

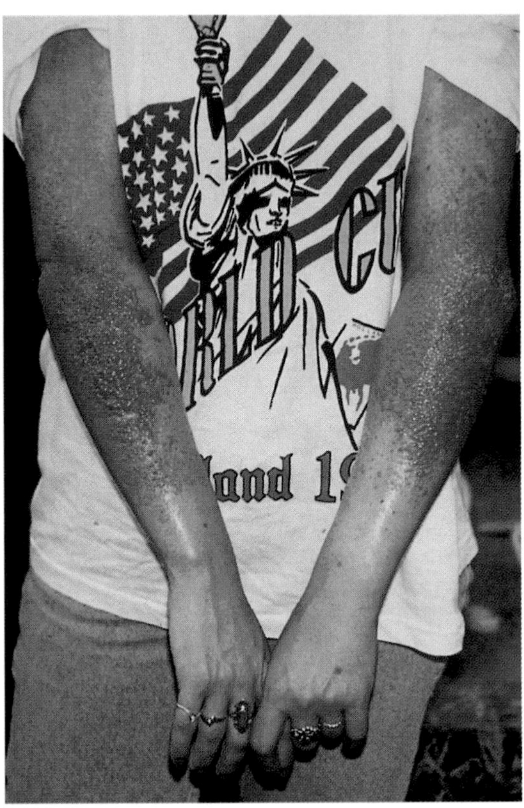

Figure 5.45 Photoallergic dermatitis occurs from substances capable of absorbing ultraviolet light. Sunscreens work by absorbing light, and paradoxically can cause photoallergic reactions, as seen here. The reaction is confined to the area of sunscreen application and subsequent sunlight exposure.

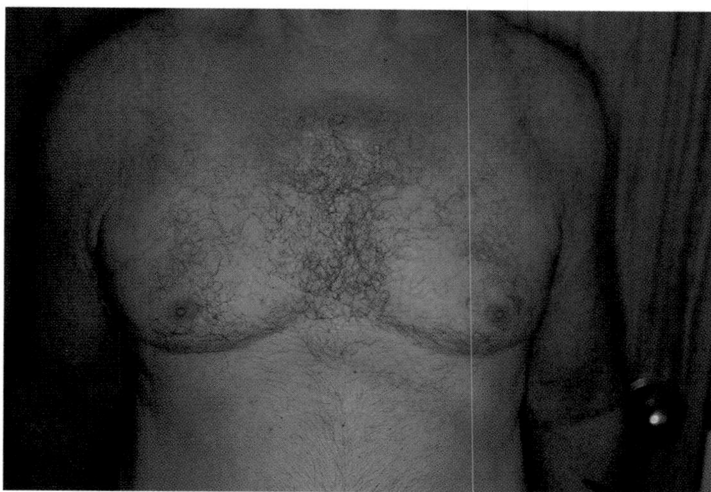

Figure 5.46 At times, the photoreaction is due to ingestion of a photosensitizing medication which may reduce the minimal erythema dose to UV-B light and cause a rapid sunburn-like reaction on exposed skin, as seen here.

Airborne Contact Dermatitis

Acute and chronic dermatoses of the exposed parts of the body and especially the face are sometimes caused by substances that are first released into the atmosphere and then settle on the exposed skin. This can occur both in occupational and in non-occupational contexts. Such allergens may be present in the air as vapours, gases, droplets or solid particles (Dooms-Goossens et al, 1986; Lachapelle, 1986; Dooms-Goossens and Deleu, 1991).

The most-common sites for contact dermatitis caused by an airborne agent are the parts of the body that are directly exposed to the air: the face, neck, upper part of the chest, hands, wrists, and underarms.

Differentiating an airborne dermatitis from a photodermatitis may pose problems. However, allergic reactions on the following sites strongly suggest an airborne dermatitis as opposed to a photodermatitis, even though the latter may extend to shadowed areas:

- covered parts of the body, such as the body folds, the genital region, and the lower legs in men, since materials may be trapped under clothing;
- anatomically shadowed portions of the body:
  - the eyelids,
  - the area behind the ears,
  - the scalp that is covered by hair,
  - the area under the chin.

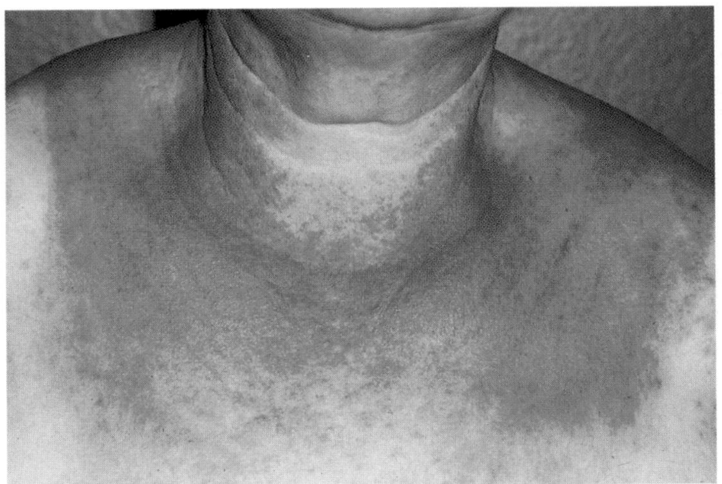

(a)

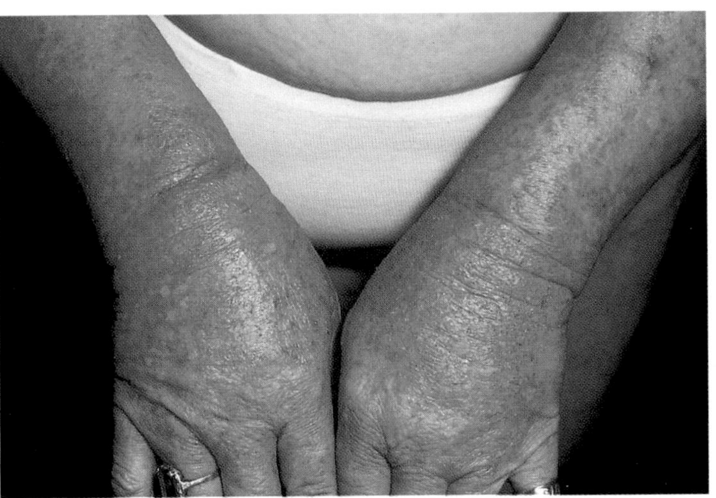

(b)

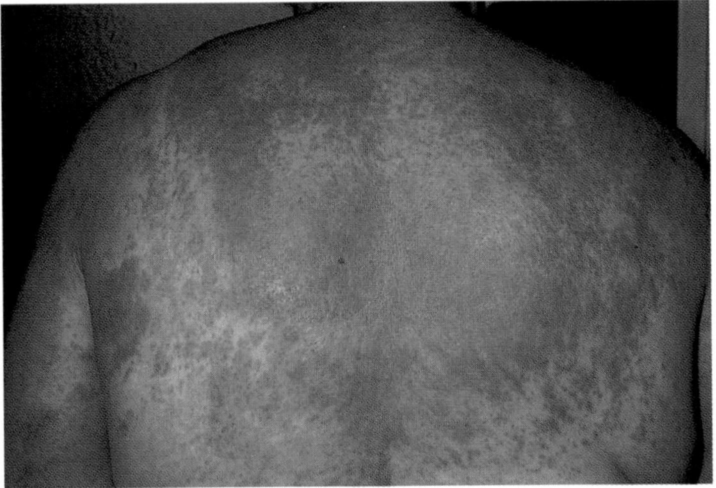

(c)

Figure 5.47 Plant material may cause photodermatitis, and when the exposure is due to plant material carried to the skin by air currents, the condition is referred to as airborne phytophoto contact dermatitis. This female gardener has a severe airborne phytophoto contact dermatitis seen on the chest (**a**), arms (**b**) and upper back (**c**). The plant substance responsible was not identified.

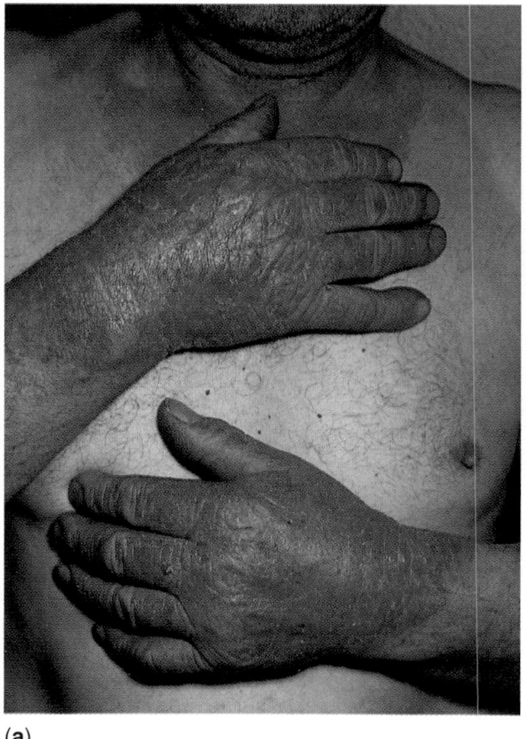
(**a**)

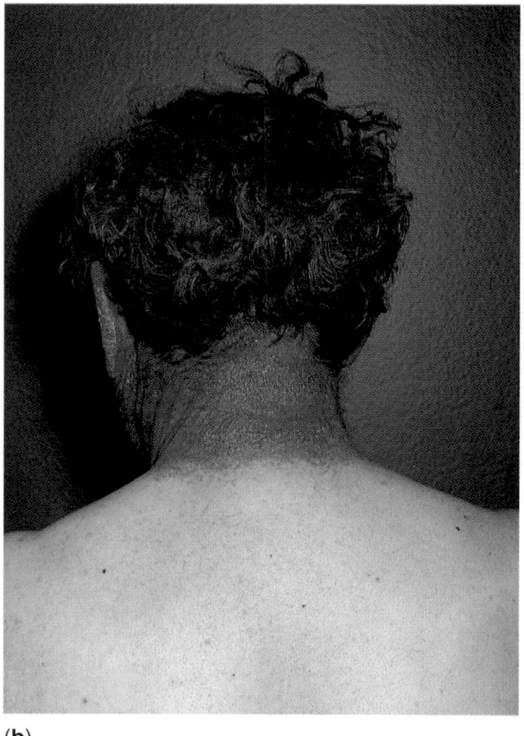
(**b**)

Figure 5.48 (**a**, **b**) Airborne contact dermatitis on the exposed areas of the body (the face was also affected) of a cement worker who was sensitive to chromates. His dermatitis recurred whenever he entered a room in which cement was being mixed.

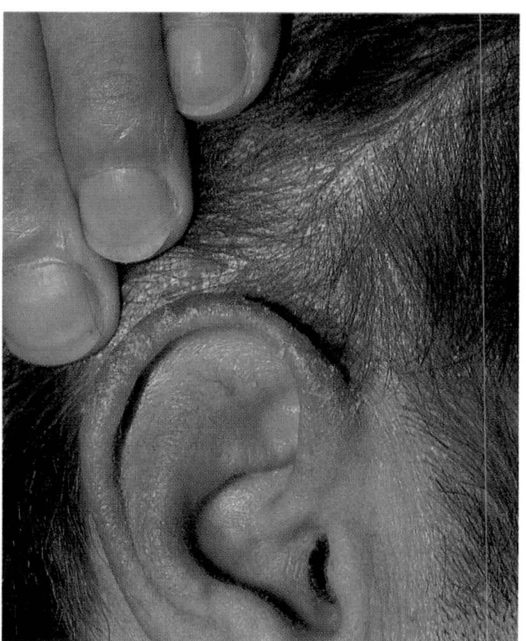

Figure 5.49 Allergic contact dermatitis of the scalp in a worker in a mirror factory who came in contact with vapour containing ethylenediamine.

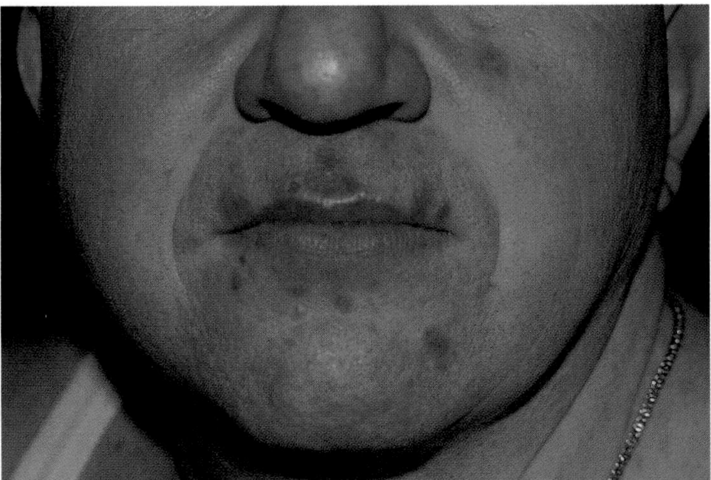

Figure 5.50 Airborne contact dermatitis due to triglycidylisocyanurate, an allergen present as a hardener in polyester powder paints. The patient also suffered from work-related asthma due to the same chemical.

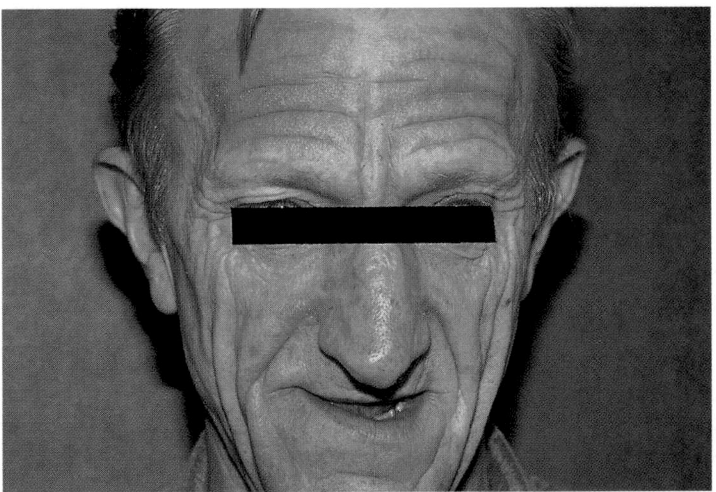

(a)

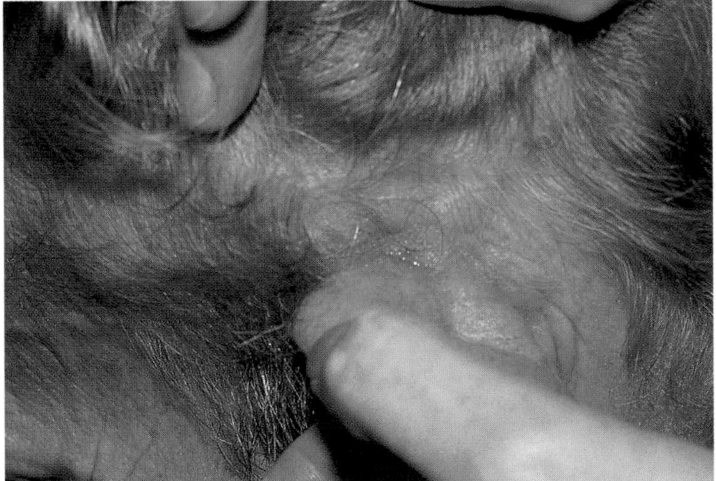

(b

Figure 5.51 Airborne dermatitis to triglycidylisocyanurate is seen in this figure. (**a**) The face shows accentuation of the skin folds in which the powder accumulated. (**b**) Demonstrates the retro-auricular involvement that is characteristic of airborne contact dermatitis. The flare-up of lesions on the forearms, which had come in contact with contaminated surfaces, is shown in (**c**). The 'work floor' is illustrated in (**d**) – this explains the localization seen in (**c**) (Dooms-Goossens et al, 1989).

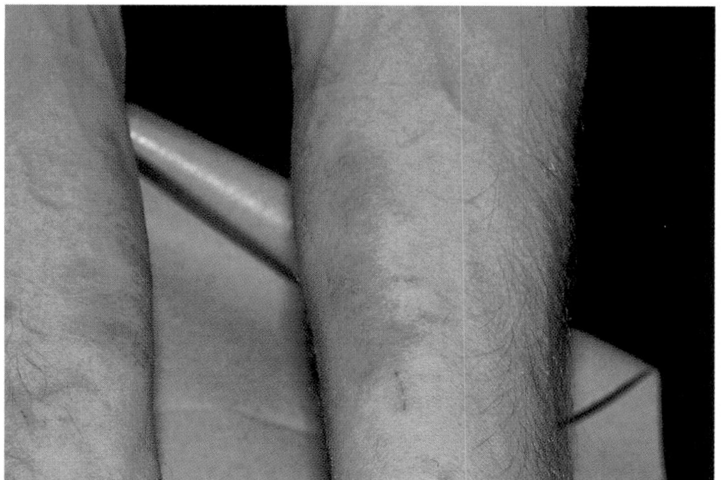

(c)

Figure 5.51 *continued*

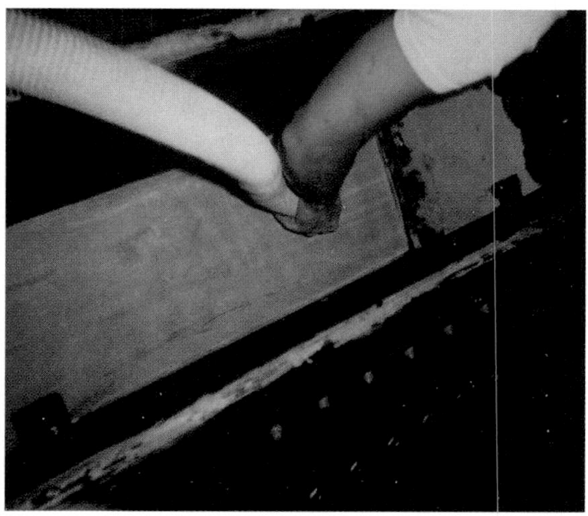

(d)

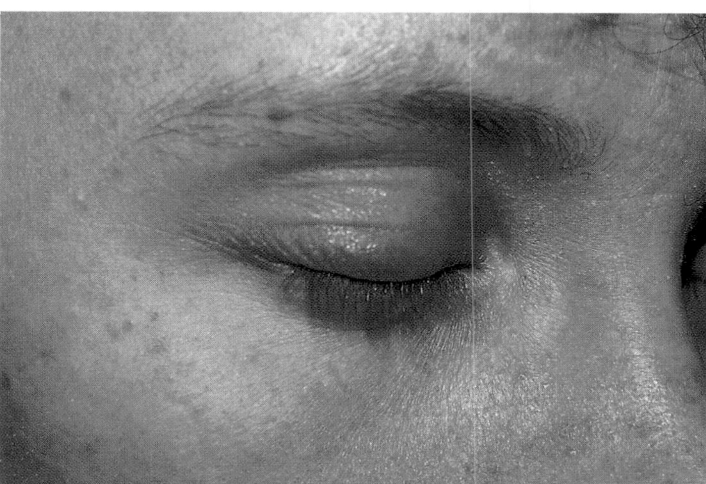

Figure 5.52 Irritant dermatitis of the eyelids due to airborne exposure to powder dust containing needle-sharp crystals. Dust is readily trapped in the folds of the eyelids.

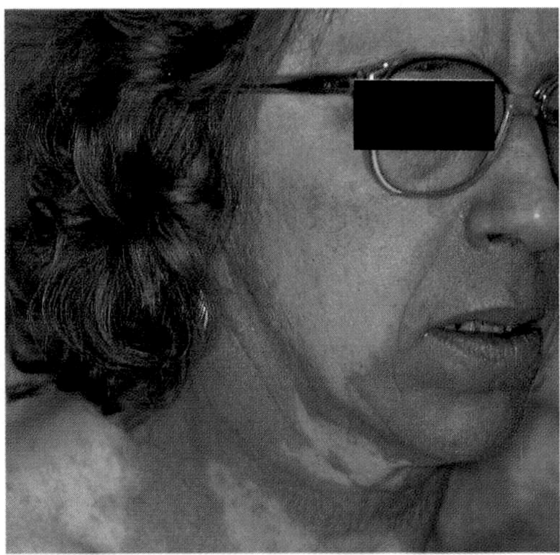

Figure 5.53 Dermatitis developed on the exposed areas of the face of this 52-year-old woman who worked as a fork lift operator in a plant where mineral fibre insulation was made. Patch testing showed a strongly positive reaction to *p-tert*-butylphenol–formaldehyde resin. This compound is used to coat the mineral fibres, and the dermatitis did not fade until she gave up her job. Although allergy to such fibres is rare, this largely refers to *users* of the product rather than those exposed to coatings that may not be fully cured. Coexistence of both immediate and delayed hypersensitivity to *p-tert*-butylphenol–formaldehyde resin used as a coating on fibreglass has been reported (Kalimo et al, 1975).

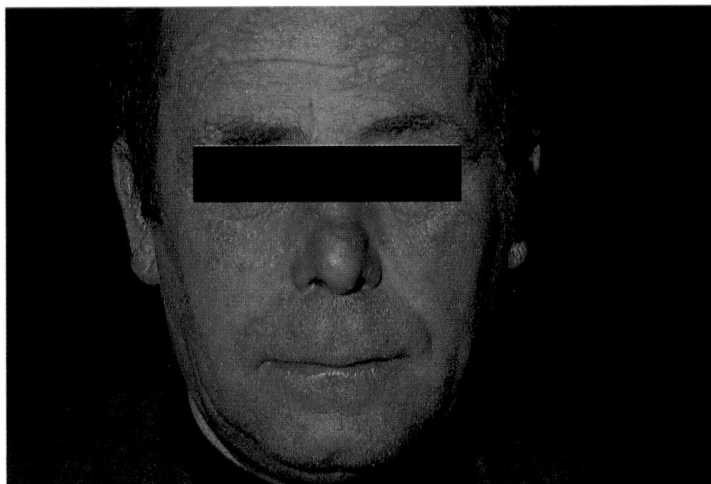

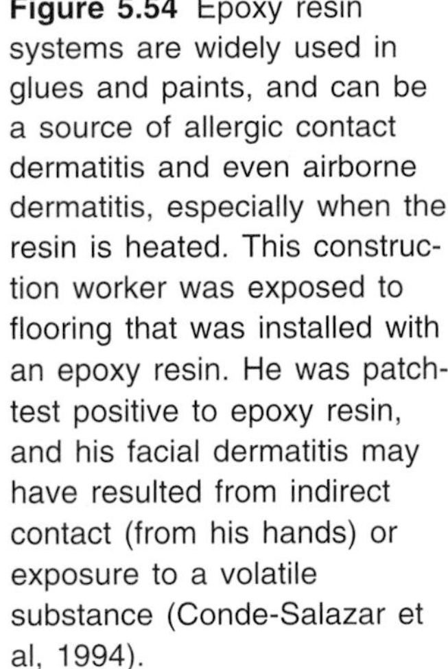

Figure 5.54 Epoxy resin systems are widely used in glues and paints, and can be a source of allergic contact dermatitis and even airborne dermatitis, especially when the resin is heated. This construction worker was exposed to flooring that was installed with an epoxy resin. He was patch-test positive to epoxy resin, and his facial dermatitis may have resulted from indirect contact (from his hands) or exposure to a volatile substance (Conde-Salazar et al, 1994).

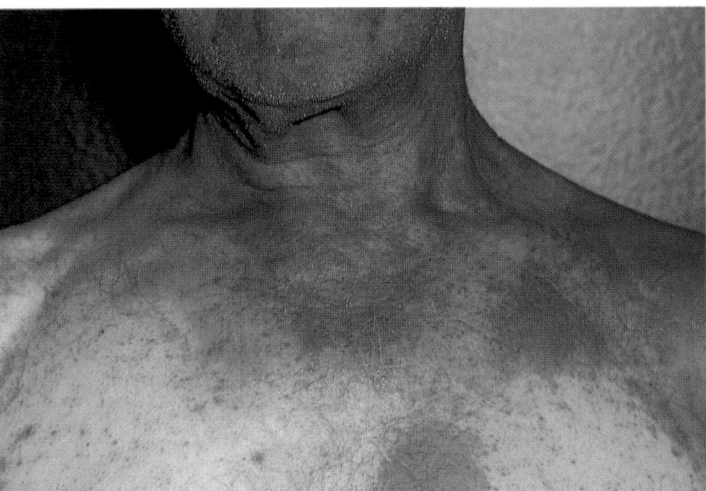

Figure 5.55 Airborne allergic contact dermatitis can occur from paints, which are frequently sprayed onto surfaces. Chloroacetamide used as a preservative in paint was responsible for this case of airborne allergic contact dermatitis.

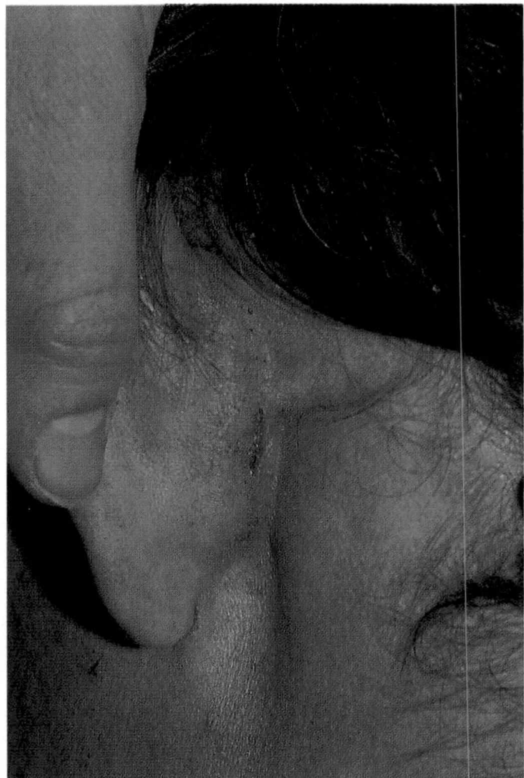

Figure 5.56 Airborne irritant contact dermatitis due to dust in an atopic metal worker. Involvement of the retro-auricular area helps to distinguish this from photocontact dermatitis.

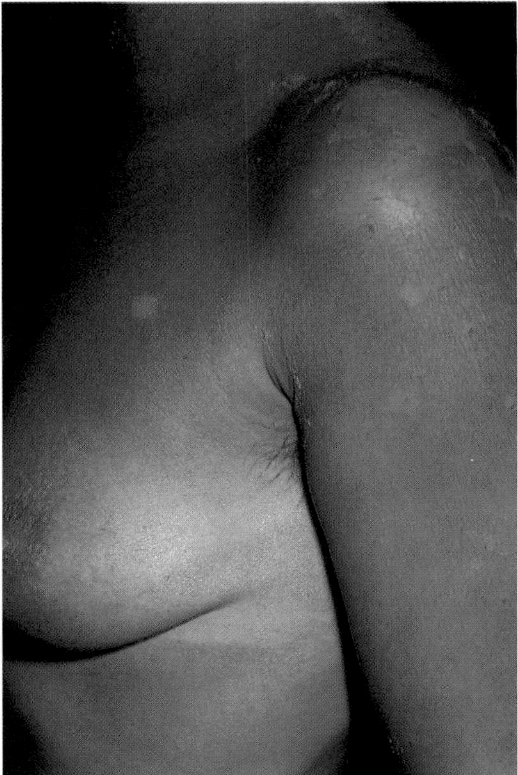

Figure 5.57 Chemical burn induced by airborne exposure to sulfuric acid vapours released when a toilet decalcifier was used abundantly. Note the sparing of the skin at the site of an adjustable nickel buckle on a brassiere strap. For once, nickel prevented dermatitis!

Contact Urticaria and Protein Contact Dermatitis

As discussed in Chapter 1, contact urticaria is of rapid onset and resolves within hours. Repeated exposure to the substance causing the urticaria often leads to protein contact dermatitis, which is clinically indistinguishable from contact dermatitis (Hjorth and Roed-Petersen, 1976).

IgE-mediated contact urticaria carries a risk of anaphylaxis. This has been described in children with spina bifida who had rubber catheters inserted in their spinal canal for prolonged periods of time and in health-care workers who wear rubber gloves for prolonged periods (Taylor and Praditsuwan, 1996; Woods et al, 1997). It has also been seen in women with seminal fluid allergy (Mathias et al, 1980; Boom et al, 1991).

Common causes of contact urticaria are given in the box.

Common causes of non-immunological contact urticaria	Common causes of immunological contact urticaria
Arthropods	Ammonium persulfate
Benzaldehyde	Amniotic fluid
Benzoic acid	Animal dander
Dimethyl sulfoxide	Apple
Formaldehyde	Beef
Histamine	Benzoic acid
Jellyfish	Cheese
Nicotinic acid esters	Chicken
Sorbic acid	Egg
Turpentine	Formaldehyde
	Latex
	Milk
	Potato
	Spices
	Wheat

CONTACT URTICARIA

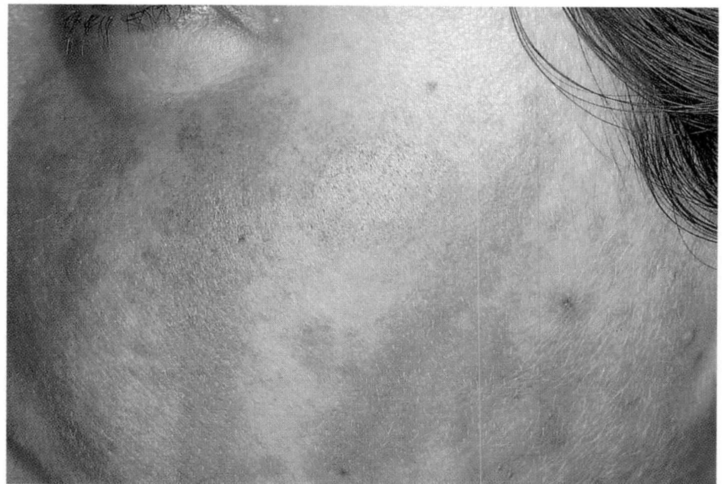

Figure 5.58 Non-immunological contact urticaria was produced on the face of this young woman by applying a 1% solution of sorbic acid to the cheek with a cotton swab. Within minutes, the figure '1%' could easily be read at the site of application. Her shampoo contained this preservative, and use of the shampoo caused urticaria of the face lasting for about 30 minutes (Rietschel, 1978).

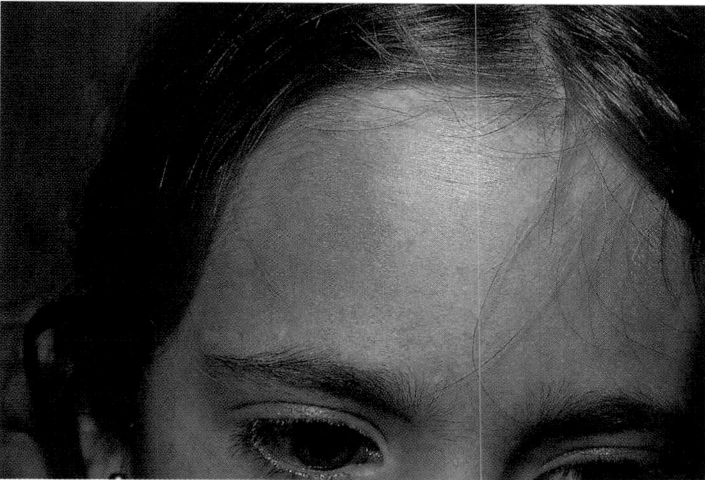

Figure 5.59 One drop of dilute cassia oil was applied to the forehead of this 8-year-old girl who experienced urticaria after contact with cinnamon-containing substances. Within minutes, a wheal-and-flare reaction occurred at the site of exposure to the cassia oil (which contains cinnamic aldehyde).

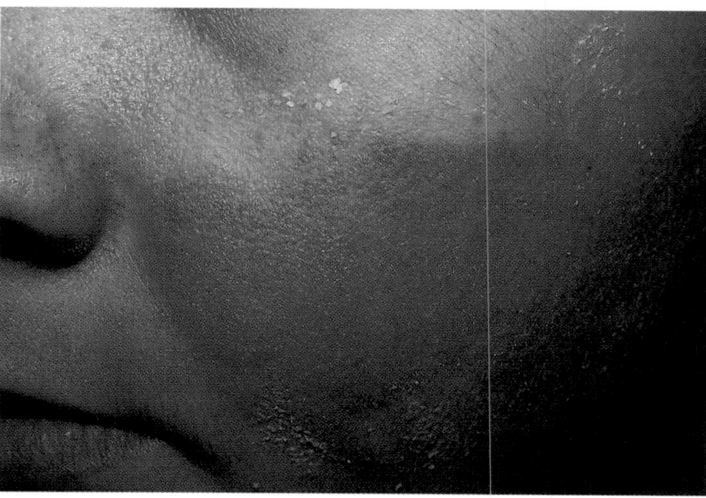

Figure 5.60 Benzoic acid can cause non-immunological contact urticaria, and is a breakdown product of benzoyl peroxide. Topical application of a 5% benzoyl peroxide acne preparation caused brisk erythema in minutes.

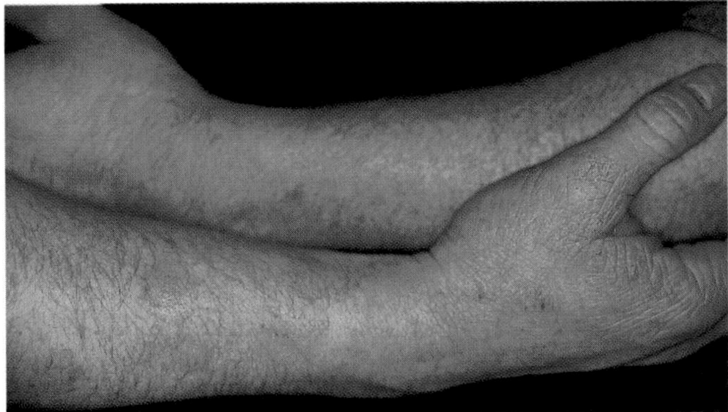

Figure 5.61 A 38-year-old man who ran a pizzeria experienced pruritus and dermatitis on his hands and forearms. The symptoms were most pronounced when he made pizzas, and he suspected a reaction to the dough. A scratch-chamber test with his own dough was strongly positive after 15 minutes. He also had a positive prick test to wheat. For economic reasons, he could not avoid contact with the dough, and the dermatitis persisted.

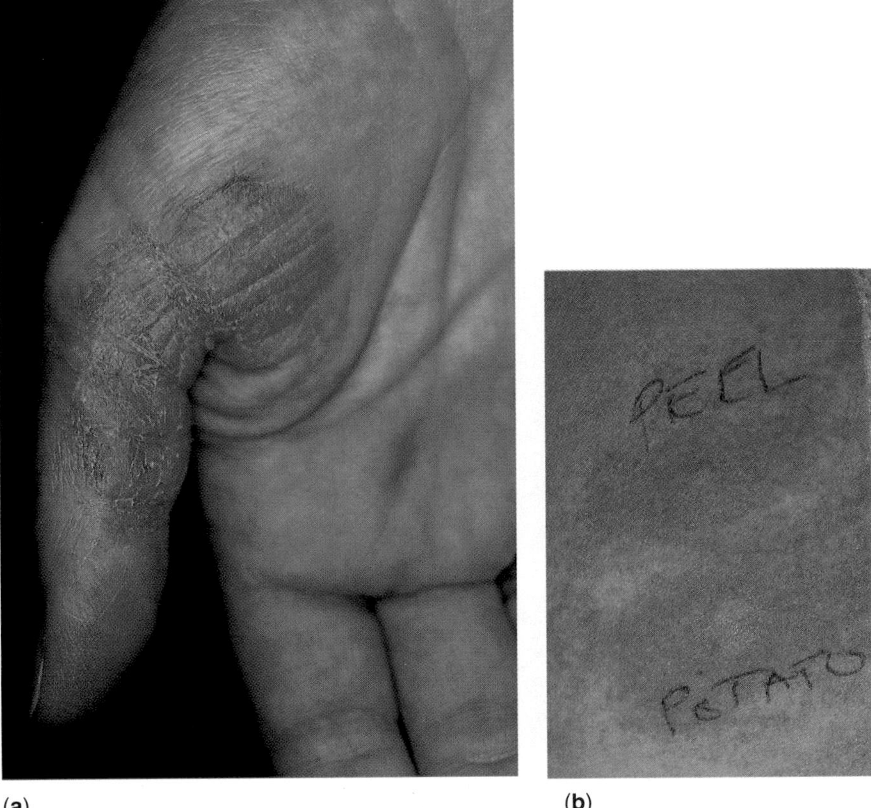

(a) (b)

Figure 5.62 (**a**) A 35-year-old woman experienced burning, stinging and pruritus when she peeled potatoes. She developed dermatitis on the left hand where she held the potatoes while peeling them. (**b**). A prick test was positive to potato skin and pulp. By wearing gloves, she was able to avoid skin contact with raw potatoes, and the dermatitis cleared. When prick testing with non-standard substances, an adequate number of controls should be tested as well.

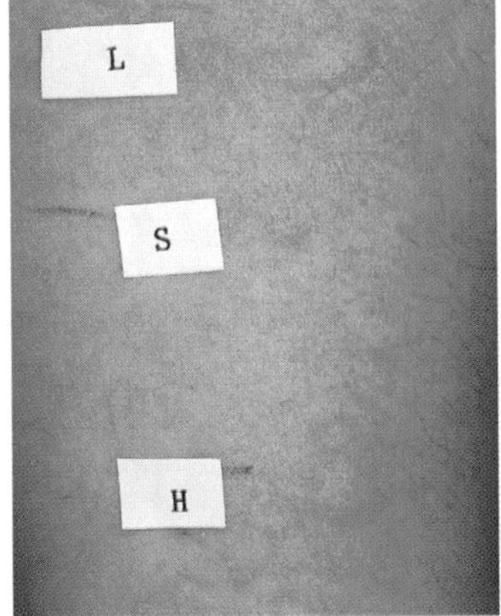

(**a**)

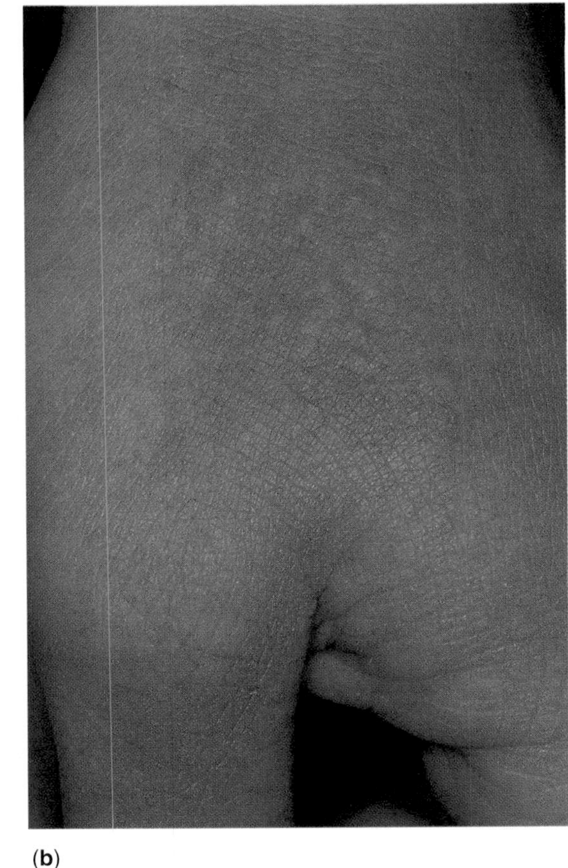

(**b**)

Figure 5.63 A 20-year-old woman who worked as a hotel maid developed an urticarial reaction immediately after putting on her rubber gloves. Patch testing was negative. (**a**) A prick test with her own gloves showed a strongly positive reaction after 15 minutes. (**b**) A challenge test with the gloves resulted in contact urticaria after 15 minutes.

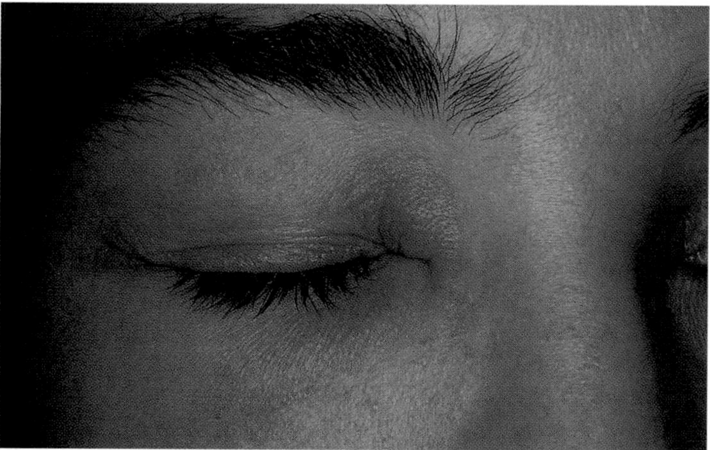

(a)

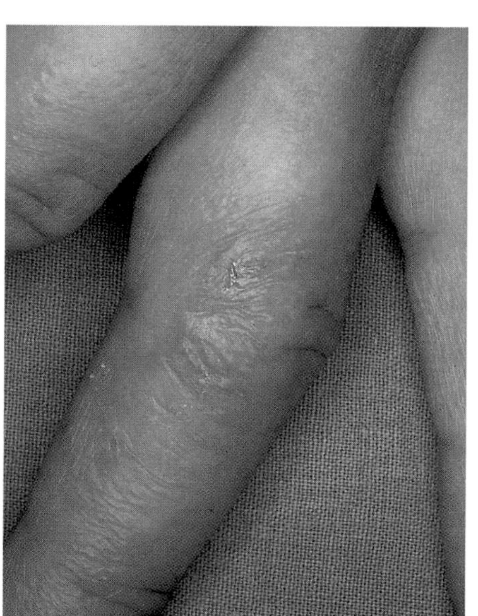

(b)

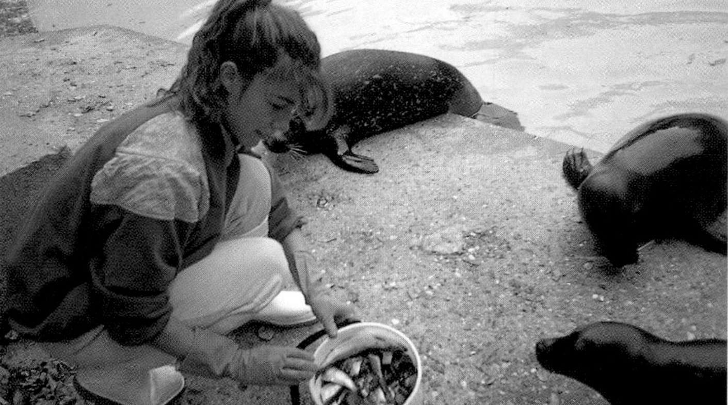

(c)

Figure 5.64 (**a**) Urticarial lesions due to protein contact dermatitis of the eyelids, appearing a short time after handling herring. (**b**) The same patient with vesicular hand dermatitis. The in vivo and in vitro test results indicated a type I allergic mechanism. In vivo cross-reactivity with fish belonging to the Clupeiform order was observed. (**c**) This patient was a marine seal-trainer at a zoo, and she fed the seals. When she used protection and stopped handling the herring, the lesions disappeared. Here she shows how she worked, protected by rubber gloves (Alonso et al, 1993).

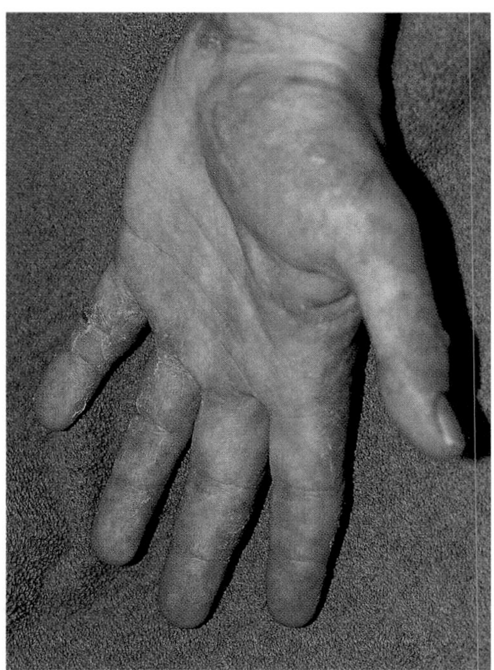

(**a**)

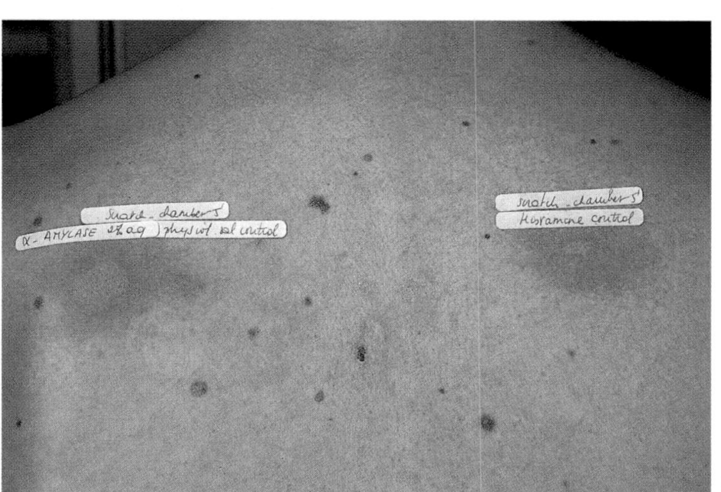

(**b**)

Figure 5.65 (**a**) Protein contact dermatitis in a baker due to α-amylase, an enzyme used in flour. (**b**) A positive scratch-chamber test to α-amylase (2% aqueous) (in comparison with histamine).

REFERENCES

Alomar A, Conde-Salazar L, Romaguera C (1985) Occupational dermatoses from cutting oils. *Contact Dermatitis* **12**:129–38.

Alonso MD, Conde-Salazar L, Cuevas M et al (1993) Occupational protein contact dermatitis from herrings. *Allergy* **48**:349–52.

Andersen KE, Hjorth N, Menné T (1984) The baboon syndrome: systemically-induced allergic contact dermatitis. *Contact Dermatitis* **10**:97–100.

Boom BW, van Toorenenbergen AW, Nierop G et al (1991) A case of seminal fluid allergy successfully treated with immunotherapy in a one-day rush procedure. *J Dermatol* **18**:206–10.

Conde-Salazar L, Gonzalez de Domingo MA, Guimaraens D (1994) Sensitization to epoxy resin systems in special flooring workers. *Contact Dermatitis* **31**:157–60.

Dooms-Goossens A, Deleu H (1991) Airborne contact dermatitis: an update. *Contact Dermatitis* **25**:211–17.

Dooms-Goossens AE, Debusschere KM, Gevers DM et al (1986) Contact dermatitis caused by airborne agents. *J Am Acad Dermatol* **15**:1–10.

Dooms-Goossens A, Bedert R, Vandaele M et al (1989) Airborne contact dermatitis due to triglycidylisocyanurate. *Contact Dermatitis* **21**:202–3.

Dooms-Goossens A, Dubelloy R, Degreef H (1990) Contact and systemic contact-type dermatitis to spices. *Dermatol Clin* **8**:89–93.

Gonçalo S, Gil J, Gonçalo M, Baptista AP (1991) Pigmented photoallergic contact dermatitis from musk ambrette. *Contact Dermatitis* **24**:229–31.

Hjorth N, Roed-Petersen J (1976) Occupational protein contact dermatitis in food handlers. *Contact Dermatitis* **2**:28–42.

Kalimo K, Saarni H, Kytta J (1975) Immediate and delayed type reactions to formaldehyde resin in glass wool. *Contact Dermatitis* **1**:181.

Lan LR, Lee JY, Kao HF et al (1994) Persistent light reaction with erythroderma caused by musk ambrette: a case report. *Cutis* **54**:167–70.

Lachapelle JM (1986) Industrial airborne irritant or allergic contact dermatitis. *Contact Dermatitis* **14**:137–45.

Lowney ED (1974) A single-step procedure for inducing partial tolerance of DNCB in human subjects. *J Invest Dermatol* **63**:260–1.

Mathias CG, Frick OL, Caldwell TM et al (1980) Immediate hypersensitivity to seminal fluid and atopic dermatitis. *Arch Dermatol* **116**:209–12.

Petrozzi JW, Shore RN (1976) Generalized exfoliative dermatitis from ethylenediamine. *Arch Dermatol* **112**:525.

Rietschel RL, Fowler JF Jr (1995) *Fisher's Contact Dermatitis.* Baltimore, MD: Williams and Wilkins.

Rietschel RL (1978) Contact urticaria from synthetic cassia oil and sorbic acid limited to the face. *Contact Dermatitis* **4**:347–9.

Saperstein H, Rapaport M, Rietschel RL (1984) Topical vitamin E as a cause of erythema multiforme-like eruption. *Arch Dermatol* **120**:906–8.

Taylor JS, Praditsuwan P (1996) Latex allergy. Review of 44 cases including outcome and frequent association with allergic hand eczema. *Arch Dermatol* **132**:265–71.

Veien NK (1989) Systemically induced eczema in adults. *Acta Derm Venereol (Stockh)* Suppl 147:1–58.

Veien NK, Hattel T, Laurberg G (1993) Low nickel diet: an open, prospective trial. *J Am Acad Dermatol* **29**:1002–7.

Veien NK, Hattel T, Laurberg G (1994) Chromate-allergic patients challenged orally with potassium dichromate. *Contact Dermatitis* **31**:137–9.

Verbov J (1989) Juvenile plantar dermatosis (JPD). *Acta Derm Venereol (Stockh)* Suppl 144:153–4.

Woods JA, Lambert S, Platts-Mills TA et al (1997) Natural rubber latex allergy: spectrum, diagnostic approach, and therapy. *J Emerg Med* **15**:71–85.

6

Specific Categories of Contact Allergens

Contact dermatitis can occur when medications are applied to treat other skin diseases, resulting in a confusing picture caused by the presence of two abnormal conditions. Contact dermatitis can also occur when medications are applied to normal skin for the promotion of health or prevention of disease. Both active ingredients and vehicle components can be responsible for contact dermatitis. Even medications prescribed to treat contact dermatitis, such as corticosteroids, can be a cause of contact dermatitis.

Medications

The list of topical preparations commonly responsible for skin sensitization varies from country to country, depending on local customs, and also with time, depending on the new products issued by the pharmaceutical industry and the recognition of the sensitizing potential of topical agents (Angelini, 1995). The most important allergens are given in the box on the following page, and those areas most typically involved are illustrated below.

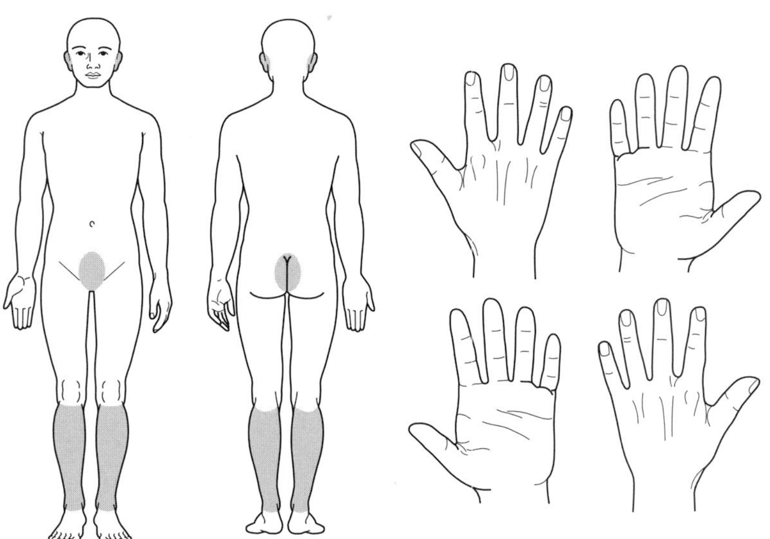

Typical distribution of topical medications

Allergens

- Antibiotics (e.g. chloramphenicol, neomycin and sulfanilamide)
- Antimicrobials
- Corticosteroids
- Local anaesthetics
- Non-steroidal anti-inflammatory drugs
- Substances derived from plants

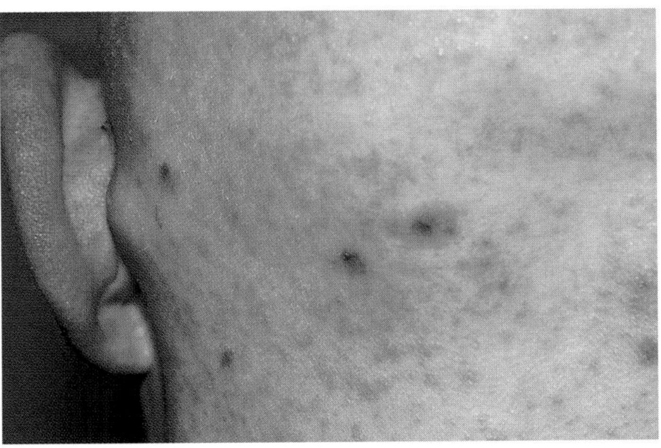

(**a**)

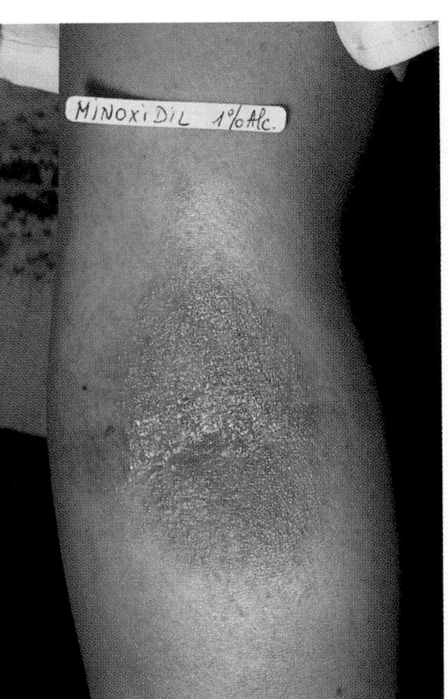

(**b**)

Figure 6.1 (**a**) Allergic contact dermatitis of the scalp due to minoxidil. (**b**) Repeated open-application test (ROAT) in the same patient with minoxidil solution (1% ethanol) was positive after two days (the patch test was negative). Patch testing for minoxidil allergy is difficult with pure material, and frequently requires that the finished product produce a positive reaction (Whitmore, 1992).

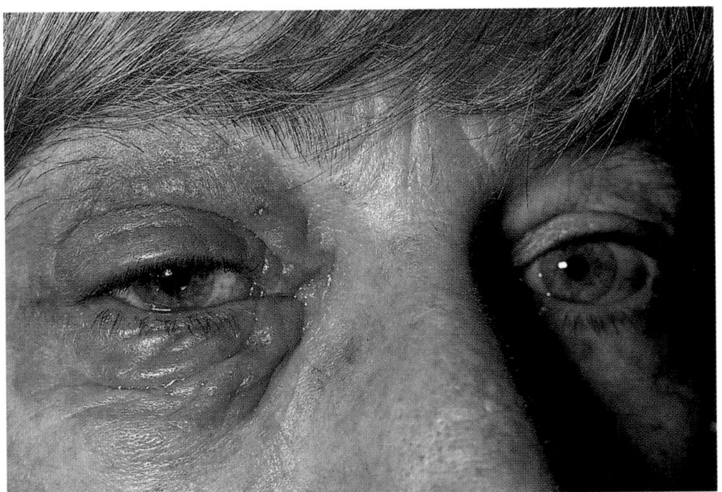

Figure 6.2 A 45-year-old woman with allergic contact dermatitis of the eyelids from chloramphenicol eyedrops.

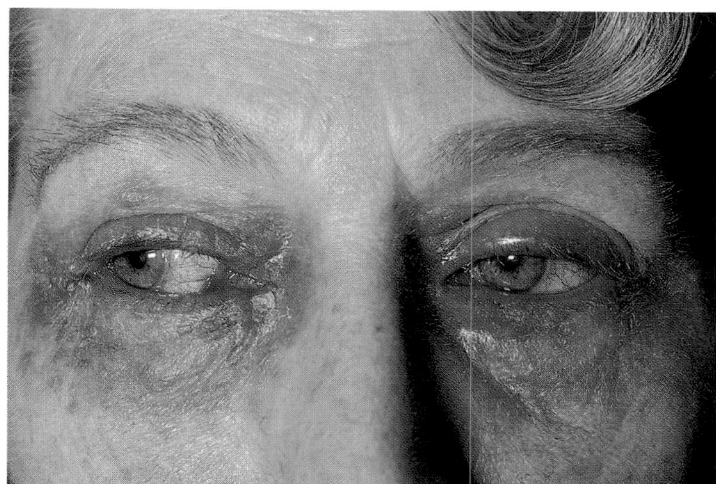

Figure 6.3 A similar picture to that seen in Figure 6.2 is seen here; however, this 64-year-old woman had an irritant reaction to benzalkonium chloride in eyedrops.

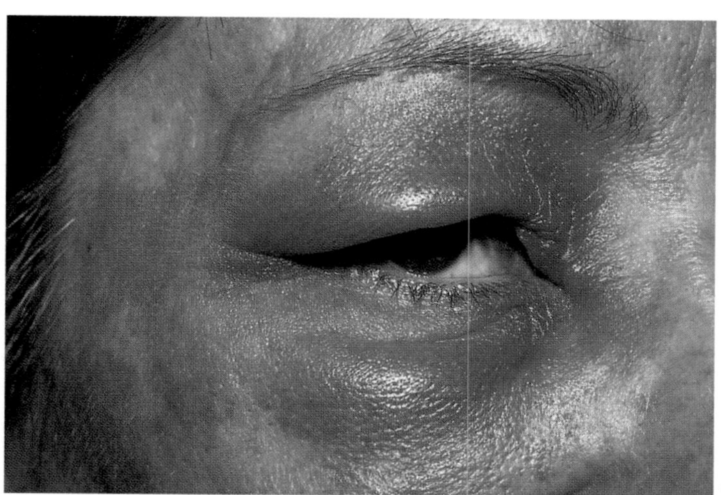

(**a**)

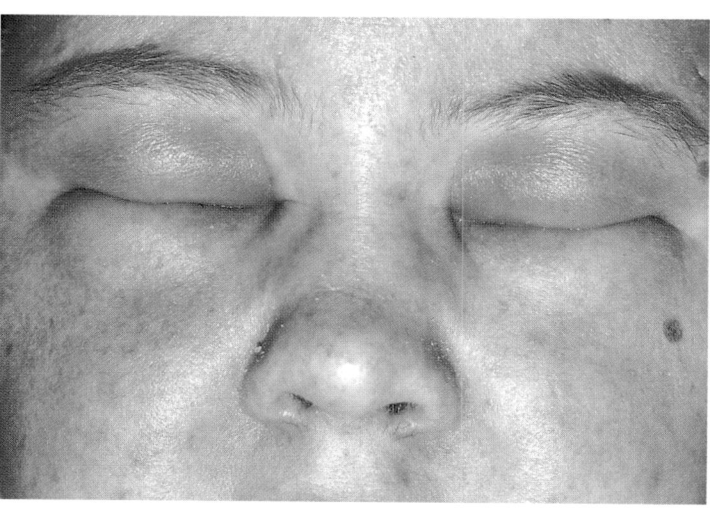

(**b**)

Figure 6.4 (**a**) A severe edematous reaction is seen on the eyelids associated with benzoyl peroxide sensitivity due to a topical acne medication used on the face. As a consequence of the loose cutaneous tissue, the condition may be so severe that it is difficult to differentiate it from angioedema (angioneurotic oedema) (**b**).

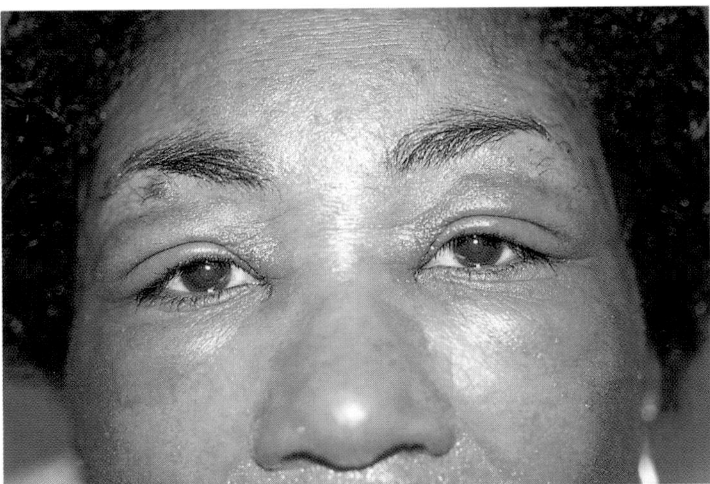

Figure 6.5 The oedema seen around this woman's eyelids was due to hydrocortisone allergy, which was detected with a patch test to tixocortol pivalate.

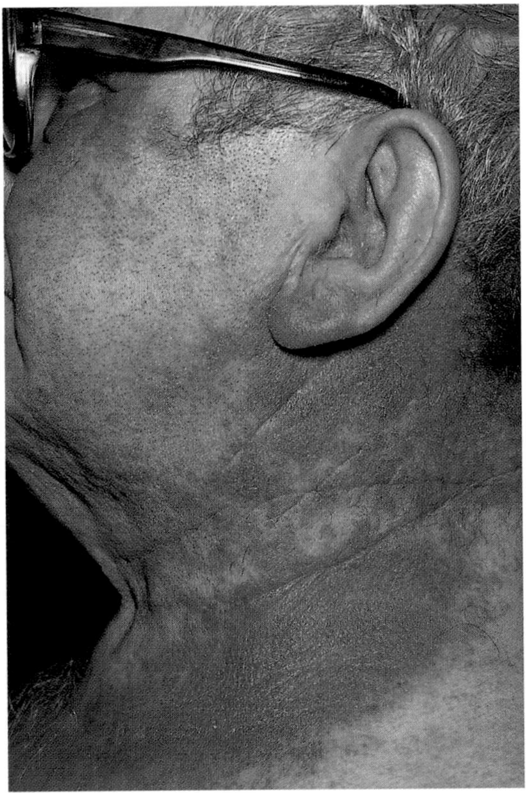

Figure 6.6 This is a 75-year-old man with allergic contact dermatitis of the ears, neck and eyelids from neomycin eardrops.

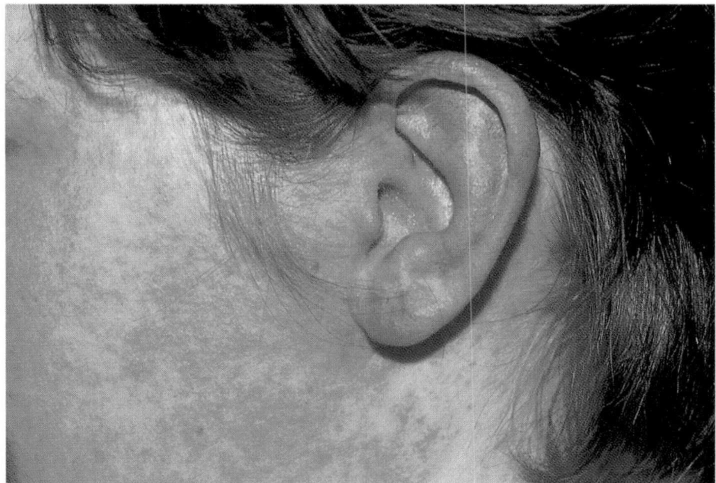

(a)

Figure 6.7 (**a**) This allergic contact dermatitis of the ears and pre-auricular area was caused by ear drops. (**b**) The positive papular patch test was due to TEA–oleylpolypeptide (5% aqueous), a protein hydrolysate found in some ear drops and some cosmetic preparations.

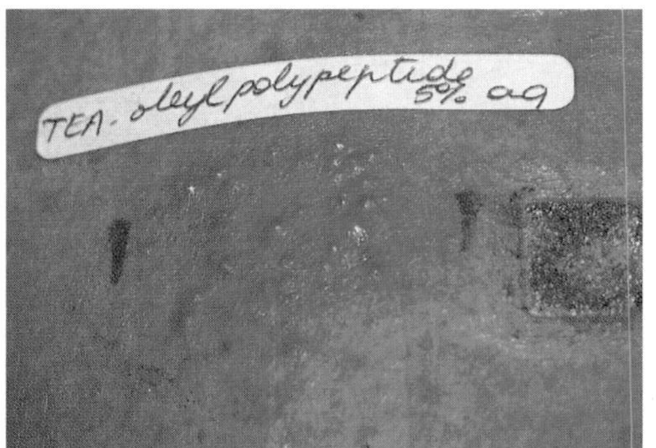

(b)

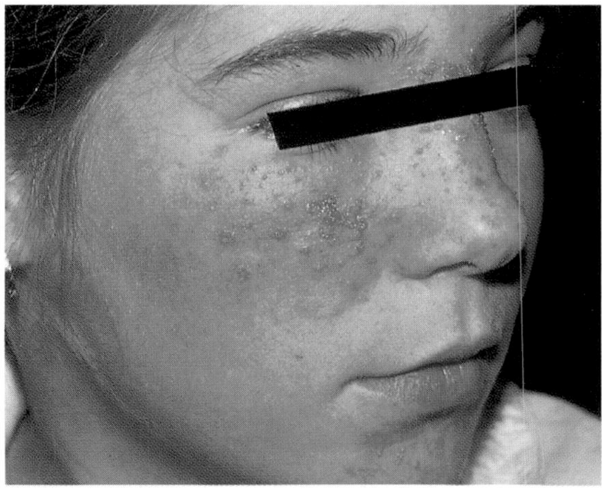

(a) (b)

Figure 6.8 (**a**) Papulovesicular contact dermatitis of the face due to hexamidine, an antiseptic agent. (**b**) This papulovesicular patch test reaction was due to hexamidine (0.15% aqueous). The patient was later exposed to a hair lotion containing hexamidine as a preservative agent, and the dermatitis reappeared.

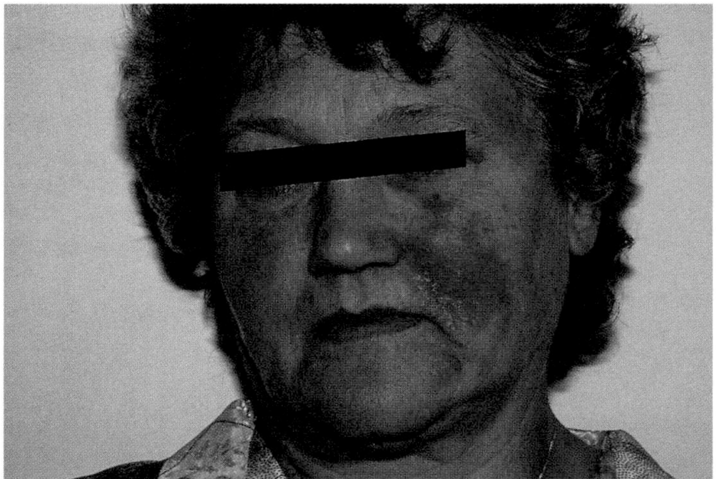

Figure 6.9 The underlying condition in this woman was rosacea. Her case was complicated by allergic contact dermatitis to her topical corticosteroid.

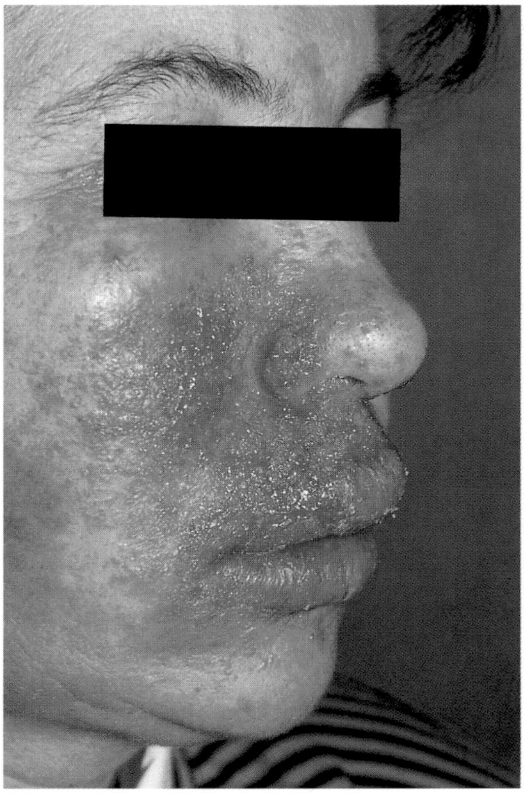

(**a**)

(**b**)

Figure 6.10 (**a**) Severe papulovesicular dermatitis on the face was induced by topical sulfanilamide. (**b**) The patch test reaction to 2% sulfanilamide in ethanol confirmed the allergy. Petrolatum dilutions may give false-negative patch test reactions – this also applies to chloramphenicol and lidocaine.

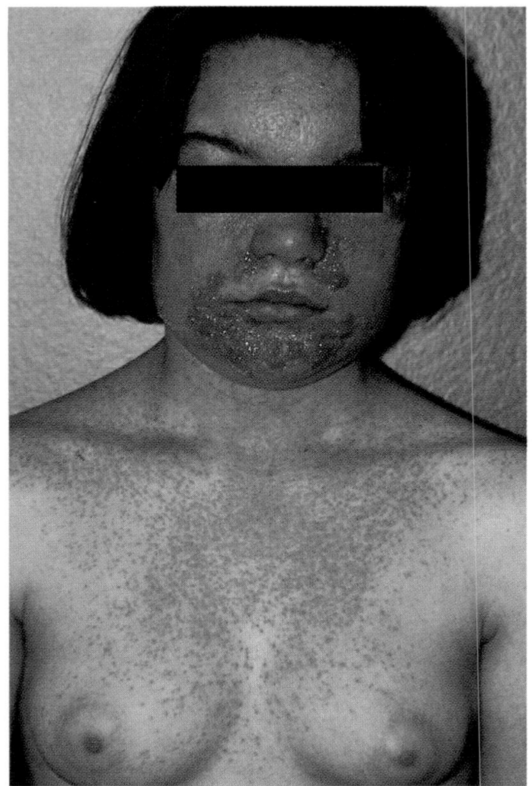

Figure 6.11 This acute allergic contact dermatitis on the face, complicated by bacterial superinfection, was due to virginiamycin with an id-like spread to the neck and presternal region.

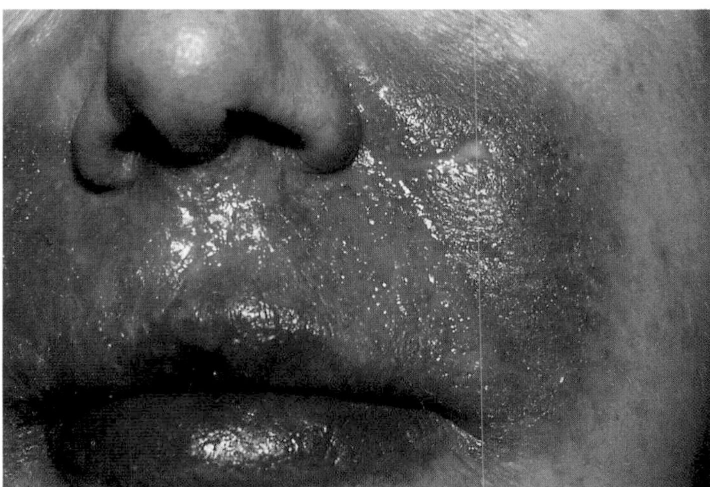

Figure 6.12 Allergic contact dermatitis due to Roman camomile flower extract in an ointment for treating radiodermatitis caused these facial lesions. Some cases of camomile contact dermatitis recur when a sensitized individual drinks camomile tea (McGeorge and Steele, 1991).

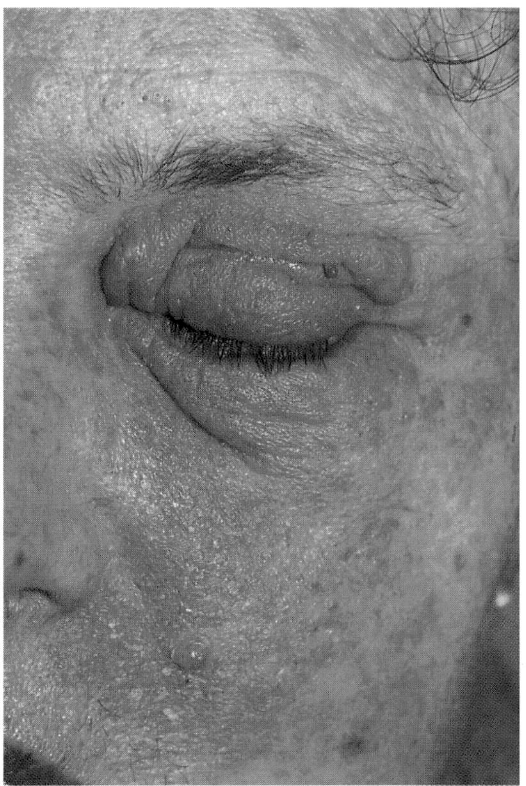

Figure 6.13 This facial dermatitis was due to an allergic reaction to parabens present as preservatives in a topical pharmaceutical product. Although widely used, parabens are a rare cause of cosmetic dermatitis.

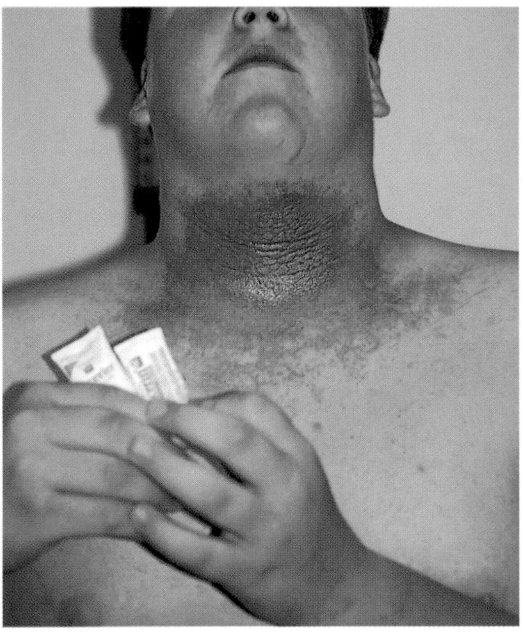

Figure 6.14 This young man was patch tested with the TRUE test, and was found to be allergic to a preservative. He was given the European name of the preservative Kathon CG, but did not correctly identify the presence of this substance in Eucerin cream under the US name methylchloroisothiazolinone–methylisothiazolinone on the label. He applied the Eucerin to the neck and produced the dermatitis seen here.

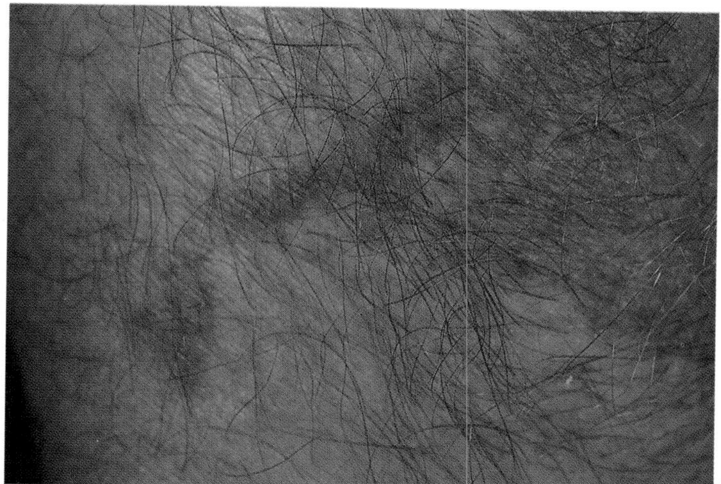

(a)

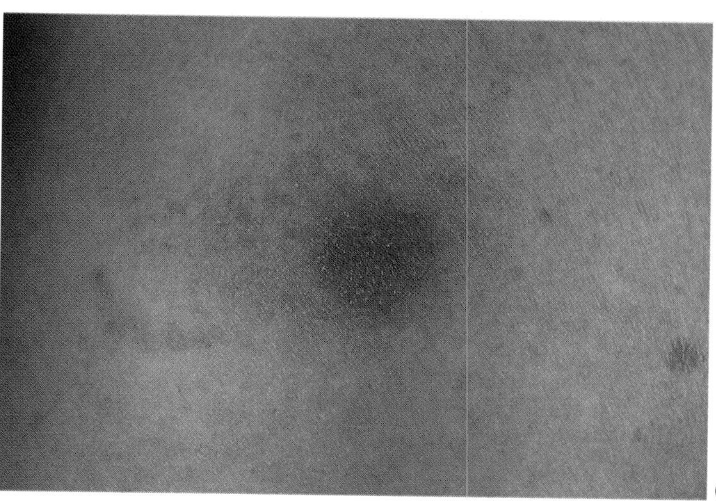

(b)

Figure 6.15 (**a**) Neosporin ointment was applied as a wound dressing to the arm of this middle-aged adult man who experienced lymphangitic spread of the allergic reaction, as seen here. This was mistakenly identified as bacterial cellulitis by his physician, and systemic antibiotic therapy and hospitalization were part of his treatment. (**b**) The correct diagnosis, however, was contact dermatitis to neomycin, and the patch test reaction was strongly positive.

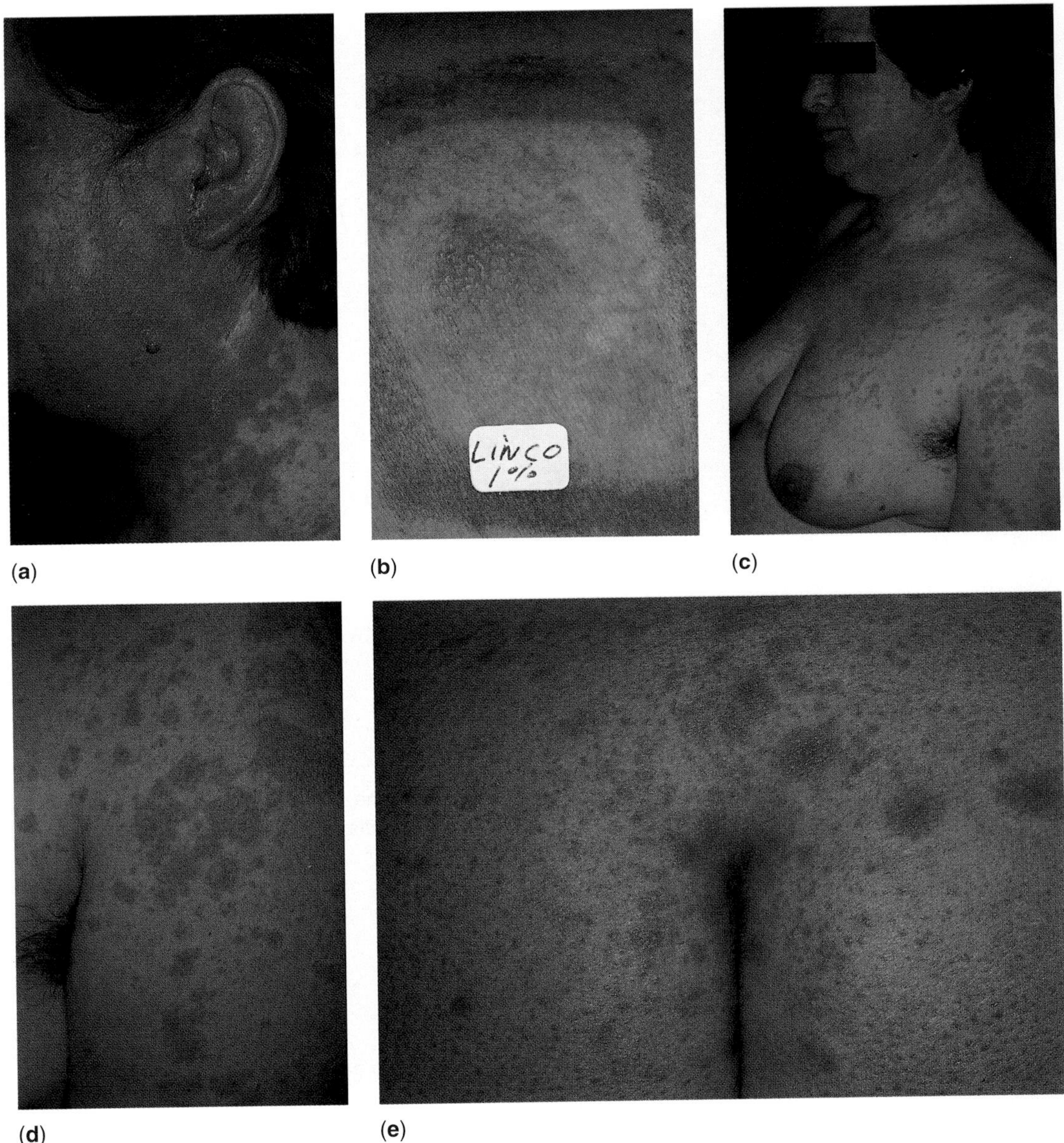

(a) (b) (c) (d) (e)

Figure 6.16 (**a**) This 36-year-old woman applied lincomycin to her ear, and developed allergic contact dermatitis, which was confirmed by a positive patch test (**b**). Persistent applications were followed by an extension of the eruption to the trunk (**c**) and upper extremities (**d**). On the buttocks lesions were seen that were consistent with systemic contact dermatitis (**e**) (Conde-Salazar et al, 1985).

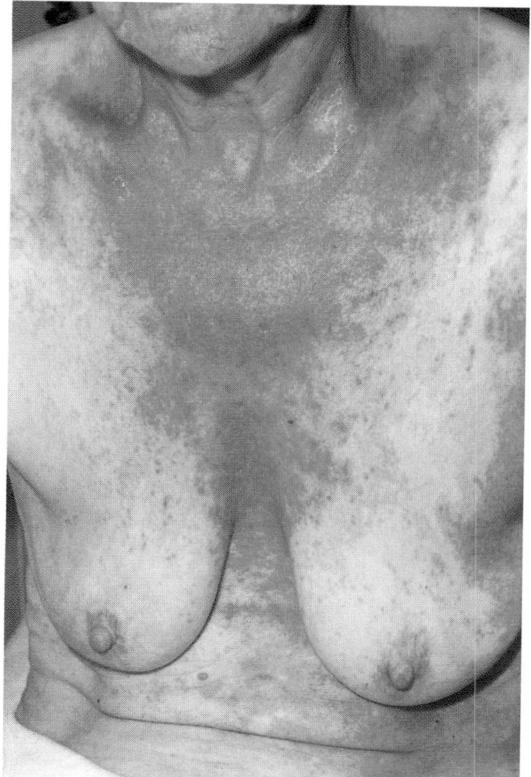

Figure 6.17 Allergic contact dermatitis was induced on the trunk by a phenylbutazone ointment applied topically.

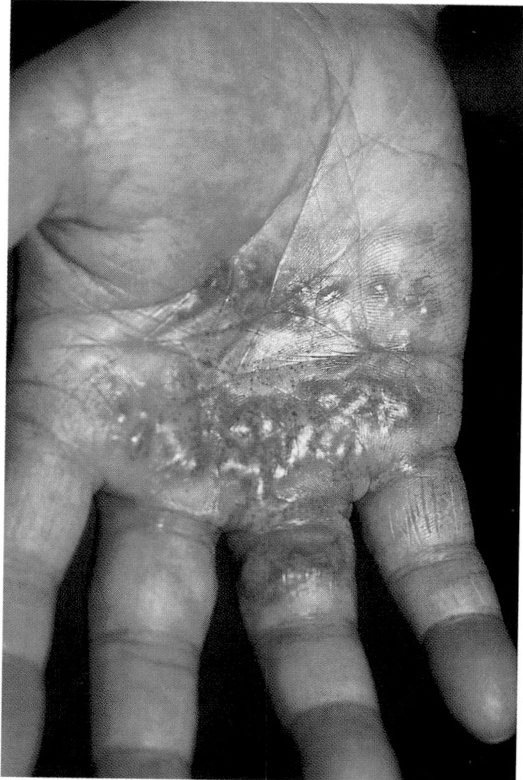

Figure 6.18 The palm can be involved in allergic contact dermatitis by application of medication to other parts of the body or as the site of direct application of a medication capable of inducing allergic reactions. This bullous reaction was due to colophony in a Chinese balsam ointment.

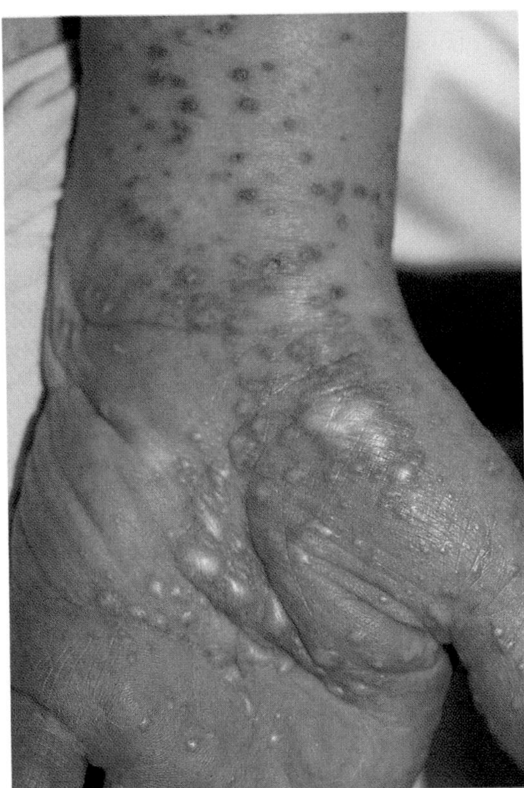

Figure 6.19 These papulovesicular changes of the palm were caused by sulfanilamide.

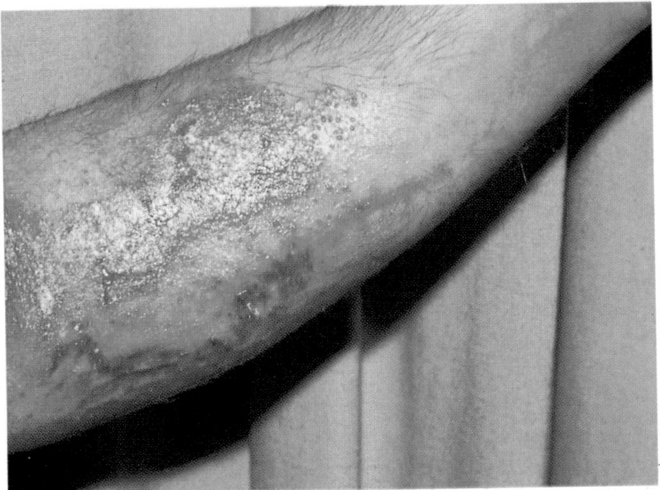

Figure 6.20 This reaction seen on the forearm of a patient with a burn was due to an antiseptic agent, cetrimide, to which the patient had become sensitized and subsequently developed allergic contact dermatitis (Lee and Wang, 1995).

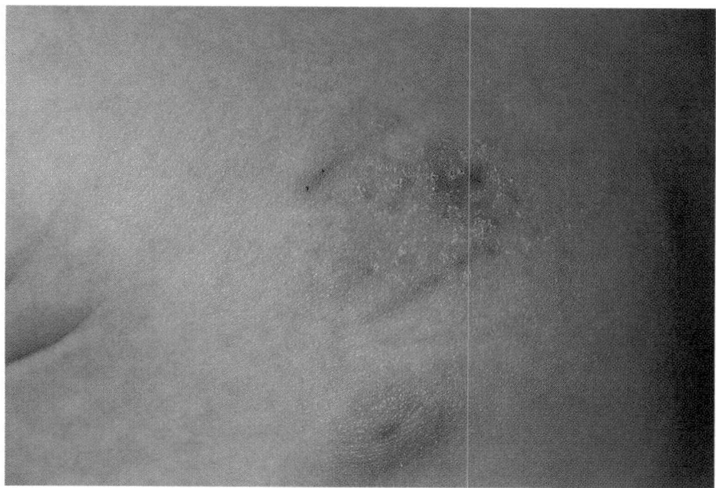

Figure 6.21 Immunizations can sometimes cause unusual cutaneous reactions. The 2-year-old boy seen here developed pruritic nodules on the right side of his chest after immunization with a combined diphtheria–tetanus–polio vaccine. The vaccine had been precipitated with aluminium hydroxide to increase its efficacy. The boy had a strongly positive patch test to 2% aluminium chloride in water (Veien et al, 1986).

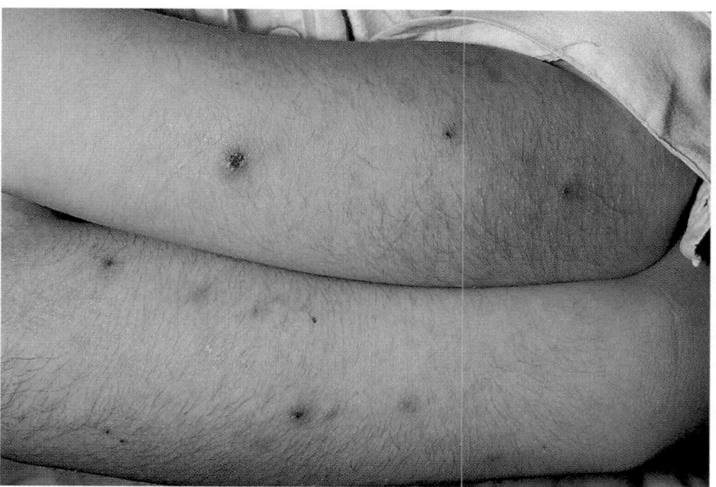

(**a**)

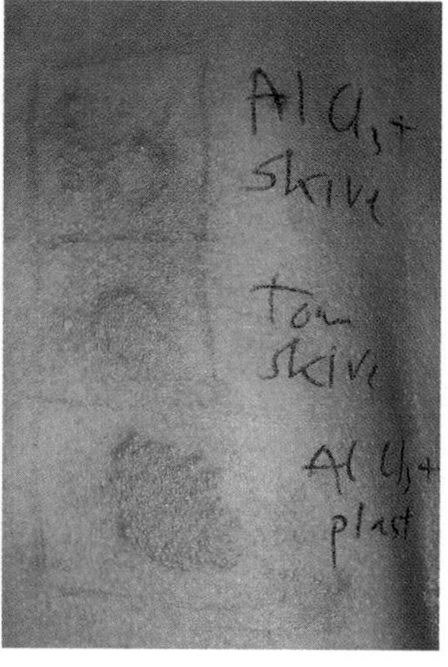

(**b**)

Figure 6.22 (**a**) A 13-year-old boy who suffered from allergic rhinitis from grass pollen was hyposensitized with a vaccine containing aluminium hydroxide. He developed pruritic nodules at the sites of hyposensitization on his forearms. He had positive patch tests to aluminium chloride, to an empty aluminium Finn chamber and to aluminium chloride occluded with plastic (**b**).

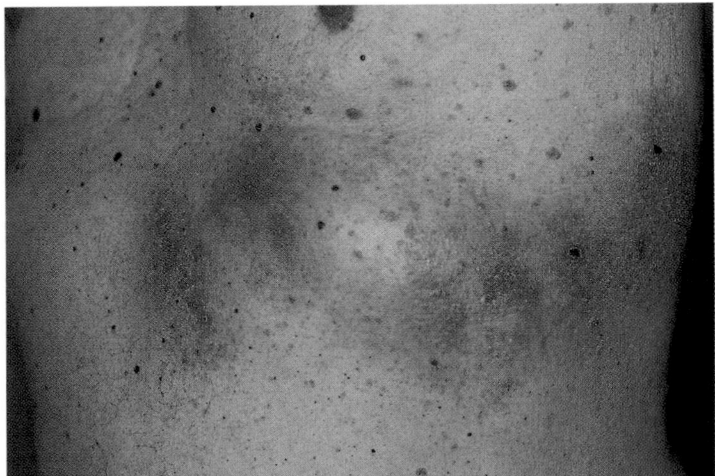

Figure 6.23 This 74-year-old man had allergic contact dermatitis from tea tree oil used to treat herpes zoster. The allergen in tea tree oil has been found to be *d*-limonene (Knight and Hausen, 1994).

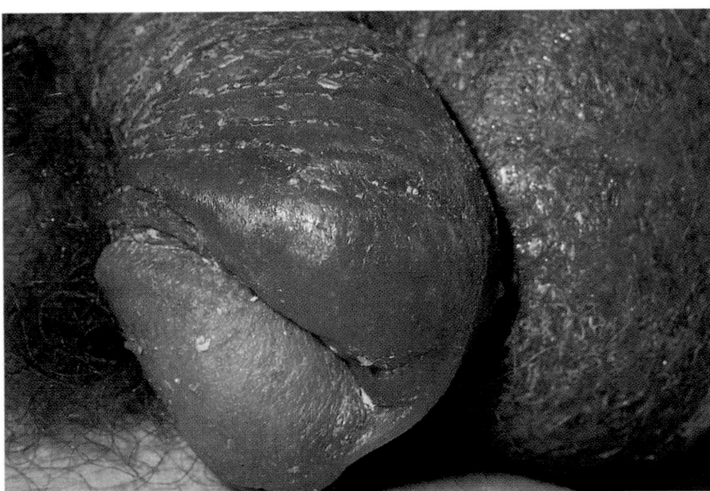

Figure 6.24 Allergic contact dermatitis of the genitalia may be accompanied by a great deal of oedema. This severely oedematous allergic contact dermatitis was due to a cream containing clioquinol, also known as chinoform or Vioform.

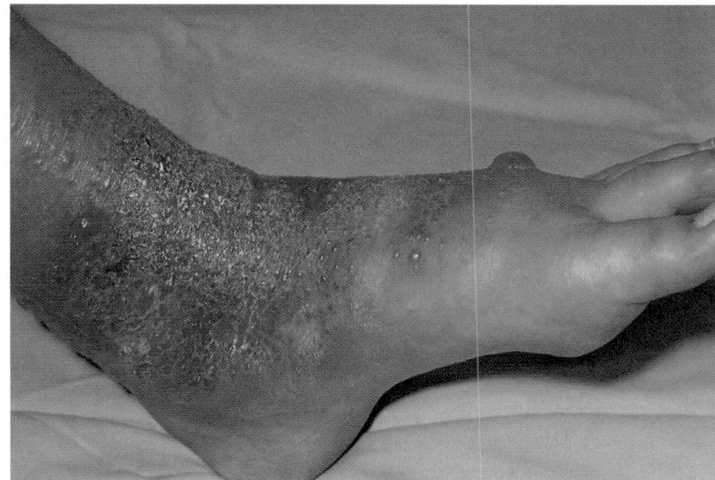

(a)

(b)

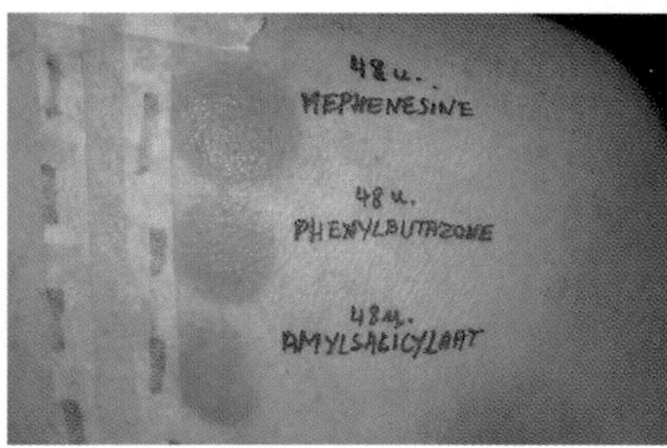

(c)

Figure 6.25 (**a**) This severe contact dermatitis of the left foot was caused by mephenesin and amyl salicylate, applied topically. (**b**) The erythema multiforme-like spread of the eruption; and (**c**) the positive patch test reactions. Compounds that cause vasodilation may enhance the penetration of allergens.

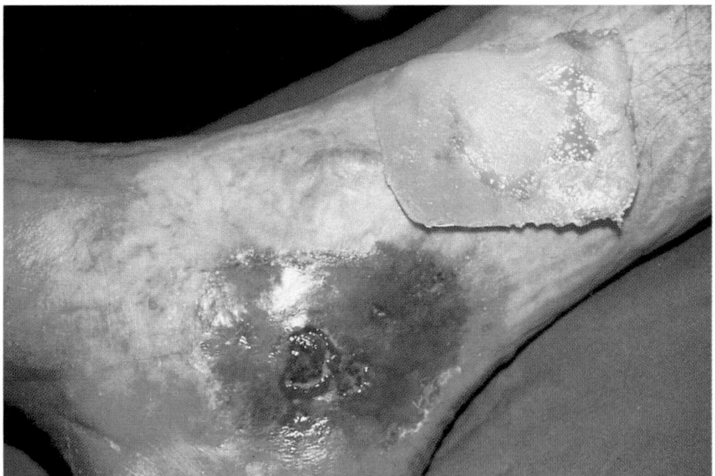
(a)

Figure 6.26 (a) Allergic contact dermatitis can be caused by wound dressings, and in this case the source of allergy was a colophony derivative. (b) Colophony contact dermatitis around a stoma.

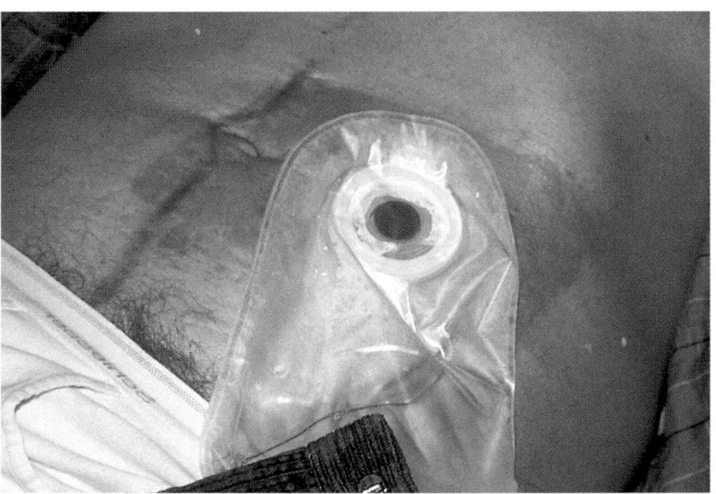
(b)

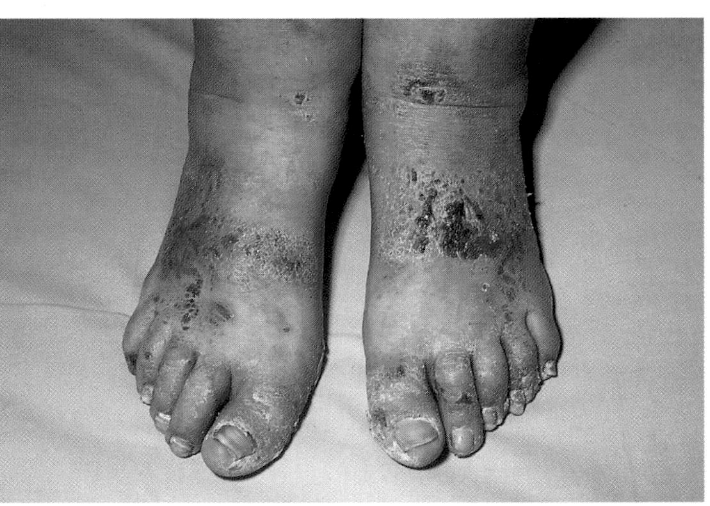

Figure 6.27 Severe allergic contact dermatitis is seen on both feet, and was caused by soaking the feet in formaldehyde to treat hyperhidrosis.

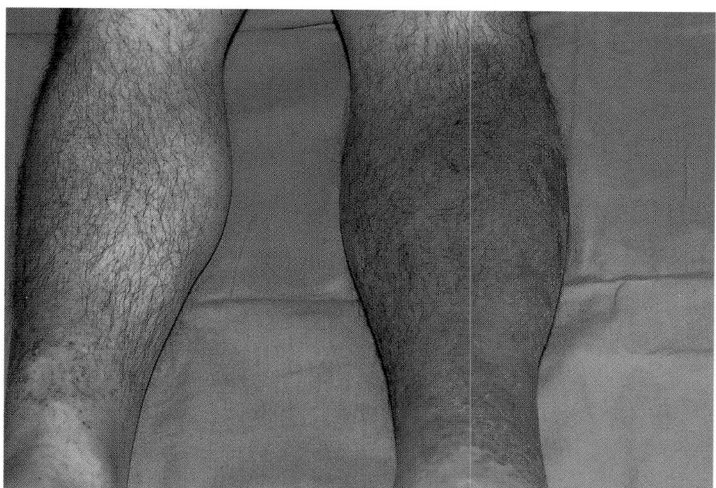
(**a**)

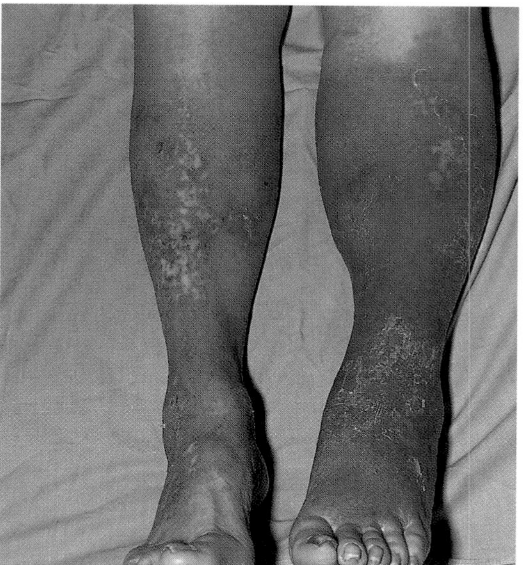
(**b**)

Figure 6.28 (**a**) Contact dermatitis frequently complicates the treatment of stasis dermatitis. Multiple sensitivities to topical pharmaceutical ingredients led to an id-like spread of contact dermatitis to the opposite leg. (**b**) An important differential diagnosis is erysipelas.

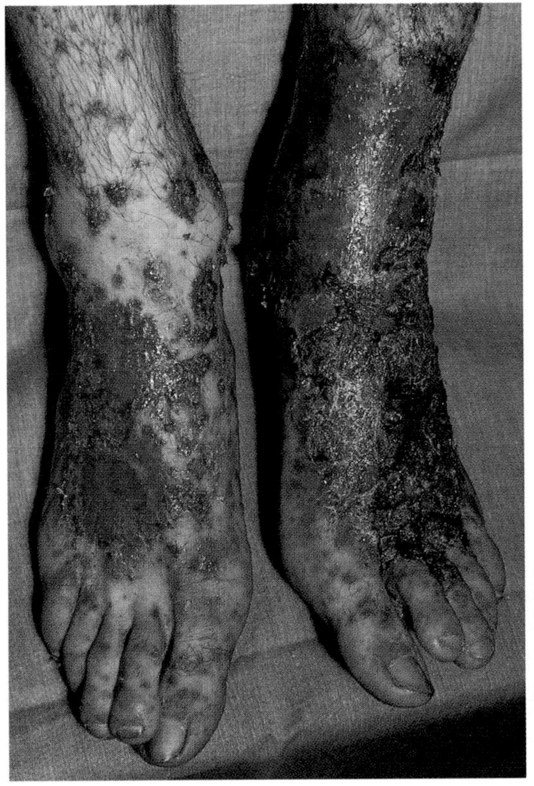

(**a**)

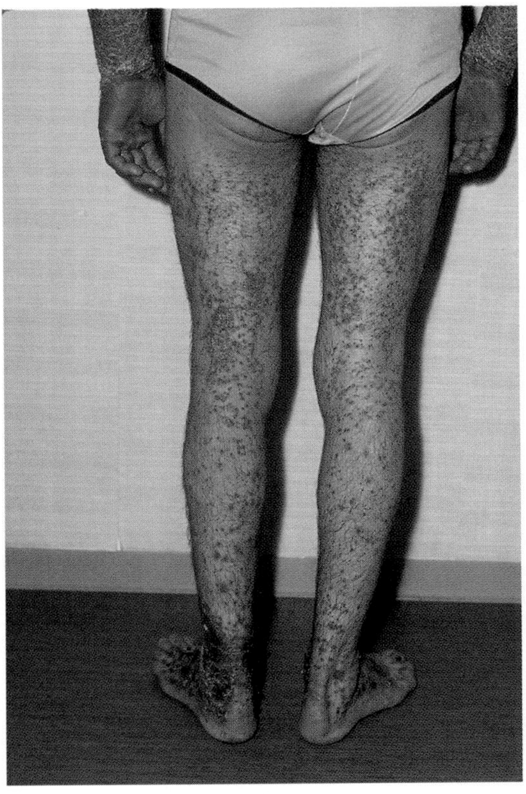

(**b**)

(**c**)

Figure 6.29 Purpuric and vasculitic allergic contact dermatitis due to topically applied sulfanilamide cream. (**a**) The original site of application was the dorsum of the feet. (**b**) Secondary lesions (an id-like spread) occurred. (**c**) This illustrates the extent to which the id-like reaction can spread, since no medication was applied to the arms or chest.

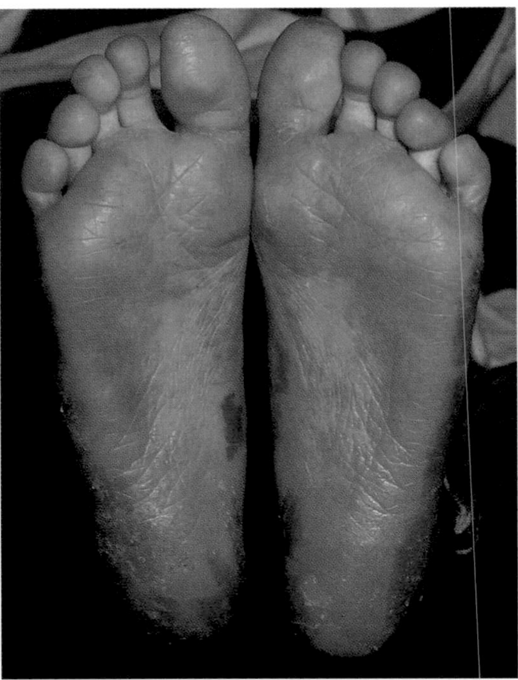

Figure 6.30 Physicians do not have a high index of suspicion that corticosteroids are part of the cause of contact dermatitis, since this class of pharmacological agent is most commonly used for the treatment of allergic reactions. It is necessary to overcome this bias and consider corticosteroids to be as suspect as any other contactants, as in this case of an atopic 6-year-old boy, who developed shoe dermatitis due to mercaptobenzothiazole, complicated by allergic contact dermatitis to triamcinolone acetonide.

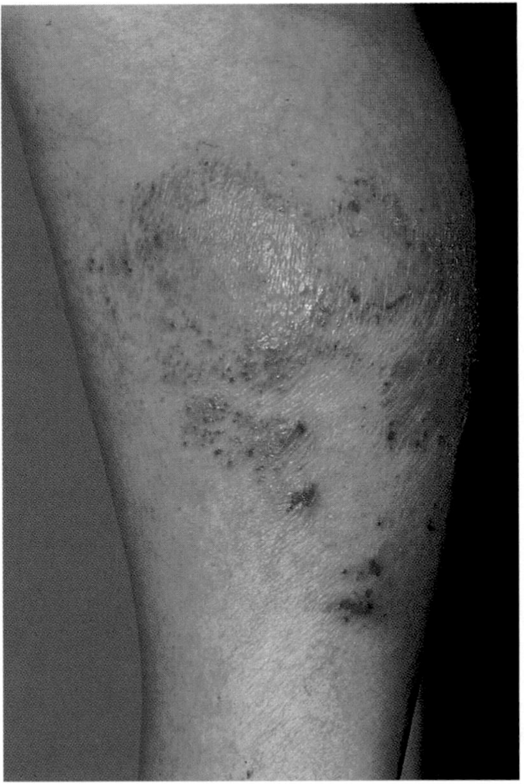

Figure 6.31 In this case, corticosteroid sensitivity complicated the treatment of stasis dermatitis.

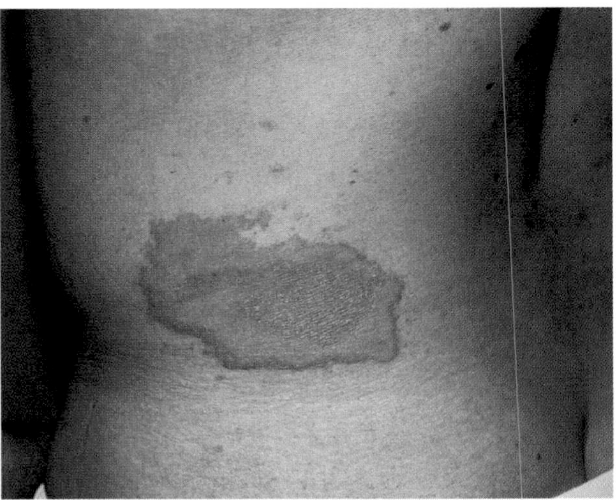

Figure 6.32 A clinical clue to the possible presence of corticosteroid allergy is the 'edge' effect. The pronounced increase in inflammation around the edge of a lesion, as seen here, can lead to the detection of corticosteroid contact dermatitis.

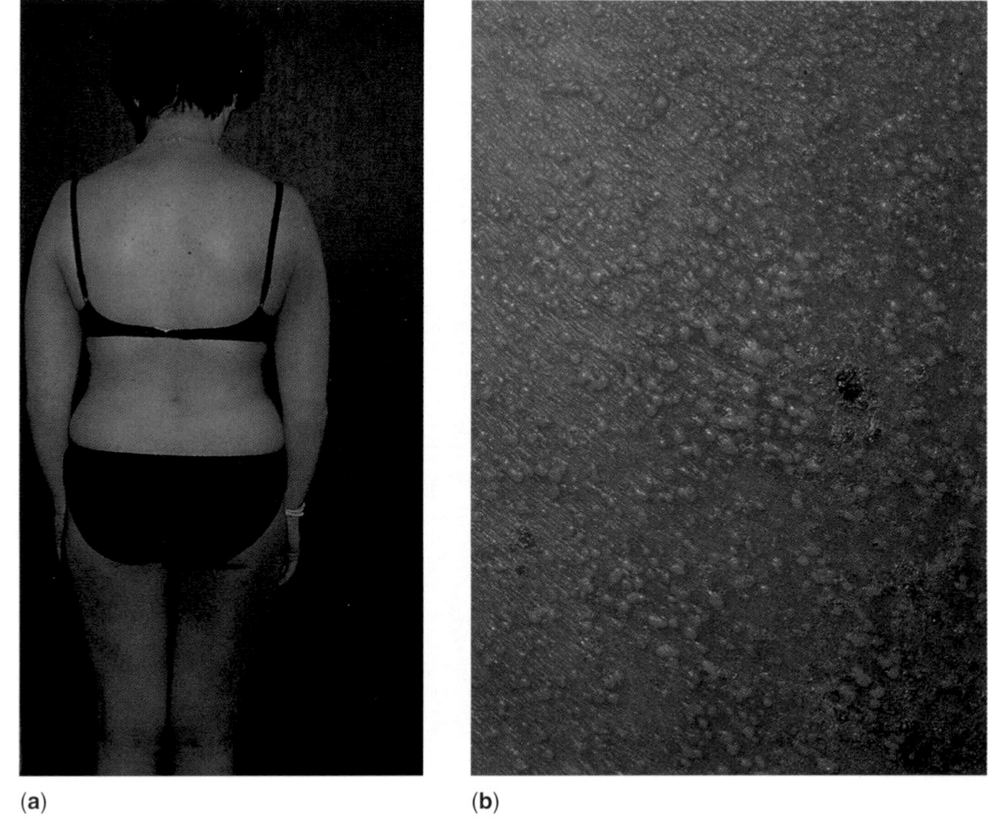

(**a**) (**b**)

Figure 6.33 Systemic reactions to corticosteroids also occur. (**a**) Here the dermatitis involved the armpits and, more strongly, the buttocks – this morphological pattern is known as the 'baboon syndrome' (Andersen et al, 1984); see also Figure 5.12. (**b**) A closer view of the thigh reveals the presence of a pustular eruption. The cause of this reaction was inhalation of a budesonide-containing corticosteroid.

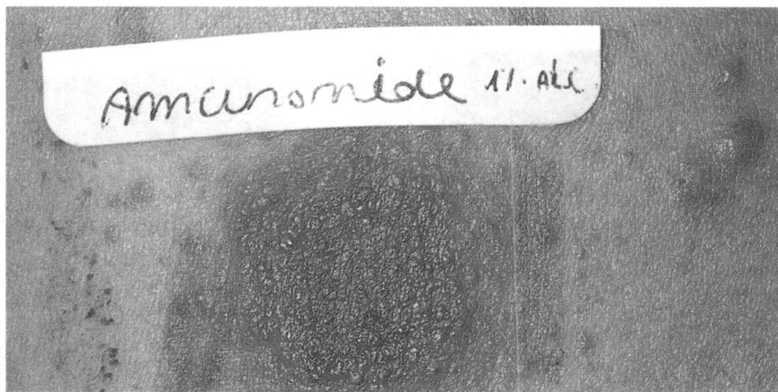

Figure 6.34 Patch test reactions can reveal the strength of an allergic sensitization. A strong reaction to the corticosteroid amcinonide tested using a 1% concentration in ethanol is seen.

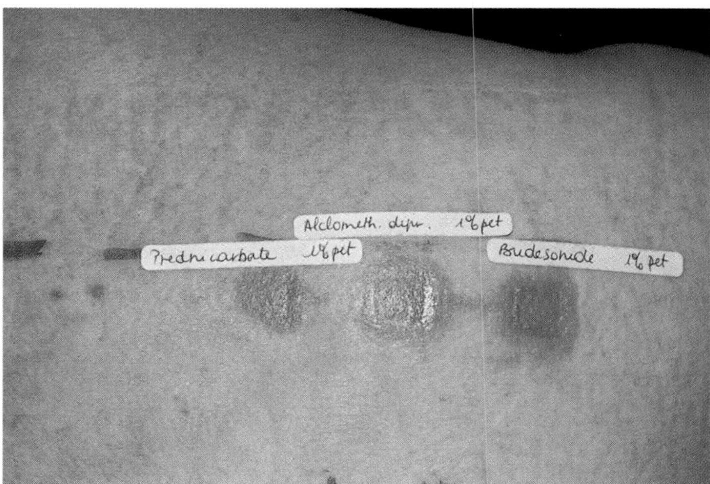

Figure 6.35 It is important to know that cross-reactions occur in corticosteroid-sensitive patients. In this patient cross-sensitivity to budesonide, the *l*-isomer of which has the same molecular configuration as esters such as prednicarbate and alclomethasone dipropionate, could be demonstrated (Lepoittevin et al, 1995).

Medical Devices

The care of sick patients brings into contact with their skin a variety of substances that may be novel and potentially allergenic; examples are given in the box on the following page. It is important to recognize and correctly modify the treatment plan when contact dermatitis occurs. Prolonged wound care and skin contact with occluded materials provides ample opportunity for induction of delayed hypersensitivity. Since the induction of new allergy generally takes 10–14 days with potent allergens, a conceptual framework can be developed as to when contact dermatitis becomes a likely diagnostic consideration. Reactions that develop more rapidly may result from a cross-reaction to preexisting sensitivity or a reaction to an allergen common to both the medical and everyday environment, such as nickel.

Allergens

Hearing aids:	Orthodontic braces:
(Meth)acrylates	Mercaptobenzothiazole
Resorcinol monobenzoate	Nickel
Injection needles	Thiurams
Epoxy resin	Orthopaedic devices:
(Meth)acrylates	Black rubber derivatives
	Prostheses and diethylthiourea

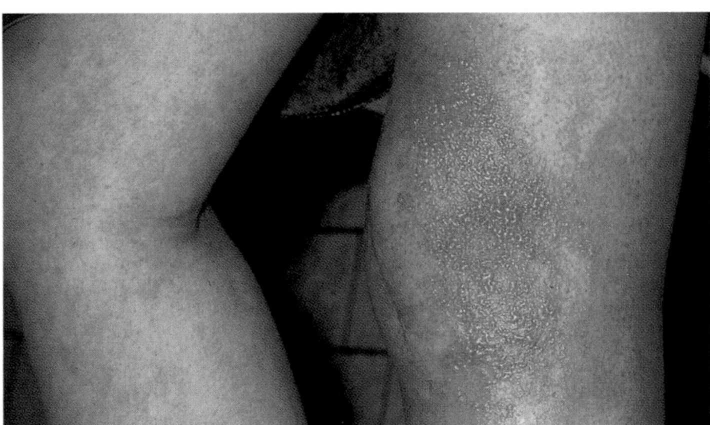

Figure 6.36 Substances applied as part of the normal preparation for medical care can lead to contact dermatitis. Here, allergic contact dermatitis of the knee developed due to benzoin tincture used as a defatting agent before putting on a plaster cast.

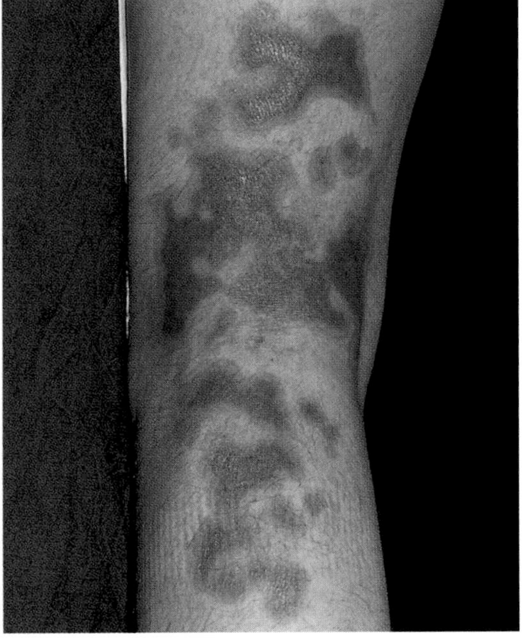

Figure 6.37 Hyperpigmented lesions occurred in the popliteal space following allergic contact dermatitis due to benzoin tincture that had been covered by a plaster cast for three weeks.

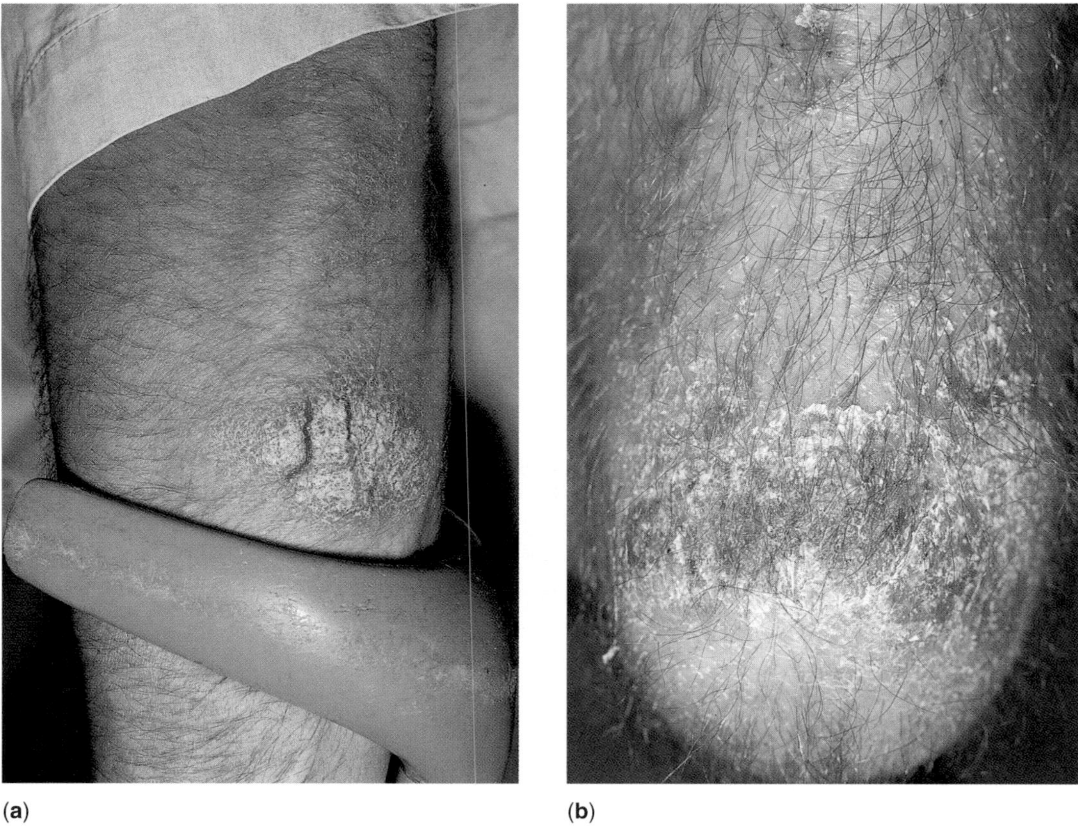

(a) (b)

Figure 6.38 (**a**) This 33-year-old man developed allergic contact dermatitis from acrylates in plastic crutches. He also reacted to his prosthesis (**b**).

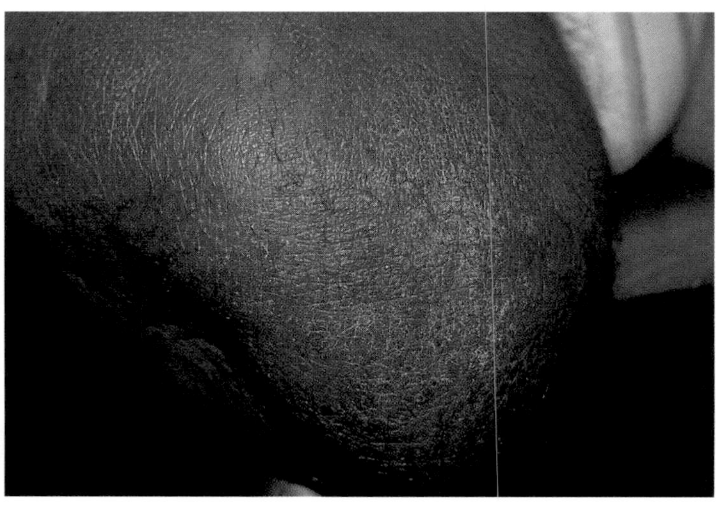

Figure 6.39 Acrylates are not the only source of problems for amputees. Allergic contact dermatitis on the amputation stump seen here was due to *p-tert*-butylphenol–formaldehyde resin in a prosthesis.

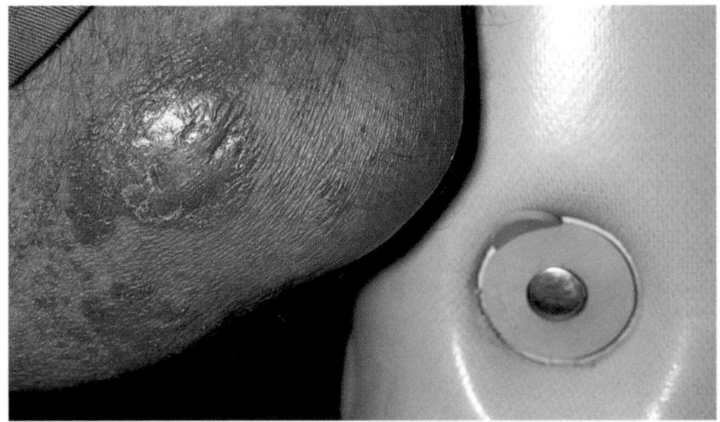

Figure 6.40 This 58-year-old man developed dermatitis under his prosthesis. A metal button in the rubber stopper used to evacuate air from the prosthesis was in contact with the skin. He had a positive patch test to nickel, and the metal button tested positive for nickel with the dimethyl-glyoxime test (see Figure 6.65) (Rietschel and Fowler, 1995, pp.857–8).

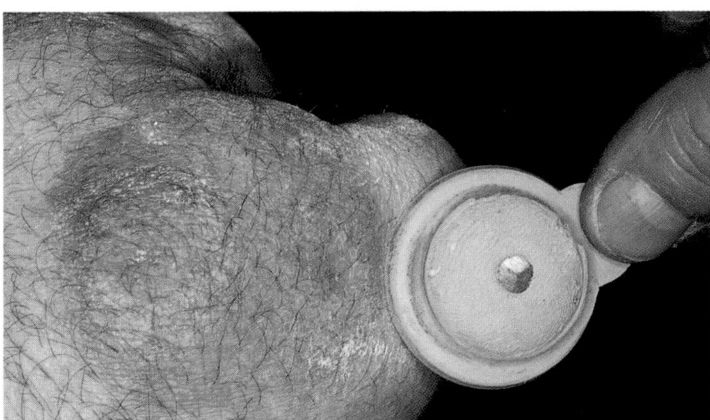

Figure 6.41 The prosthesis worn by this amputee was a suction type of device with a rubber stopper (Conde-Salazar et al, 1988). The allergen was mercaptobenzothiazole.

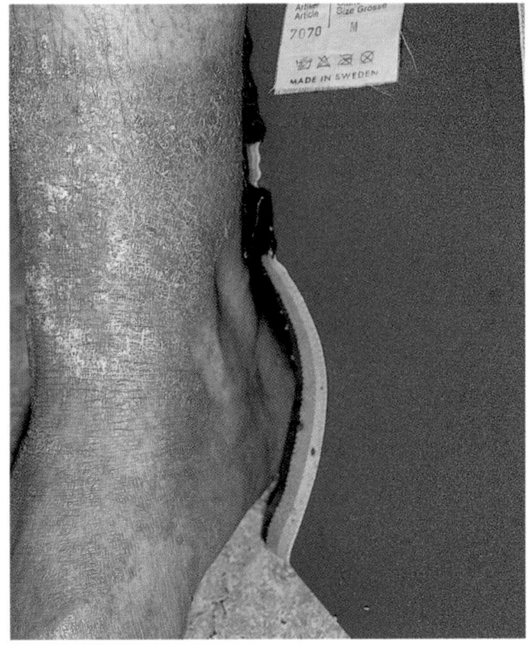

Figure 6.42 A 19-year-old man used a support bandage on his right ankle because of ligament damage. He developed pruritic dermatitis under the support, and he had positive patch tests to the black rubber mix and *p-tert*-phenol–formaldehyde resin from a screening patch test series. The dermatitis cleared when the bandage was discontinued and he was treated with topical corticosteroids.

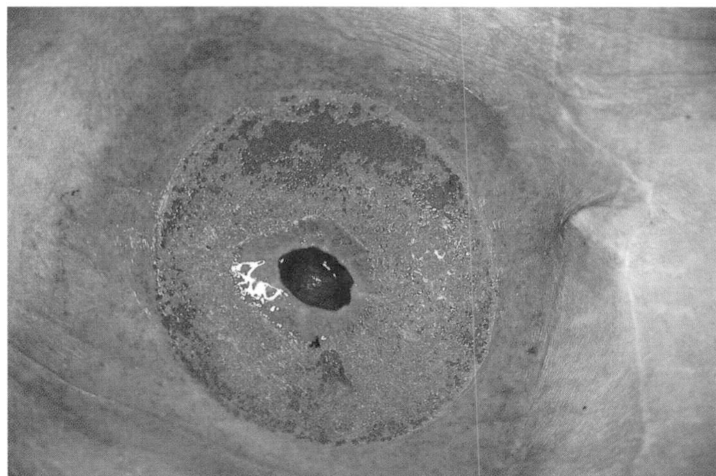

Figure 6.43 A 69-year-old woman developed irritant contact dermatitis around the stoma of a Bricker bladder.

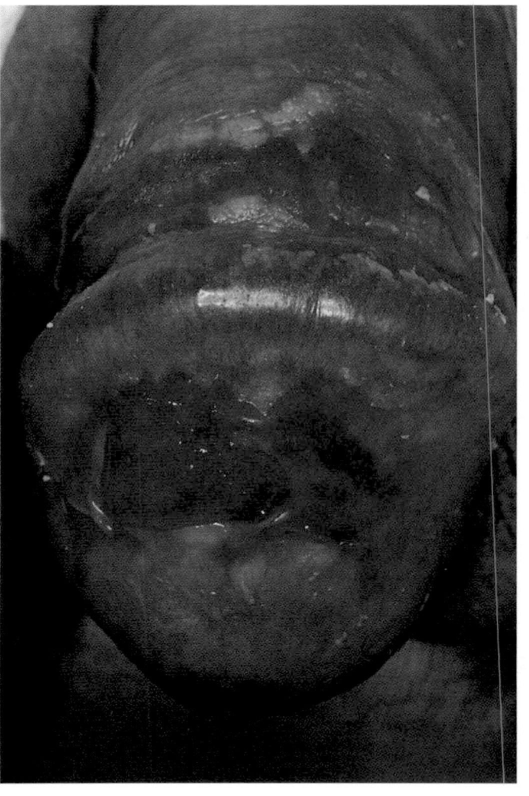

(**a**)

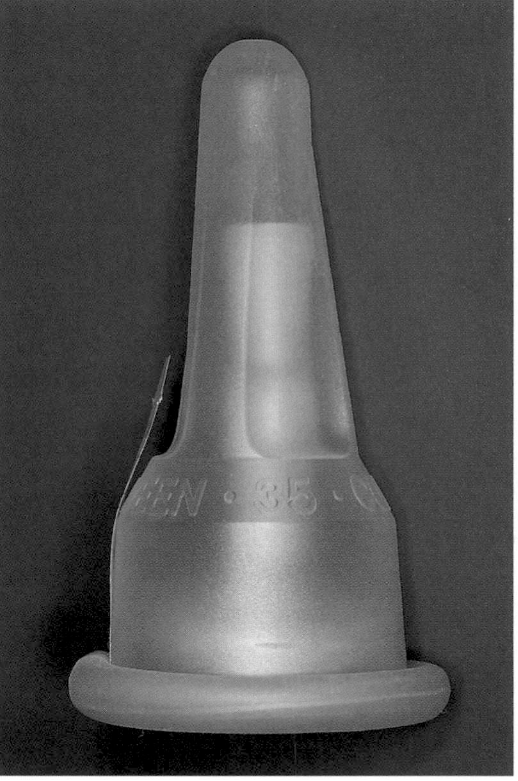

(**b**)

Figure 6.44 (**a**) This 69-year-old man had severe balanitis and dermatitis of his scrotum and penis. (**b**) He had used a rubber urinal condom for several years. Unlike the case of the irritant contact dermatitis shown in Figure 6.43, this patient had a positive patch test to the sheath device. The composition of the rubber could not be determined, but changing to a different brand was curative.

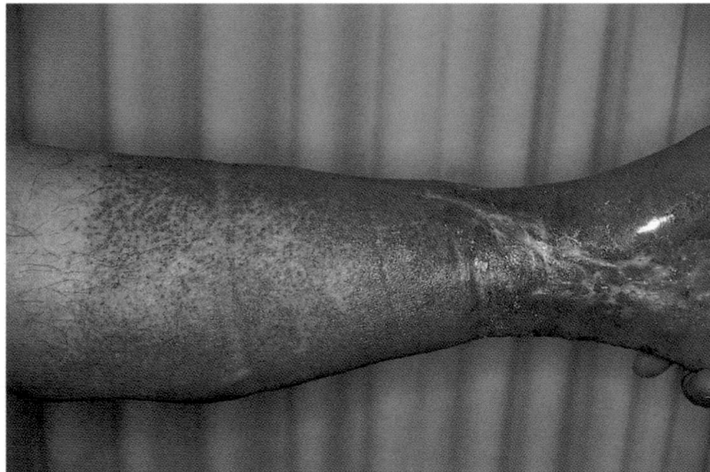

Figure 6.45 This 72-year-old man was treated with Unna boots for his varicose leg ulcer. Pruritic dermatitis developed under this bandage. He had a positive patch test to the paraben mix, and paraben preservatives were indeed used in the bandage.

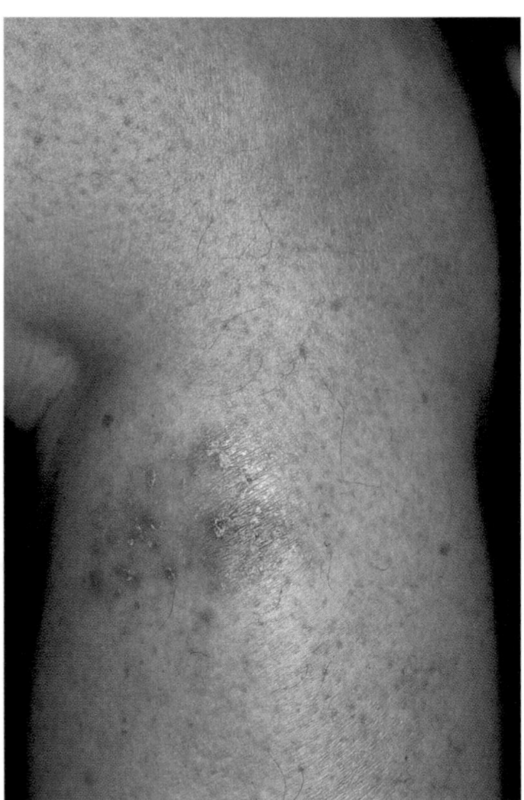

Figure 6.46 A 61-year-old woman developed dermatitis at the site of an electronic stimulator of the peroneus nerve. The device was used to treat foot drop. The allergen was not identified.

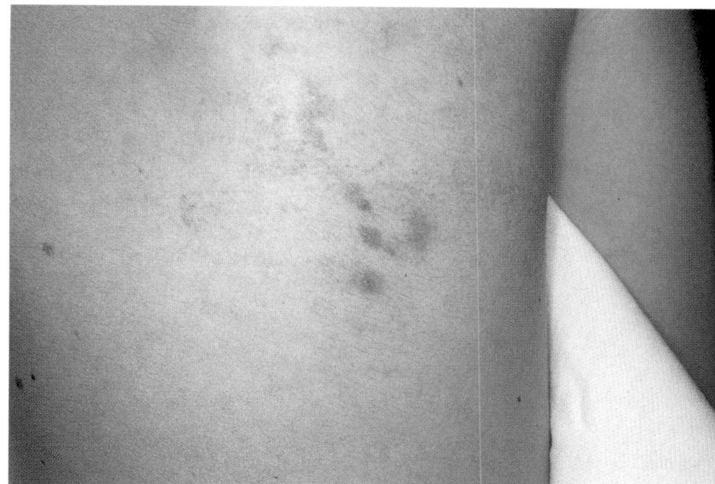

(a)

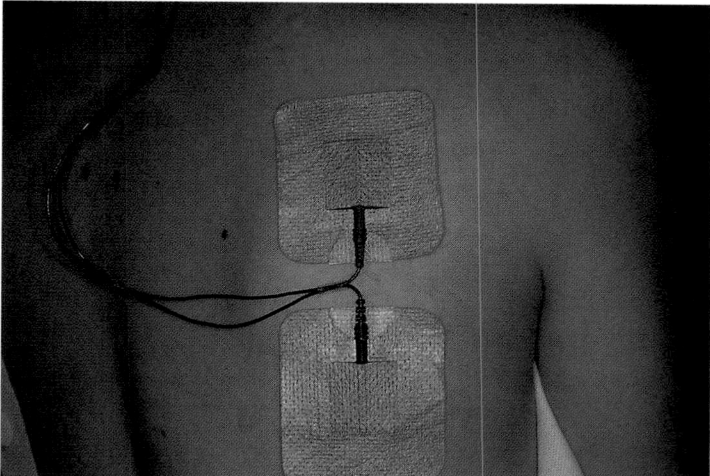

(b)

Figure 6.47 (**a**) Contact dermatitis caused by TENS (transcutaneous electrical nerve stimulation), used by a female patient for three months for a spinal problem. Standard allergy tests and tests for acrylates and methacrylates were negative. (**b**) The way in which TENS is applied. Although tests with patches used by the patient were negative, when an electrical charge was applied to the patches, irritative lesions were observed (Fisher, 1978).

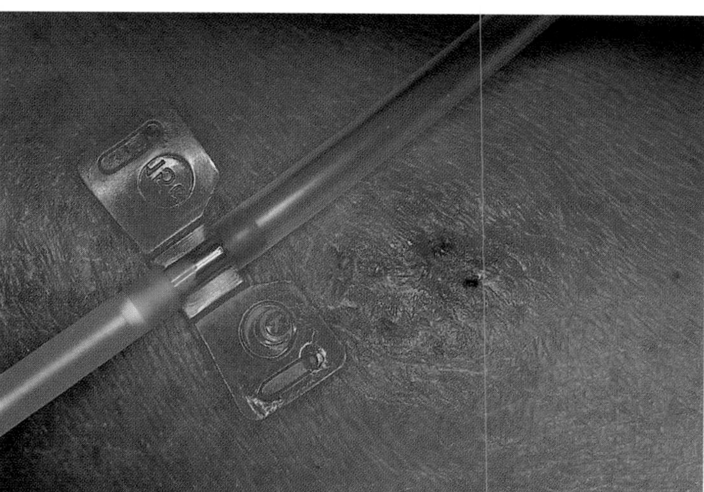

Figure 6.48 Allergic contact dermatitis due to epoxy resin and BisGMA in a female patient undergoing haemodialysis. The allergens were present in the epoxy resin of the 'butterfly' clamp, as confirmed by the manufacturer.

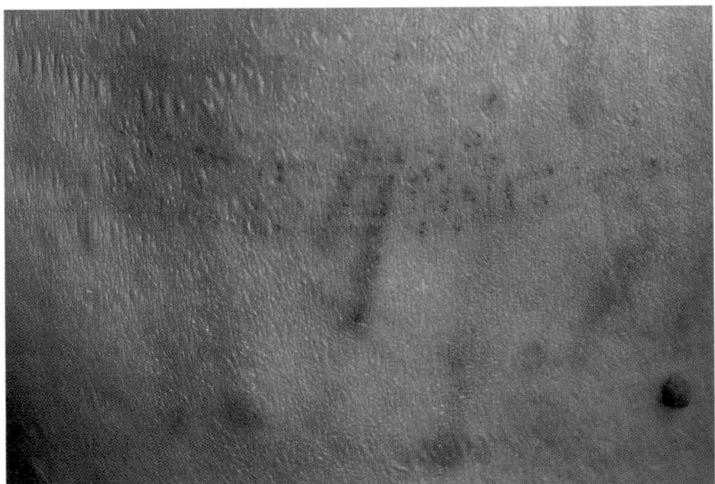

(a)

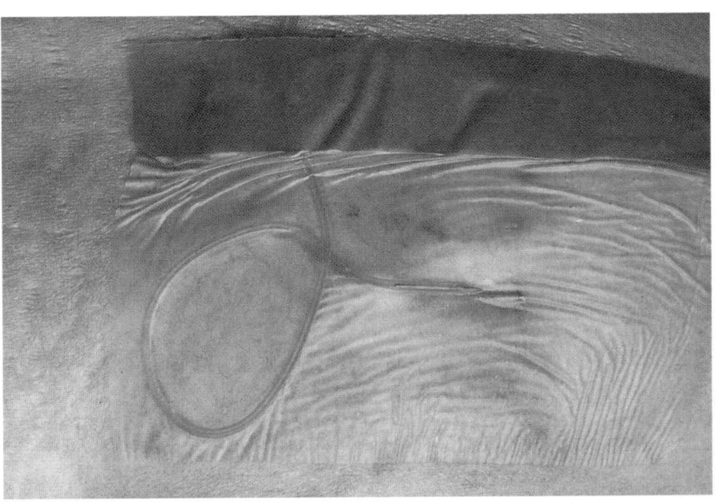

(b)

Figure 6.49 Allergic contact dermatitis due to epoxy resin in a needle linked to an insulin pump. (**b**) The method of needle placement on the skin explains the linear lesions.

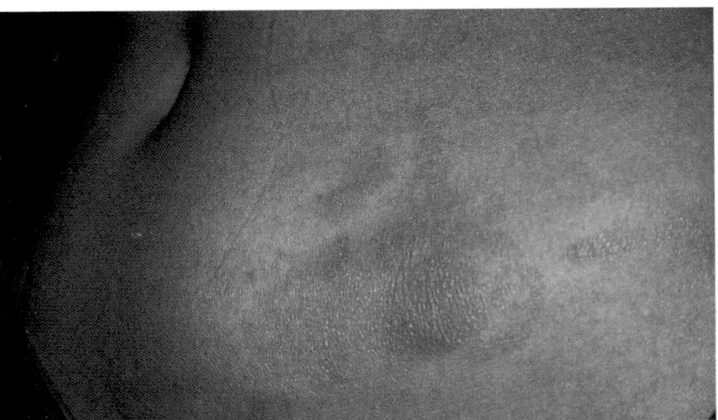

Figure 6.50 Allergic contact dermatitis due to several acrylates in the glue used to fix a needle into the plastic butterfly of an insulin pump infusion set.

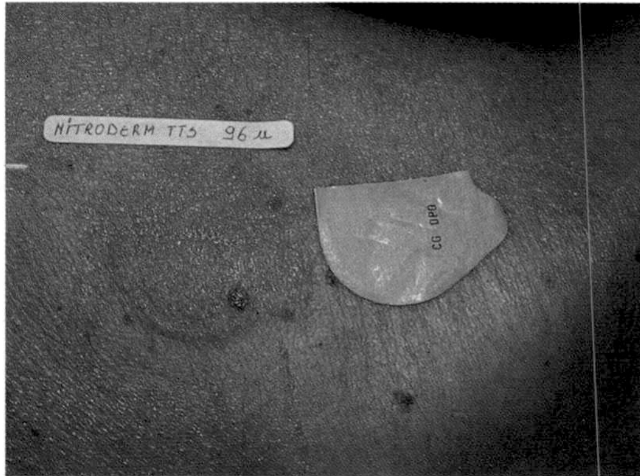

Figure 6.51 Transdermal delivery systems have been associated with contact dermatitis. In this example nitroglycerin was the allergen; a placebo device without the nitroglycerin gave a negative patch test.

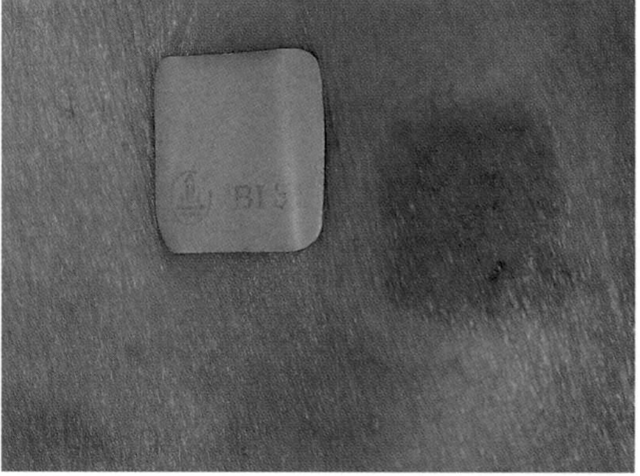

Figure 6.52 Transdermal reactions tend to be shaped like the device. This reaction was to clonidine. While cutaneous reactions to clonidine are not rare in transdermal devices, systemic reactions to oral clonidine in individuals with this skin sensitivity remain extremely rare (Maibach, 1987).

Cosmetics

The overall incidence of skin reactions to cosmetics is difficult to assess. In general, when mild and transient reactions occur, consumers do not report them to the manufacturer, nor do they consult a physician (Dooms-Goossens, 1993). Few epidemiological studies of such adverse effects have been conducted. In 1978, the UK Consumers' Association reported a roughly 10% incidence in the adult population (Consumers' Association, 1979), which is comparable to Dutch (de Groot et al, 1987) and Swedish (Berne et al, 1994) reports of an incidence of 12% of mostly mild adverse cosmetic effects in the general population. As in the Westat Report from the USA (Westat Inc, 1975), irritant reactions were more common than contact allergic reactions, and the products most commonly involved were soaps, deodorants, face and body-care products, shampoos and eye make-up in women, and soaps, aftershave lotions, deodorants and shower products in men.

There are two common causes of contact dermatitis from cosmetics: preservatives and fragrances (Adams and Maibach, 1985). While any ingredient is a potential suspect, the categories of preservatives and perfumes (fragrances) constitute more than half of the causes of contact dermatitis due to cosmetics.

The most commonly used preservatives are the parabens, followed by imidazolidinyl urea, quaternium-15, butylhydroxyanisole, methylchloroisothiazolinone–methylisothiazolinone (Kathon CG), formaldehyde, bronopol, diazolidinyl urea and DMDM hydantoin (Rietschel and Fowler, 1995, p.269). Fragrance allergy is most commonly investigated by patch testing with a fragrance mix of eight substances and the biological balsam of Peru. This combination is thought to detect about 75% of fragrance-sensitive patients (Rietschel and Fowler, 1995, p.449). Hair-care products can also cause contact dermatitis: the main allergens are dyes based on paraphenylenediamine and permanent wave solutions based on glyceryl thioglycolate. The most common cause of contact dermatitis in nail polish is the substance now known as tosylamide–formaldehyde resin, which was formerly known as toluene sulfonamide–formaldehyde resin.

PRESERVATIVES

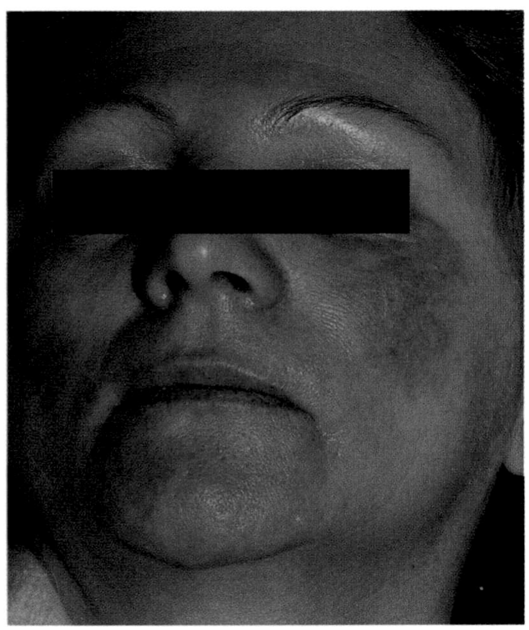

(a)

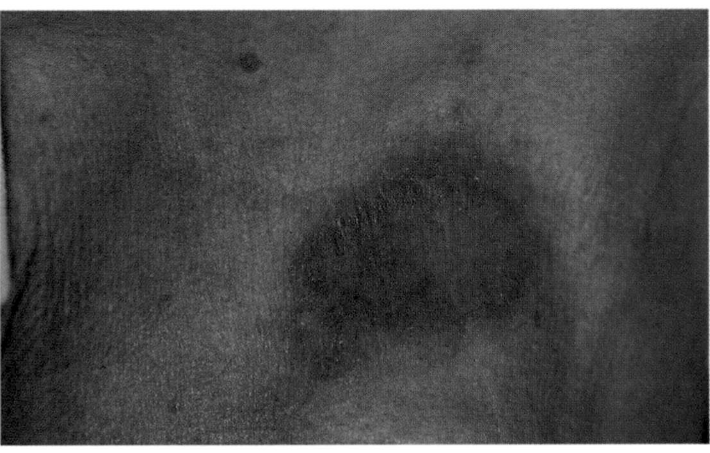

(b)

Figure 6.53 Sharply demarcated oedematous lesions on the cheek (**a**) of a middle-aged woman. (**b**) A similar lesion, in close up, on the neck of another patient. The cause of these reactions was methylchloroisothiazolinone–methylisothiazolinone (Kathon CG, Euxyl K100), a popular preservative found in make-up.

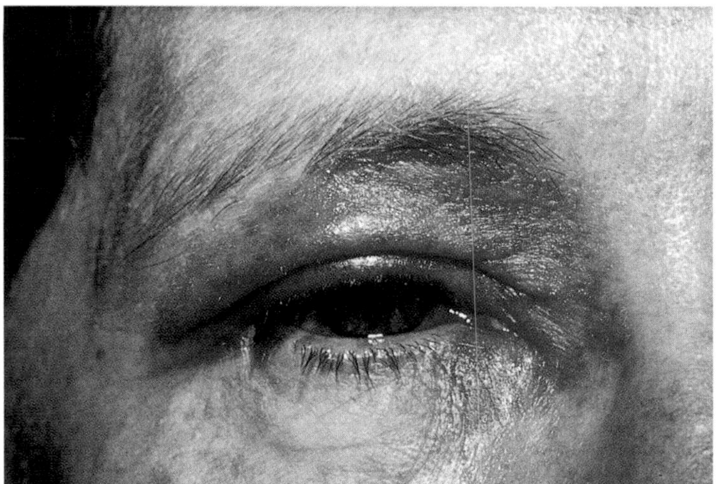

(c)

Figure 6.53 *continued*
(**c**) This same preservative was also found in the eye make-up of this patient. Clinically, a differential diagnosis of benign lymphocytic infiltration had been considered.

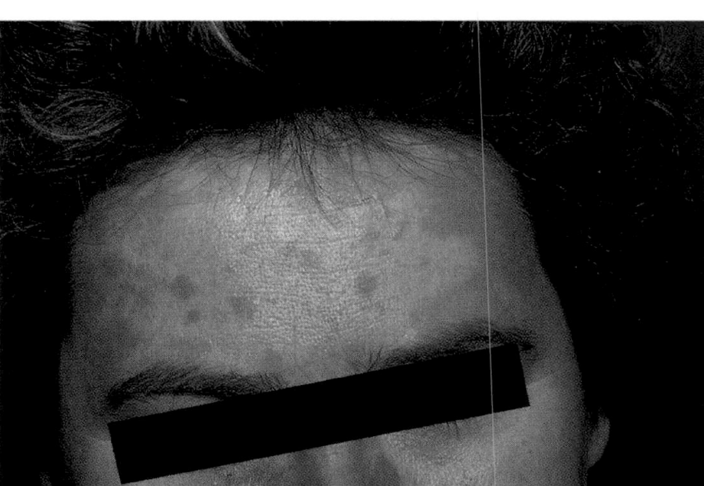

Figure 6.54 This dermatitis of the face was due to a cosmetic that contained the preservative methyldibromoglutaronitrile (i.e. dibromodicyanobutane)–phenoxyethanol (Euxyl K400). In this case, a differential diagnosis of seborrhoeic dermatitis was considered.

PERFUME

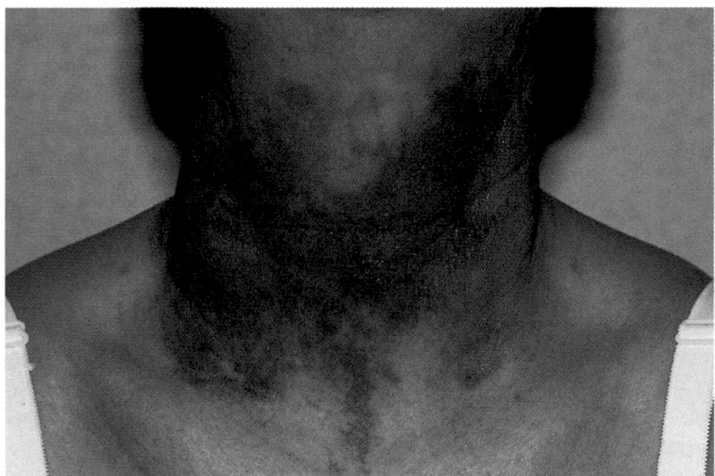

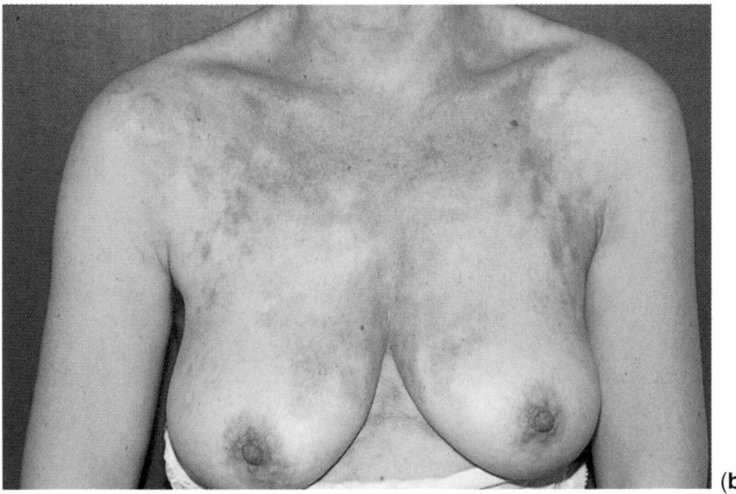

Figure 6.55 (**a**) Allergic contact dermatitis caused by a perfume spray resulted in chronic lesions on this patient's neck. (**b**) A spray perfume was also responsible for the neck and presternal dermatitis seen in this case.

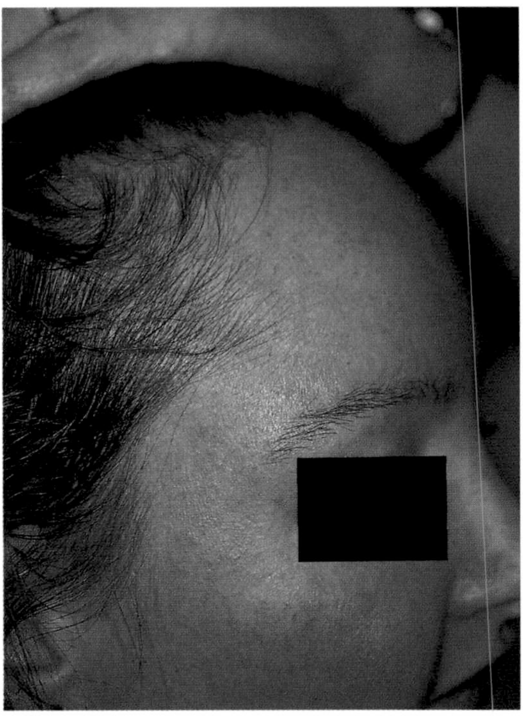

Figure 6.56 This facial dermatitis mimicked mild sunburn. The cause was traced to a photo-allergic reaction to atranorin. This fragrance chemical is commonly found in perfume with a woody scent, and is a component of oak moss (Thune et al, 1982).

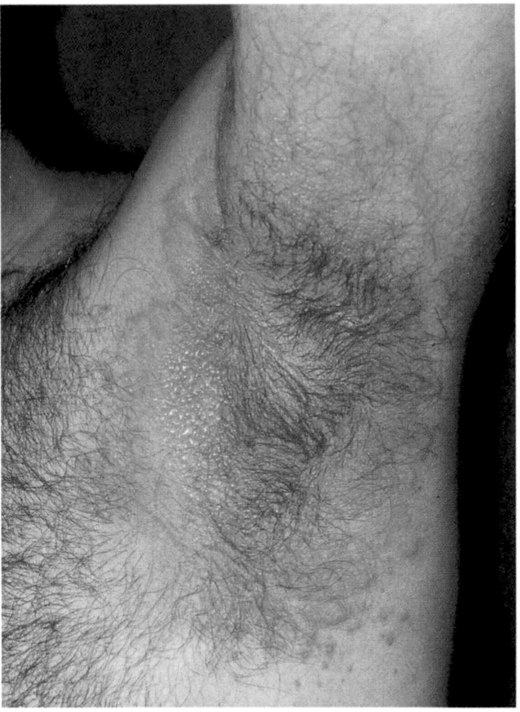

Figure 6.57 Seborrhoeic dermatitis of the axillae was complicated by allergic contact dermatitis to a musk deodorant. The patch test reaction to a 1% musk mix in petrolatum was positive.

VEHICLE INGREDIENTS

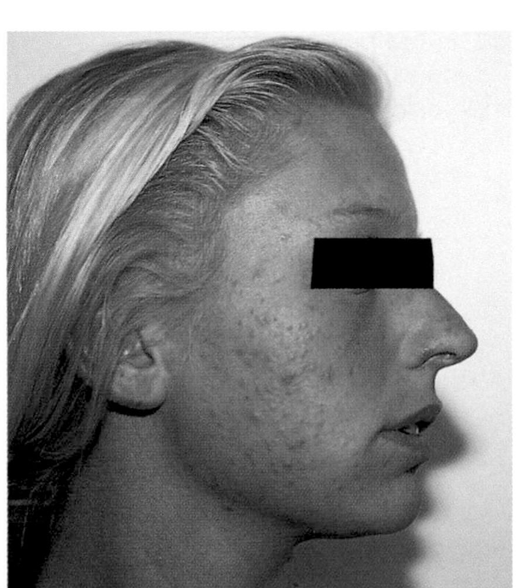

Figure 6.58 This case illustrates how seemingly innocuous ingredients present in cosmetics can sometimes be the source of problems. The dermatitis was follicular and acneiform, and was due to a cosmetic cream that contained maleated soybean oil, which proved to be the allergen.

HAIR-CARE PRODUCTS

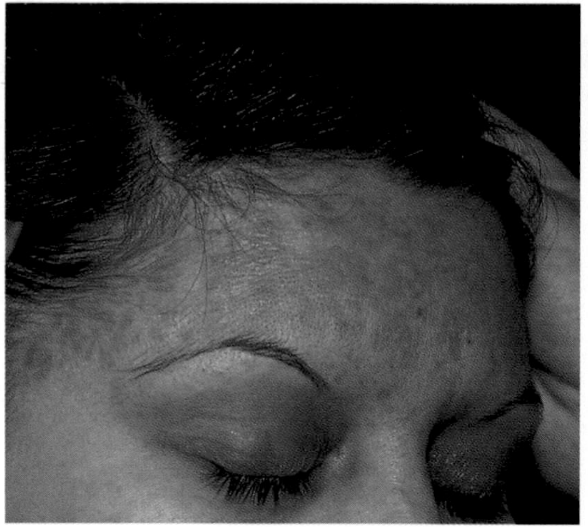

(**a**)

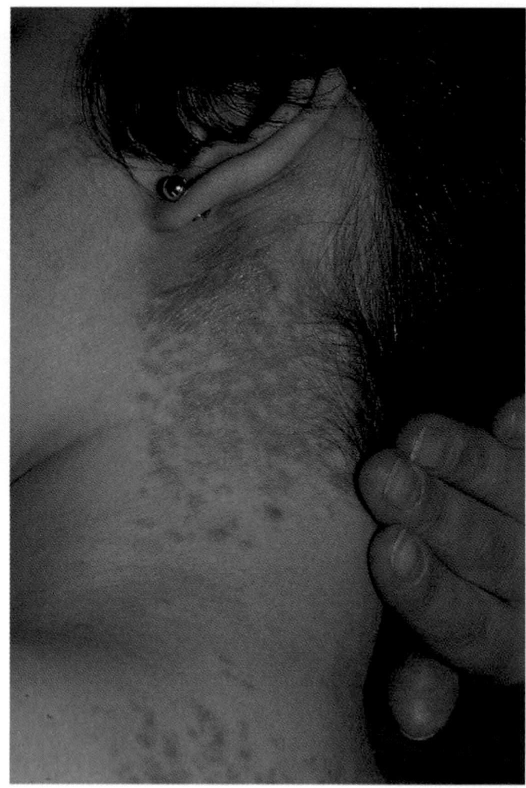

(**b**)

Figure 6.59 This reaction was due to paraphenylenediamine allergy from a hair dye. The eruption is typically more pronounced on the skin surrounding the scalp rather than on the scalp itself. (**a**) The face; (**b**) the post-auricular area.

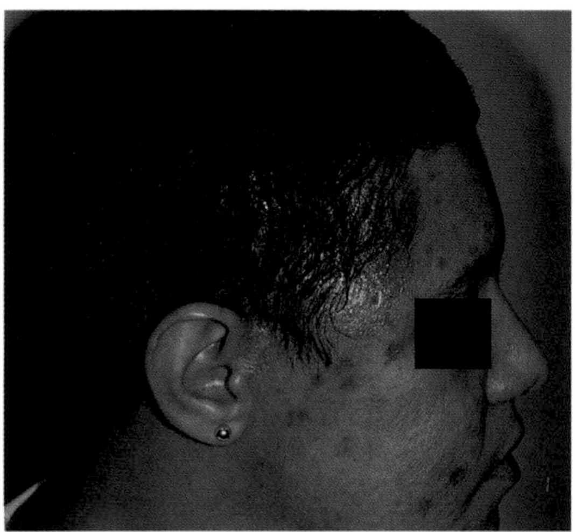

Figure 6.60 In this paraphenylenediamine reaction, scalp involvement was seen in the frontoparietal region.

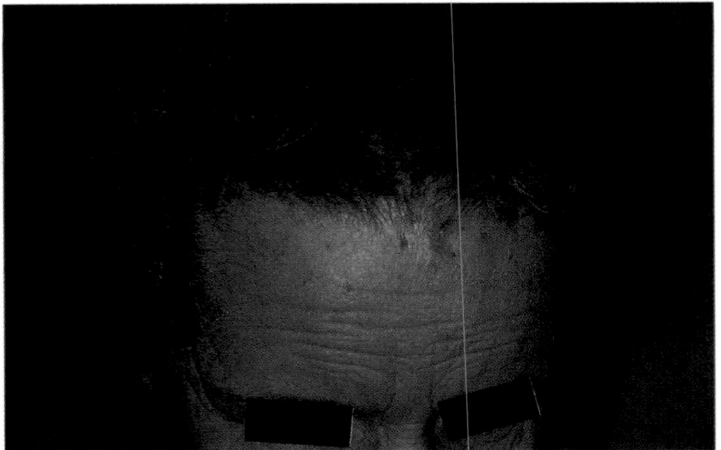

(a)

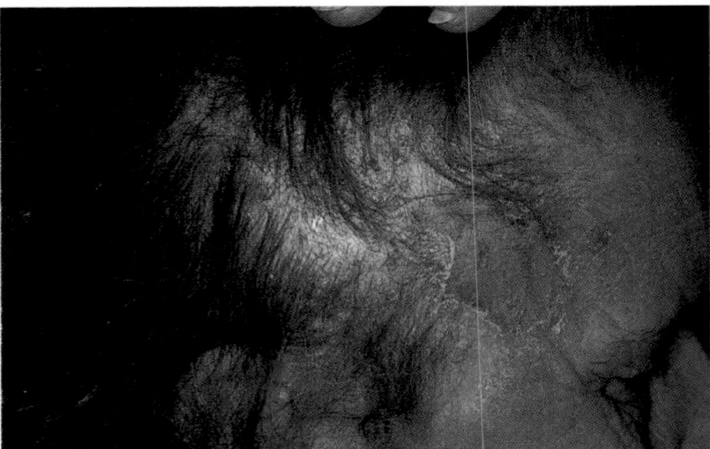

(b)

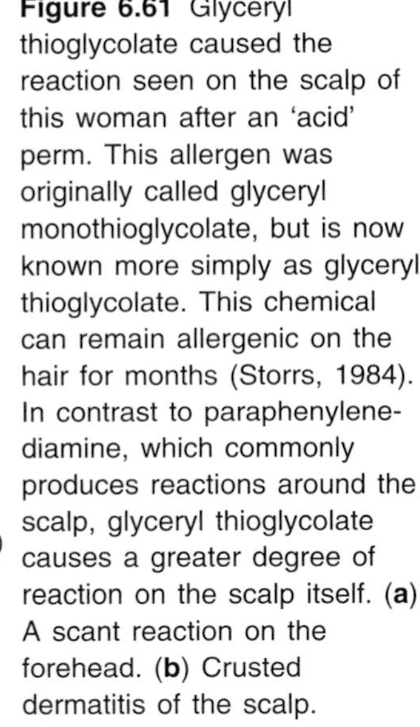

Figure 6.61 Glyceryl thioglycolate caused the reaction seen on the scalp of this woman after an 'acid' perm. This allergen was originally called glyceryl monothioglycolate, but is now known more simply as glyceryl thioglycolate. This chemical can remain allergenic on the hair for months (Storrs, 1984). In contrast to paraphenylene-diamine, which commonly produces reactions around the scalp, glyceryl thioglycolate causes a greater degree of reaction on the scalp itself. (**a**) A scant reaction on the forehead. (**b**) Crusted dermatitis of the scalp.

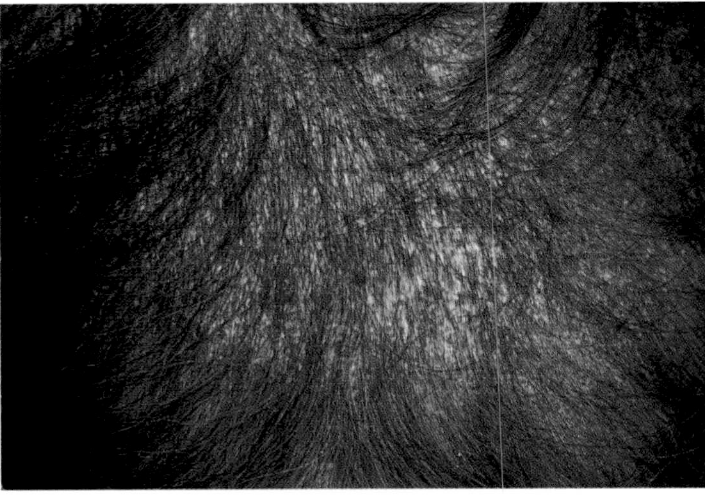

Figure 6.62 Irritant contact dermatitis of the scalp is seen in this patient who presented with tinea amiantacea accompanied by hair loss. However, this dermatitis was induced by a setting lotion containing too much of a quaternary ammonium compound.

Metals

Standard screening series of allergens include tests for nickel, chromate and cobalt. These are the most commonly tested and most commonly identified sources of allergic contact dermatitis among the metals. However, when other metals are tested, the frequency of positive reactions can often be found to be similar to that of some of the metals used in screening series. Gold (Fowler 1987) and palladium (Camasara et al, 1991) are examples of metals that when used for testing produce frequent positive reactions. Unlike the screening metals, the relevance of these noble metal reactions can be difficult to ascertain. The traditional teaching that reactions to jewellery are due to nickel may be correct when based on the magnitude of nickel sensitivity, but it is a flawed teaching based on the many exceptions found when additional metals are tested. Nickel sensitivity has been doubling every 10 years among women, and prevalence rates of 30% of women screened with the standard patch test series have been reported (Romaguera et al, 1988). Ear piercing has been blamed for the high prevalence of nickel sensitivity among women and the low prevalence among men. A study of men in the Swedish army found that men who had pierced ears had a higher prevalence of nickel allergy, which suggests that the difference between the sexes as to rates of nickel sensitivity can be explained by cultural rather than biological factors (Meijer et al, 1995). The typical distributions of allergic contact dermatitis from nickel and chromate are illustrated below and on the facing page. Common metal allergens are given in the box.

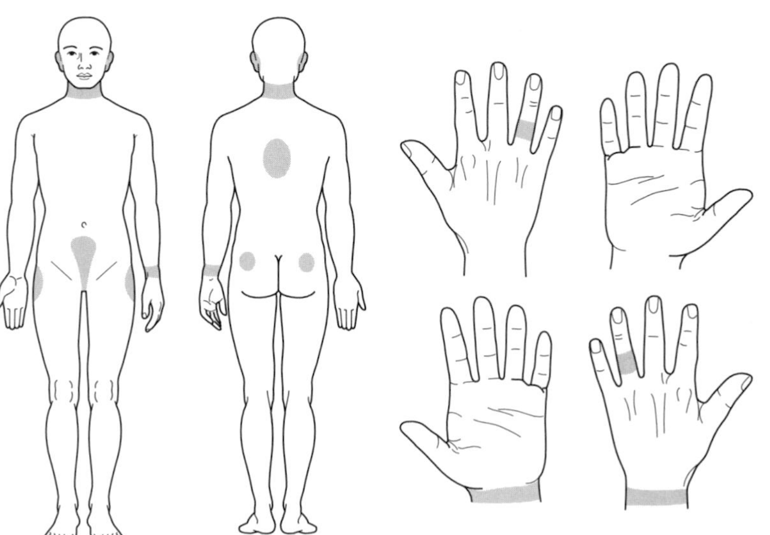

Typical distribution of nickel dermatitis

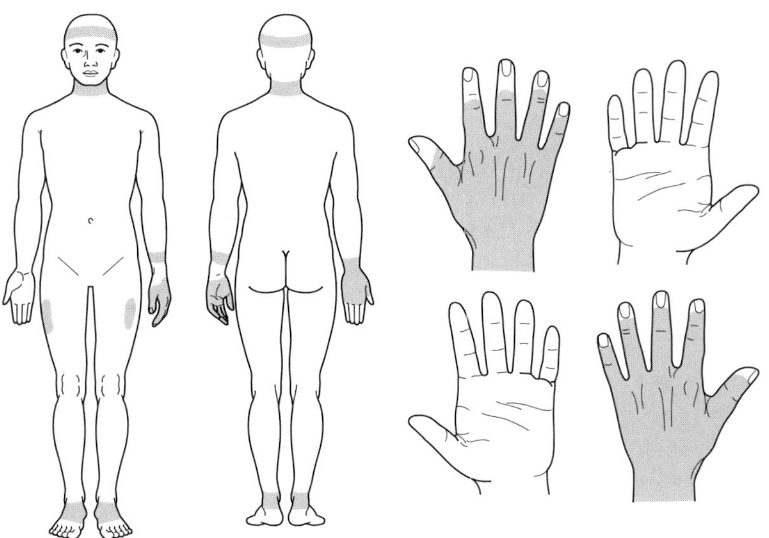

Typical distribution of chromate dermatitis

Allergens	
Chromium salts	Mercury
Cobalt	Nickel
Gold salts	Palladium

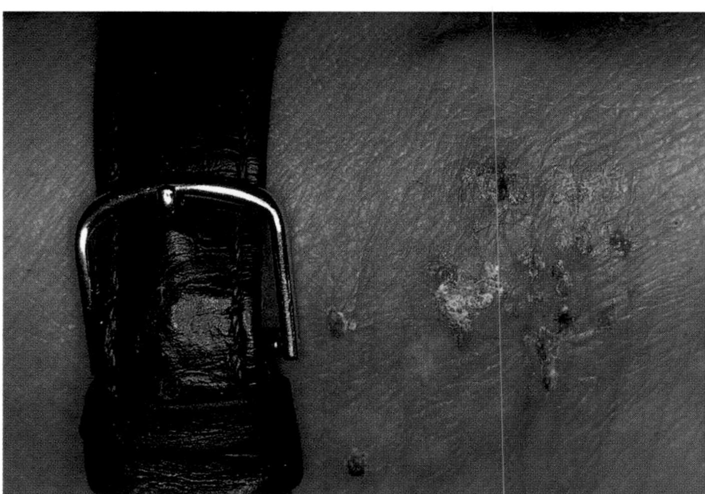

Figure 6.63 This 66-year-old woman developed nickel dermatitis under the metal buckle of her watch-strap.

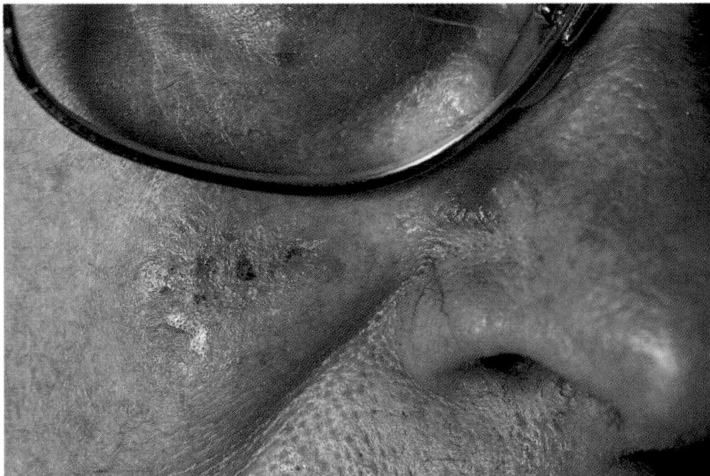

Figure 6.64 A 64-year-old woman had nickel dermatitis under the metal of her spectacle frames. Such frames may have a coating that initially protects the patient against this type of eruption, but over time the coating wears off and the nickel-containing metal comes in contact with the skin, causing dermatitis.

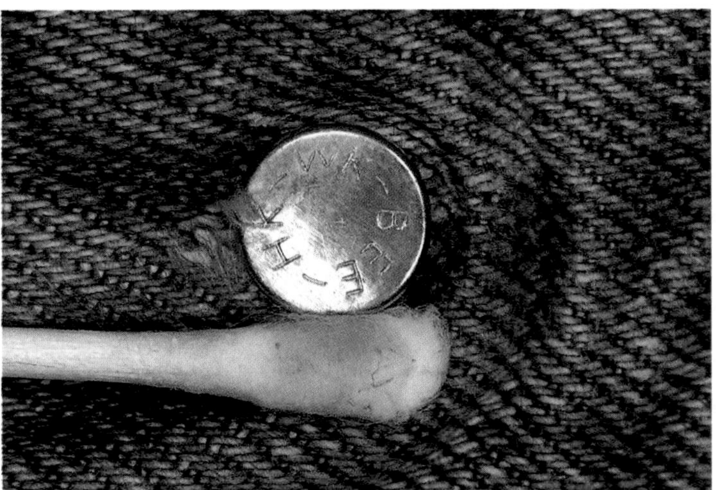

Figure 6.65 The dimethylglyoxime test can identify the presence of nickel in metal objects. The solution turns pink in the presence of nickel, as seen here. The solution is a combination of two components: 1% dimethylglyoxime in alcohol and 10% ammonium hydroxide solution. The test can detect nickel in concentrations as low as 1:10 000 (Rietschel and Fowler, 1995, p.857). The object tested here was a jeans button.

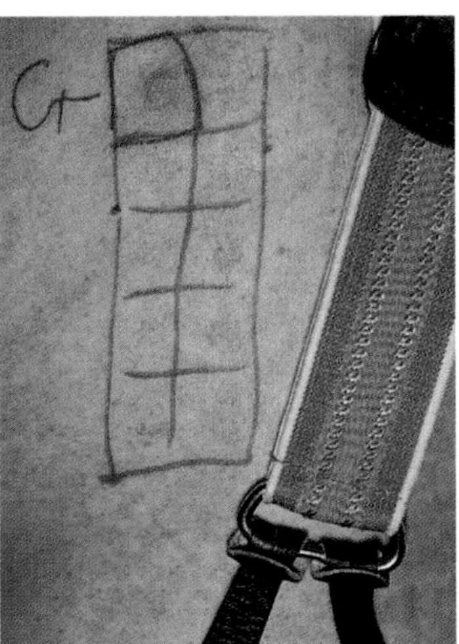

Figure 6.66 This 71-year-old man had dermatitis on his back caused by the leather straps of his braces. The allergen in the leather was identified as potassium dichromate by patch testing.

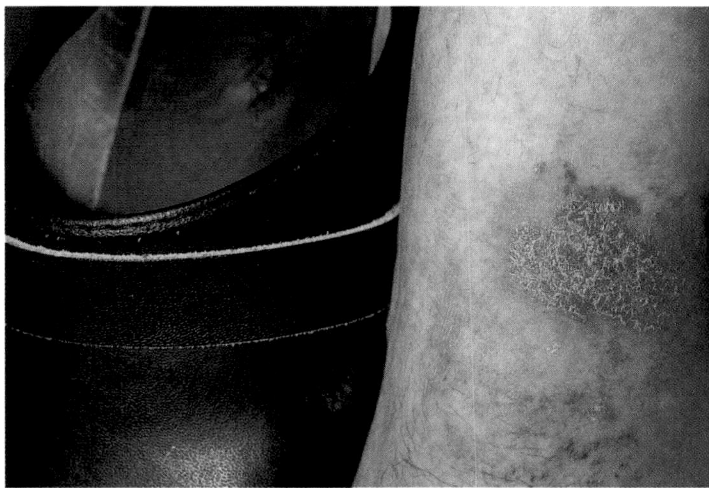

Figure 6.67 Leather is commonly tanned with chromates. This 72-year-old man wore wooden shoes with leather tops. He developed dermatitis from the leather component of his shoes on the dorsal aspects of his feet because of the chromate content of the leather.

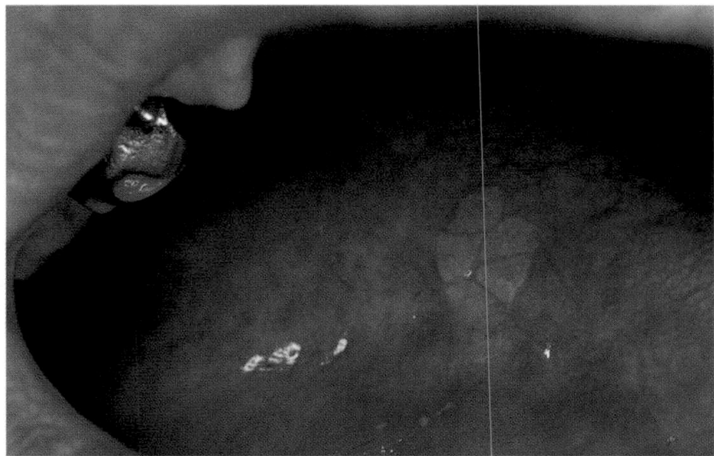

(**a**)

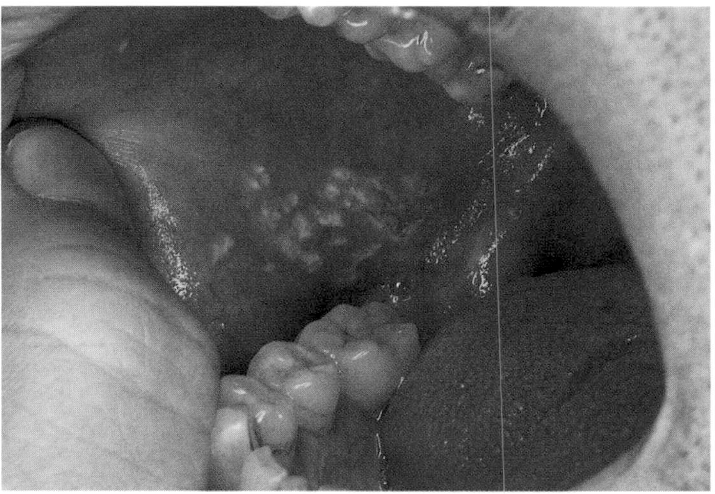

(**b**)

Figure 6.68 Intraoral reactions to dental metals may occur, and when the reaction is in close proximity to the dental metal and a positive patch test is found, removal of the metal is usually curative. (**a**) This 56-year-old woman, with glossitis and soreness of the mouth, was identified as mercury-sensitive by patch testing. The association of non-oral dermatitis with intraoral mercury amalgams and positive patch tests to mercury is more controversial, and removal of the mercury is not always beneficial (Laine et al, 1992). (**b**) Lichen planus should be considered as a differential diagnosis. Typical lichen planus lesions on the mucous membrane are illustrated here.

Plants and Woods

Vegetation varies widely among different geographical areas. The most notorious allergy-causing plant in Europe is the primrose (*Primula obconica*), while in the USA it is poison ivy (*Toxicodendron radicans*). The allergens in the *Toxicodendron* genus are urushiols, which are found in poison ivy, poison oak and poison sumac. The allergen in primrose is primin. There are numerous plants capable of causing contact dermatitis. Some of these plants are also used as foods, and can cause oral symptoms. Other plants are used as medications, and can cause contact dermatitis as an unwanted side-effect.

The frequency of plant dermatitis depends on the local flora and the occupation, lifestyle, including leisure activities, and cutaneous sensitivity of the patient (Benezra et al, 1985).

Tests are performed with the patient-supplied plant, which should be identified by a botanist wherever possible. Different parts of the plant are used. When the suspect plant is not known to be a sensitizer, the tests should also be performed on at least 10 control subjects. However, the most practical method is to use not the plant itself but rather an extract, since extracts are often commercially available all year round. Alcohol-, ether- or acetone-based extracts are preferable to aqueous extracts, which are prone to bacterial contamination, and also degrade and lose their sensitizing capacity rapidly. However, with time and evaporation of the more-volatile solvents, the allergen concentration and its sensitizing and sometimes irritant properties increase. Indeed, as with the plants themselves, irritant or false-positive reactions to extracts are frequent. Moreover, testing has given rise to primary sensitization to plants, woods, or their extracts and oleoresins (Mitchell and Rook, 1979; Benezra et al, 1985; Hausen, 1988).

The most important allergens are given in the box.

Allergens

Alstroemeria
Chrysanthemum and other members of the Asteraceae (Compositae) family containing sesquiterpene lactones[a]
Exotic woods
Garlic
Juniperus species
Laurel
Lichens
Poison ivy, oak and sumac
Primula
Tulip

[a] The sesquiterpene lactone mix as used in the European Standard Patch Test Series is a screening agent for many such plants, as well as for other plant materials containing the same allergens, such as costus and laurel oil.

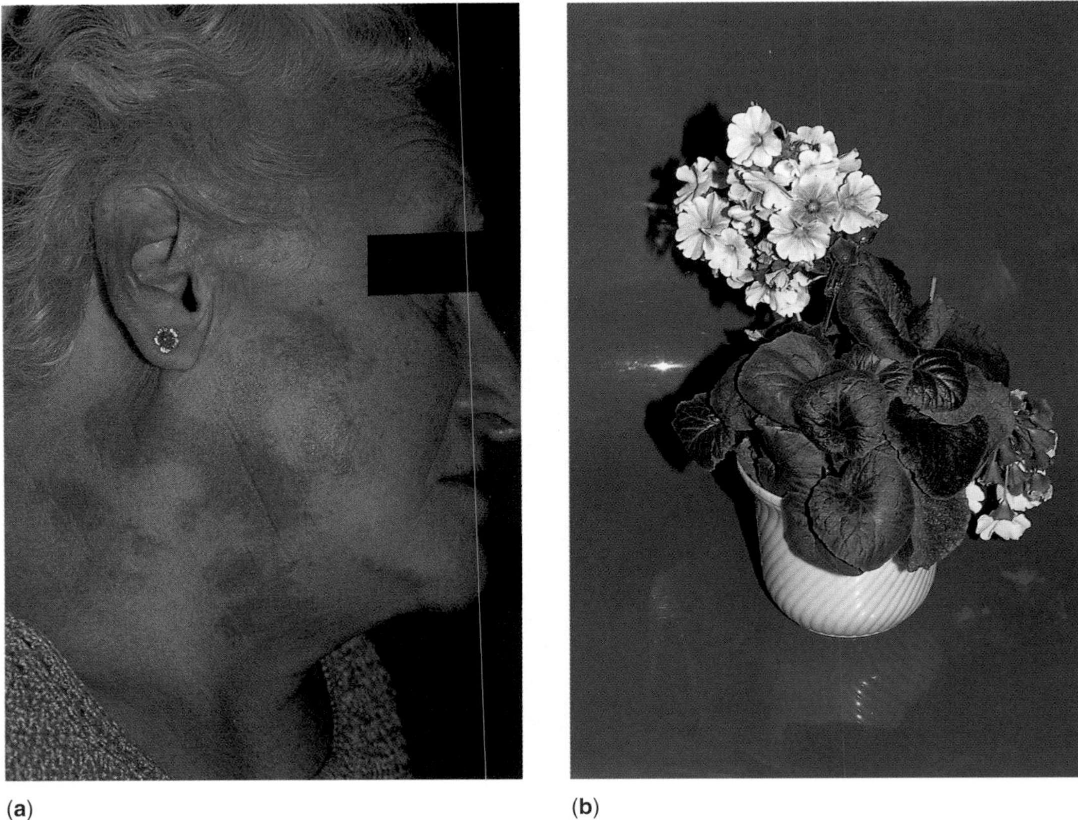

(a) (b)

Figure 6.69 (**a**) A patchy dermatitis may occur with unintentional transfer of allergen to the face. This is an example of ectopic dermatitis due to transfer of the primula allergen by the hands after contact with the plant *Primula obconica* (**b**). Primin is the allergen found in the primrose plant, which is more commonly a problem in Europe than the USA. Rosewood may cross-react with primula (Hjorth et al, 1969).

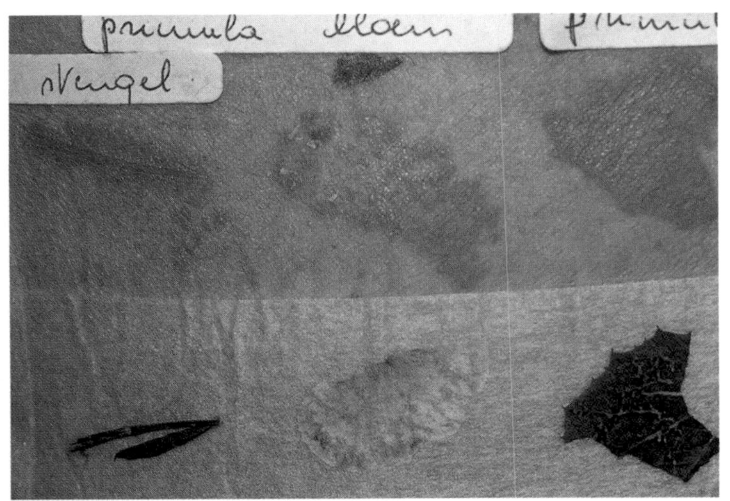

Figure 6.70 Positive reactions to different parts of the primula plant are shown here.

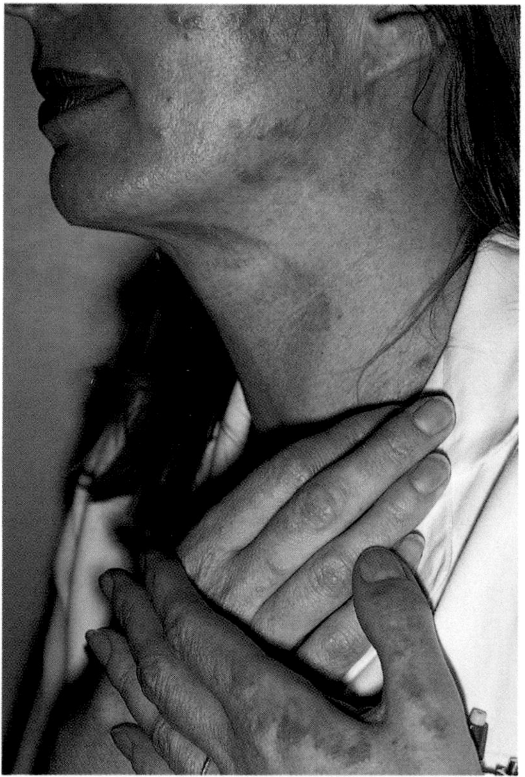

Figure 6.71 Another example of primula dermatitis. This 43-year-old woman had touched a primula plant with her left hand. Ectopic dermatitis was seen on her neck and face.

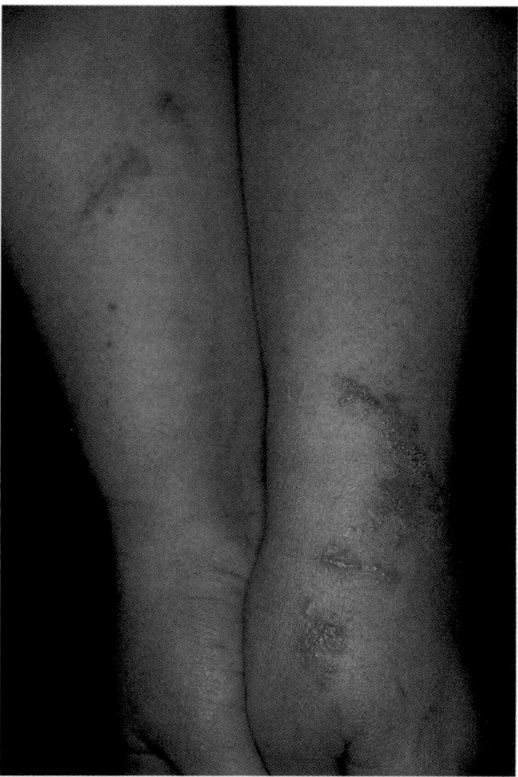

Figure 6.72 Linear lesions consisting of erythema, vesicles and bullae are typical of plant-induced contact dermatitis. Identification of the specific plant responsible is not always possible. This 40-year-old woman illustrates the characteristic clinical presentation of plant contact dermatitis.

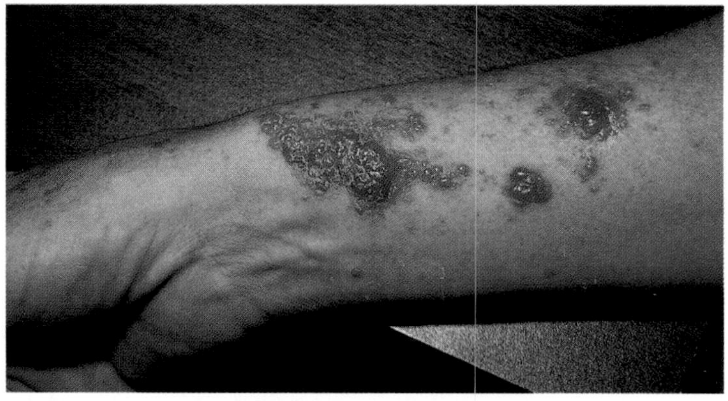

(**a**)

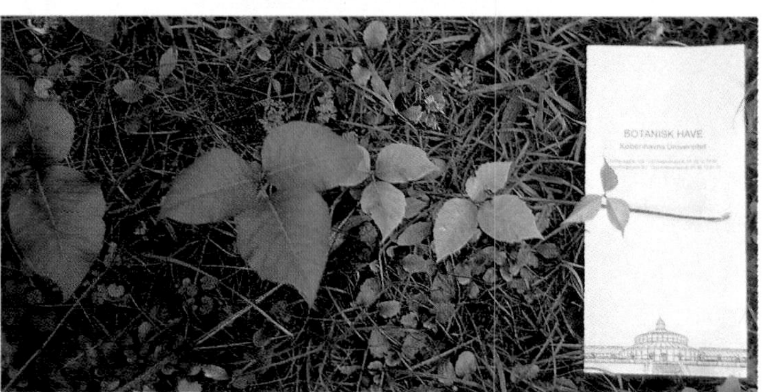

(**b**)

Figure 6.73 (**a**) In the USA, a linear pattern of vesicular dermatitis, as seen here, would lead to a presumptive diagnosis of poison ivy in the eastern states and poison oak in the western states.
(**b**) Poison ivy, showing the leaves of three leaflets and a runner.

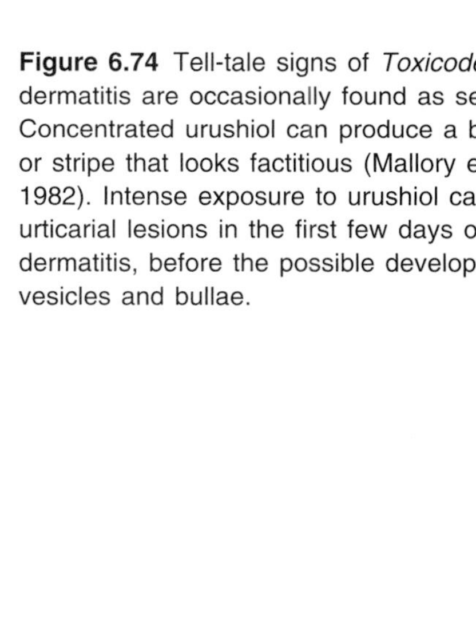

Figure 6.74 Tell-tale signs of *Toxicodendron* dermatitis are occasionally found as seen here. Concentrated urushiol can produce a black spot or stripe that looks factitious (Mallory et al, 1982). Intense exposure to urushiol can produce urticarial lesions in the first few days of dermatitis, before the possible development of vesicles and bullae.

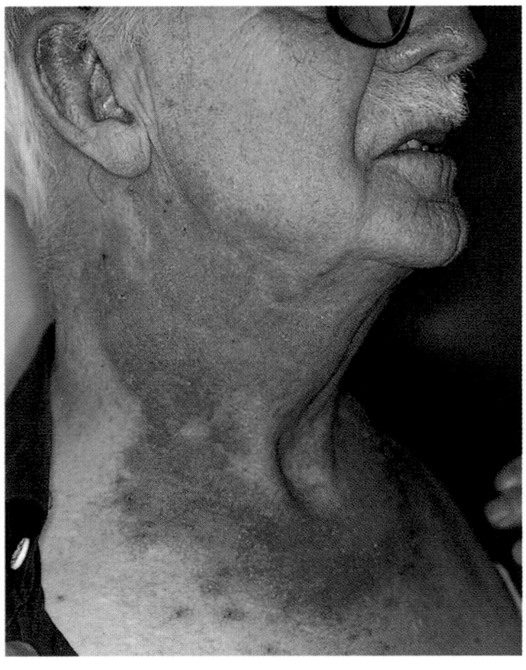

(**a**)

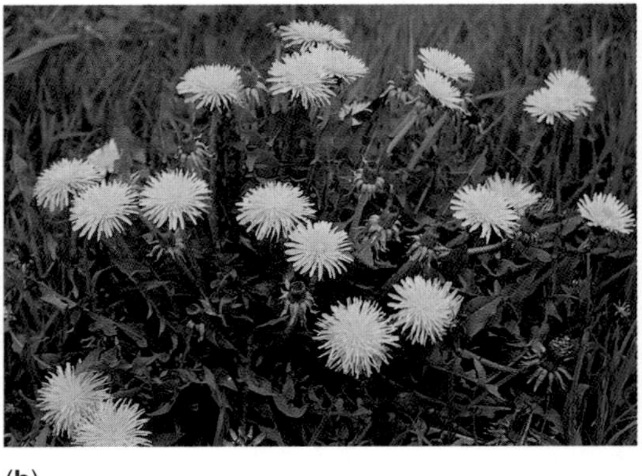

(**b**)

Figure 6.75 Plants of the Compositae family contain sesquiterpene lactones that are allergenic. A commercially available patch test known as the sesquiterpene lactone mix is used to detect allergy to this family of plants. The Compositae family includes ragweed and other common weeds, chrysanthemums, and parthenium. Foods that contain sesquiterpene lactones include laurel oil, chicory, artichoke, camomile and lettuce (Rietschel and Fowler, 1995, p.486). (**a**) This 82-year-old man had intense dermatitis of the neck and chest from Compositae and a positive patch test to the sesquiterpene lactone mix. (**b**) Dandelion is a Compositae.

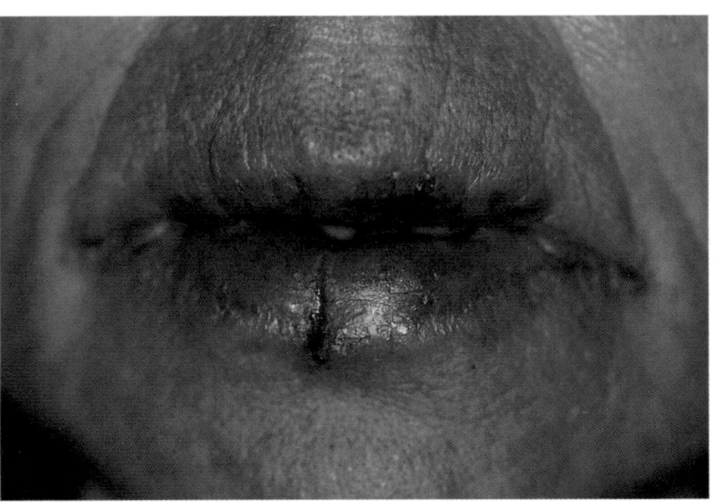

Figure 6.76 A 61-year-old sesquiterpene lactone-sensitive woman developed cheilitis from eating lettuce (Oliwiecki et al, 1991).

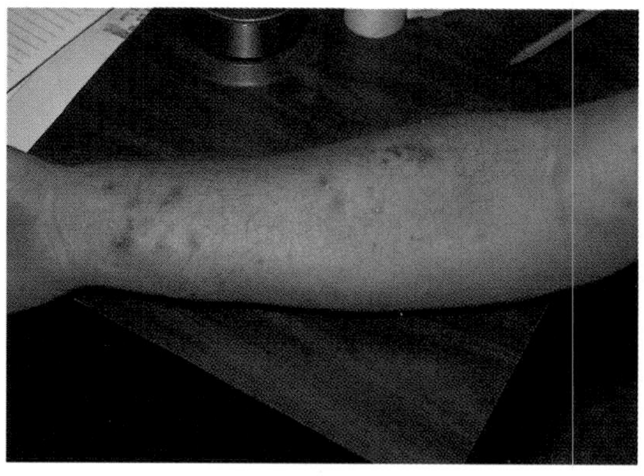

(**a**)

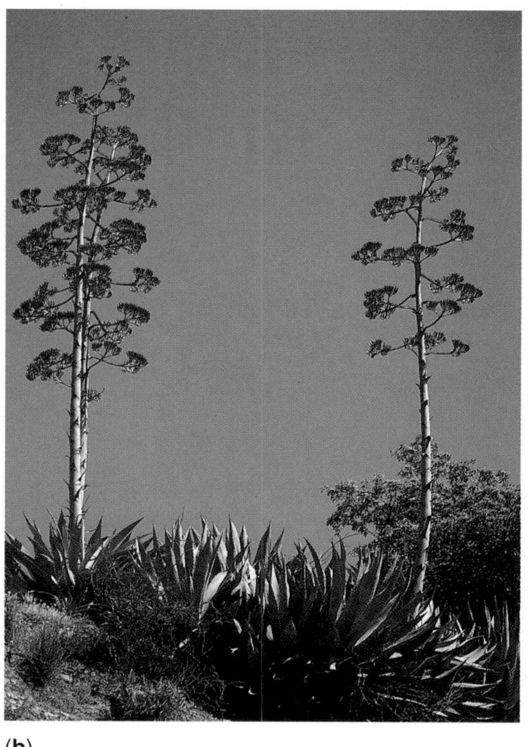

(**b**)

Figure 6.77 (**a**) This young man developed this dermatitis after chopping down a century plant, *Agave americanus* (**b**). (The common name of this cactus is derived from the folklore that the plant only blooms every 100 years). Once again, the pattern of reaction is the same as for other vegetation.

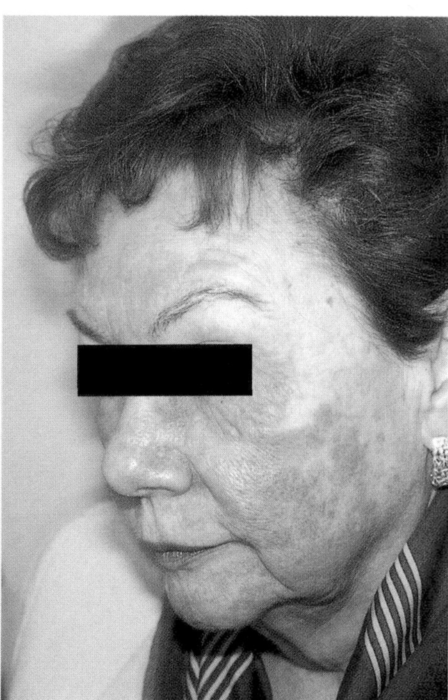

Figure 6.78 Spread of plant material from fingers to face occurred in this woman after work with her philodendrons.

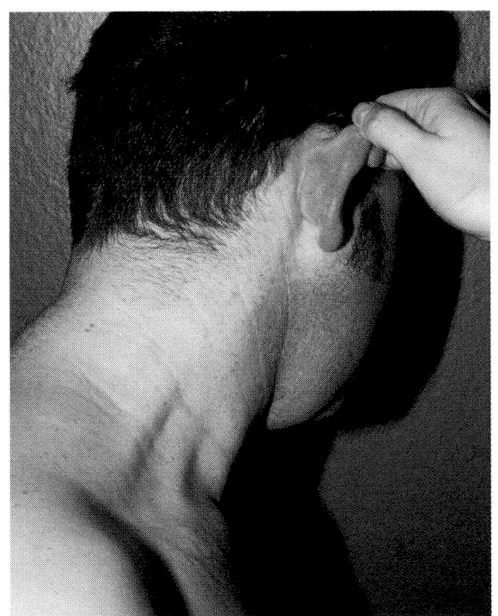

(**a**)

Figure 6.79 This man developed airborne allergic contact dermatitis (see Chapter 5) to the *Juniperus* species. He was sensitive to colophony and wood tar. (**a**) The lesions on his face and retro-auricular area – an area characteristically involved in airborne dermatitis, but which is spared in photodermatitis. (**b**) The involvement of the forearms. (**c**) A patch test to the plant *Juniperus chinensis herzii* was positive.

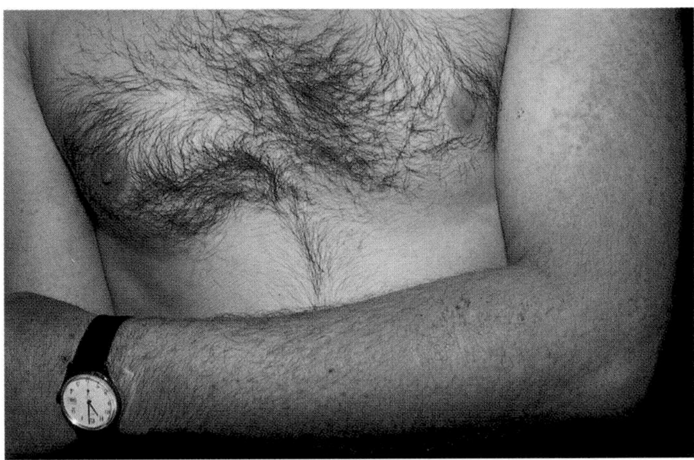

(**b**)

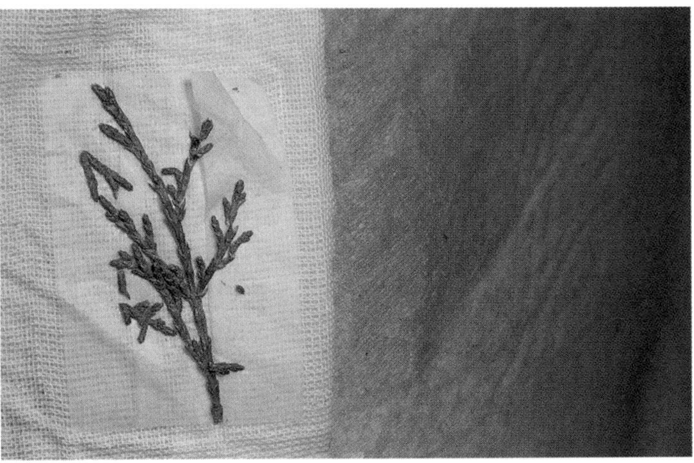

(**c**)

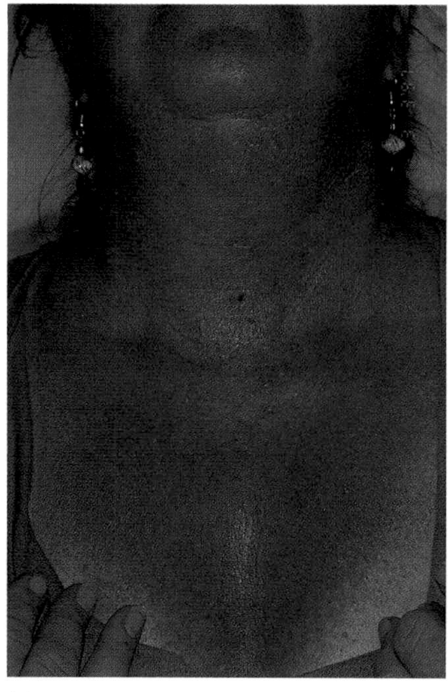

(**a**)

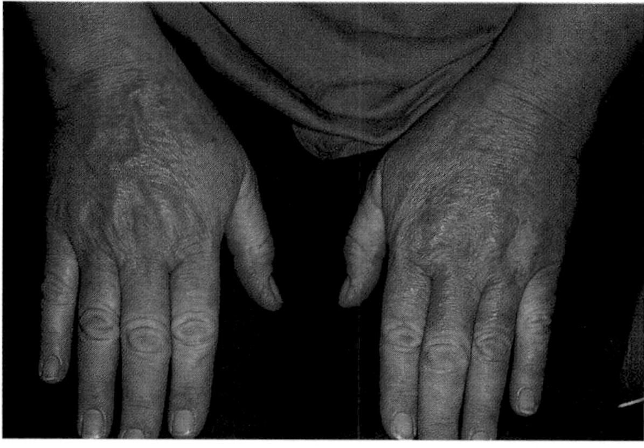

(**b**)

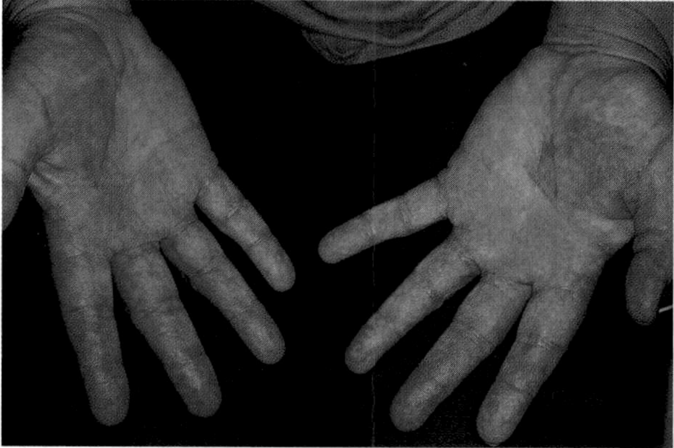

(**c**)

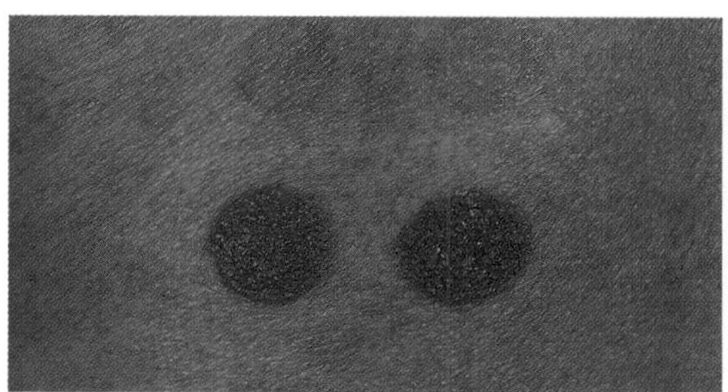

(**d**)

Figure 6.80 This woman owned a greenhouse and worked on a daily basis with plants in pots decorated with Spanish moss (a type of lichen). She had persistent dermatitis of the face and neck (**a**), as well as the hands (**b**, **c**). She had a positive patch test to colophony, to the lichen mix, and to the lichen allergen, usnic acid: (**d**) shows the patch test reactions to the lichen mix (left) and to usnic acid (right). To make matters worse, she was treating herself with a herbal product that contained colophony in the form of tree resin.

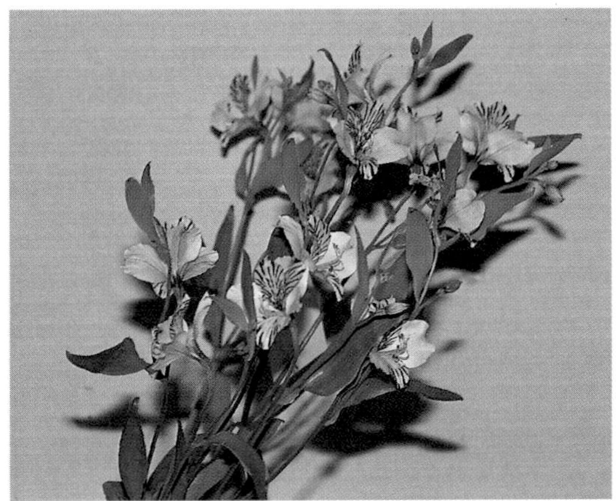

(**a**)

Figure 6.81 (**a**) *Alstroemeria*, which is also known as the Peruvian lily, can cause contact dermatitis with a distinctive hyperkeratotic component (**b**). The allergen is known as tulipalin A, or α-methylene γ-butyrolactone. The hyperkeratosis seen in patients with allergy to this material is shown in (**c**).

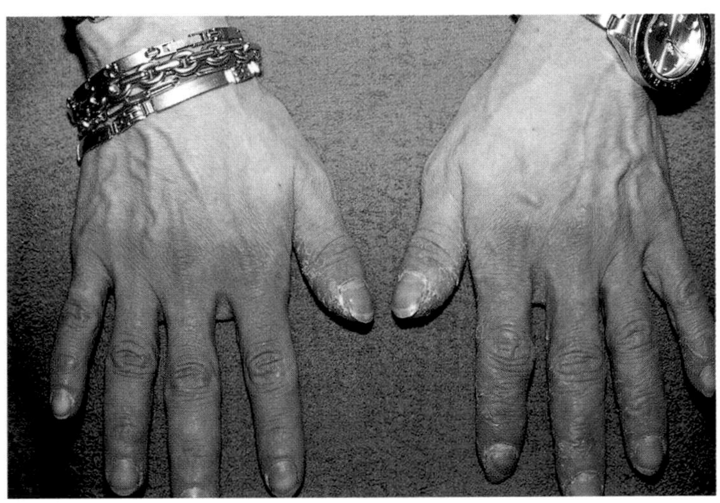

(**b**)

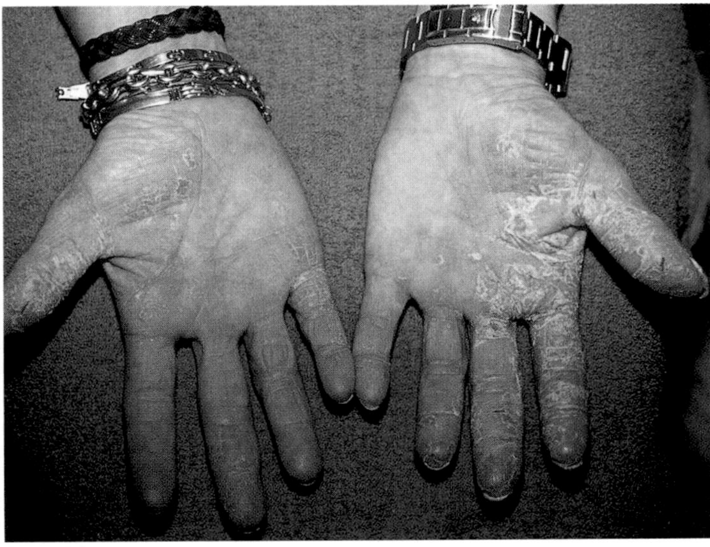

(**c**)

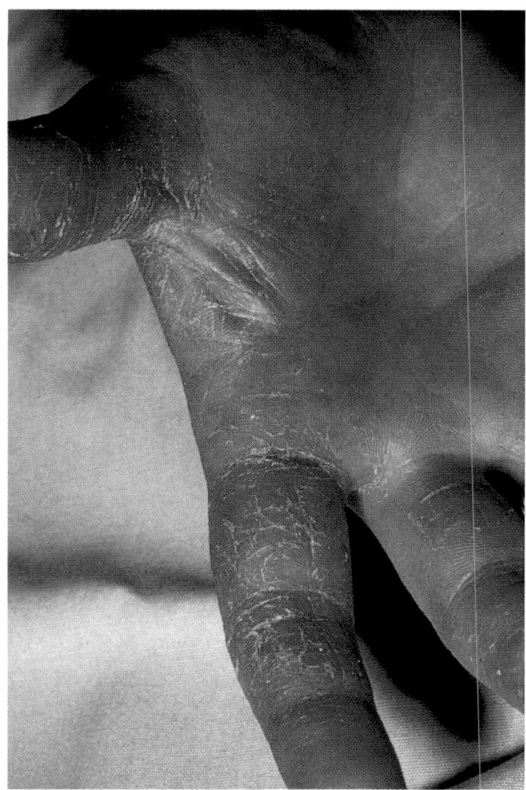

Figure 6.82 Allergic contact dermatitis to *Alstroemeria* is common among florists who work with this plant.

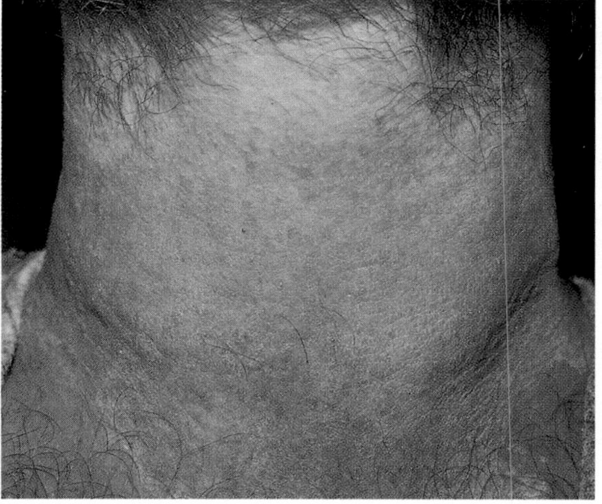

(**a**)

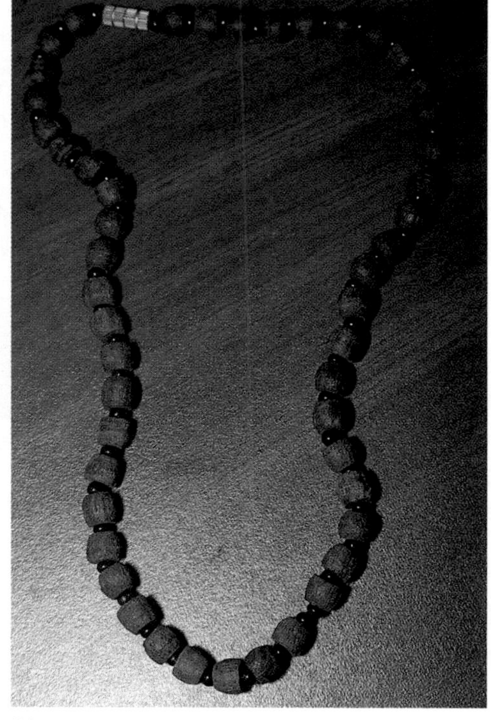

(**b**)

Figure 6.83 Exotic woods can cause contact dermatitis. The usual allergens are quinones. This young man developed dermatitis of the neck (**a**) due to the necklace (**b**). The nature of the wood was not identified, but his rash disappeared when he gave the necklace to a friend!

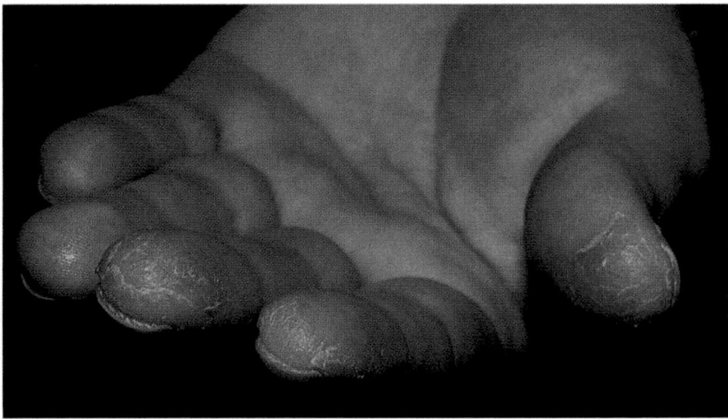

Figure 6.84 Another plant capable of inducing hyperkeratosis as a manifestation of allergic contact dermatitis is garlic. The allergic pulpitis of the left thumb and middle and index fingers seen in this right-handed cook was due to garlic.

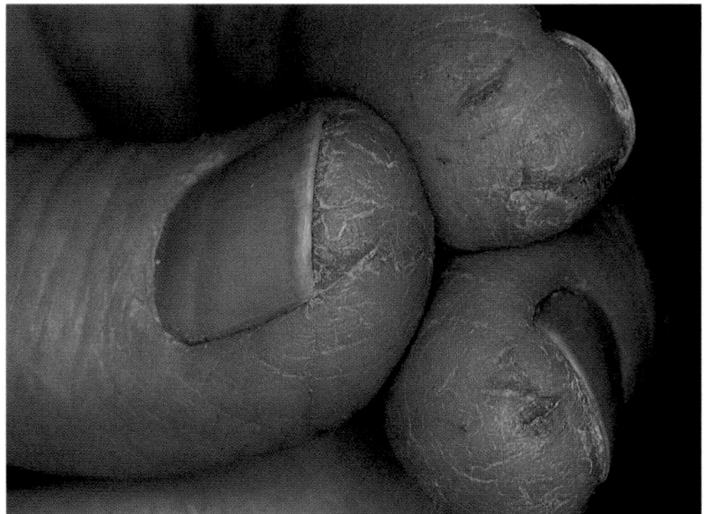

(**a**)

Figure 6.85 (**a**) This 75-year-old woman was very fond of garlic. She prepared considerable amounts almost daily, and developed fissured fingertip dermatitis on the thumb, index and middle fingers of her left hand, which held the garlic while it was chopped. (**b**) A further example of allergic contact dermatitis caused by garlic in a female restaurant cook. (**c**) Her positive test reaction to garlic and diallyl disulfide.

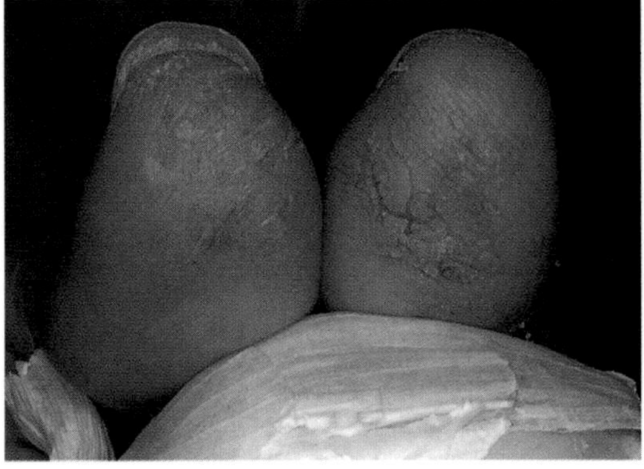

(**b**)

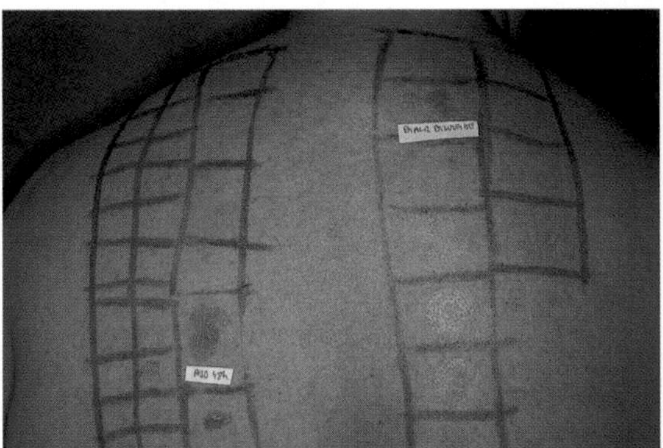

(**c**)

Textiles, Clothing and Shoes

Contact dermatitis due to clothing or textiles has been reported from dyes, finishes and additives such as flame retardants. Permanent press clothing finishes have been the focus of attention since the 1960s, when formaldehyde was found to be a problem in clothing treated to resist wrinkles (Schorr et al, 1974). Of additional interest were related compounds that replaced formaldehyde, such as dimethyldihydroxyethylene urea–formaldehyde resin (Foussereau, 1995). Features that suggest clothing dermatitis include sparing of the face, hands and feet, and increased dermatitis in areas of tight clothing such as the waist, the shoulder, around the axillae and on the thighs. The typical distribution of textile dermatitis is illustrated below. Patients sensitive to textile finishes commonly also react to formaldehyde-releasing preservatives. Natural fibres such as cotton are known for their absorbency, and hold on to higher levels of formaldehyde than many artificial fibres (Schorr et al, 1974).

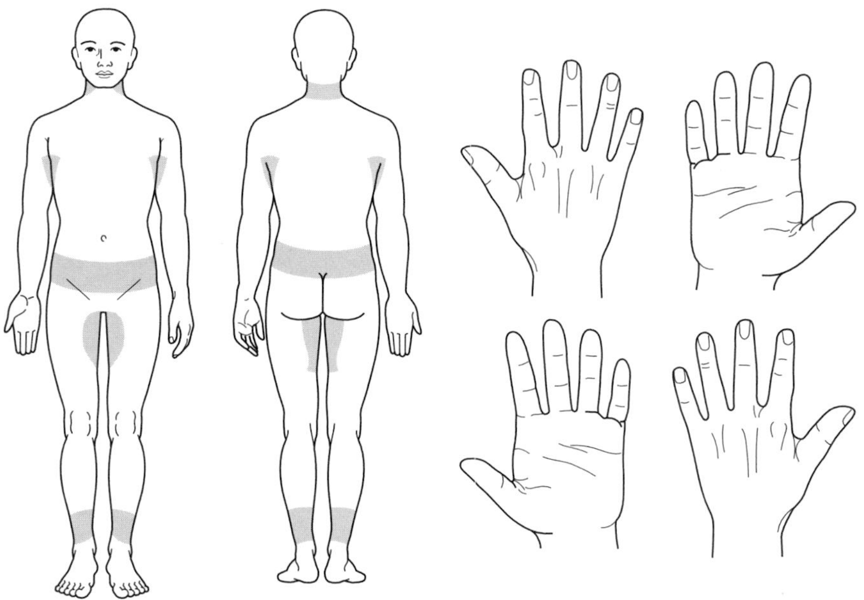

Typical distribution of textile dermatitis

Dyes are the most common allergens in textiles. In the case of shoes, many chemicals are used in their production (Podmore, 1995). The allergens are present in the leather (chromium salts), glues, (PTBP resin, colophony, diaminodiphenylmethane, mercaptobenzothiazole), rubber additives (thiurams, carbamates, mercaptobenzothiazoles), and various plastic materials. The spectrum of the allergens identified may vary from country to country. For example, rubber additives are frequent allergens in Canada and the USA, while chromium salts have a high incidence as allergens in Europe. Shoe dermatitis affects women more often than men, and frequently on the dorsal aspects of the feet (60% of the cases). Generally, the areas between the toes are spared. Chromium salts and *p-tert*-butylphenol–formaldehyde resin frequently cause dermatitis on the dorsal aspects of the feet, while mercaptobenzothiazole is often the cause of plantar dermatitis. One should also keep in mind that a dermatitis on the foot may also be due to ingredients of locally applied medications.

Specific allergens are given in the box.

Allergens

Shoes:
- Chromium salts
- Cobalt
- Colophony
- Diaminodiphenylmethane
- Mercaptobenzothiazoles
- Nickel
- *p-tert*-butylphenol–formaldehyde resin
- Thiourea
- Thiurams

Textiles and clothing:
- Disperse orange 3
- Disperse yellow 3
- Disperse blue 106
- Disperse blue 124
- Formaldehyde resins

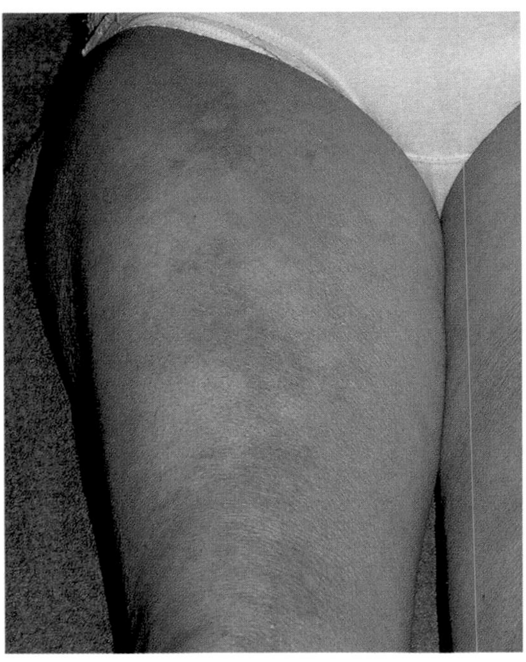

(a)

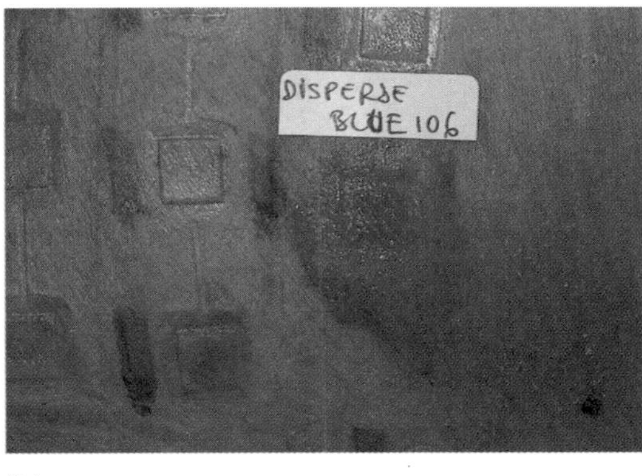

(b)

Figure 6.86 (**a**) Dermatitis of the thighs due to a textile dye in a skirt. (**b**) The allergen was identified as disperse blue 106 by patch testing.

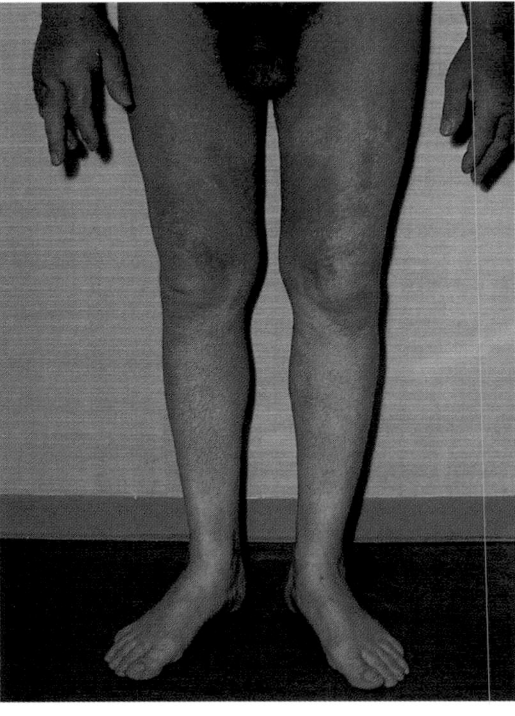

(a)

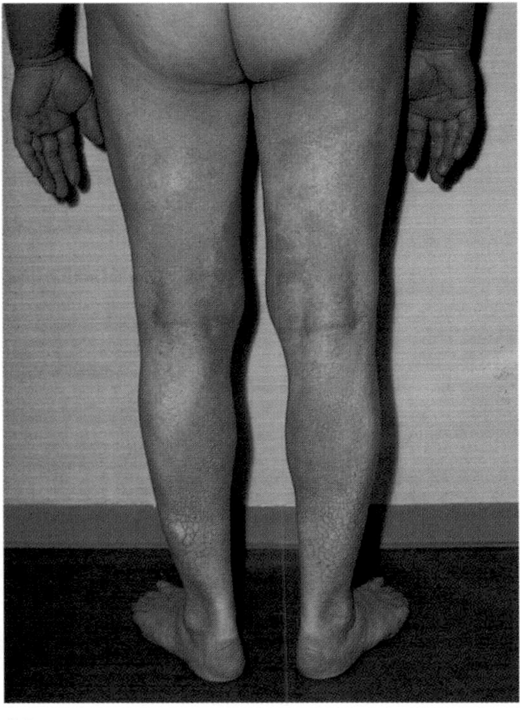

(b)

Figure 6.87 (**a**, **b**) Textile dermatitis due to dark-blue trousers caused the eruption seen here. An azo dye was responsible.

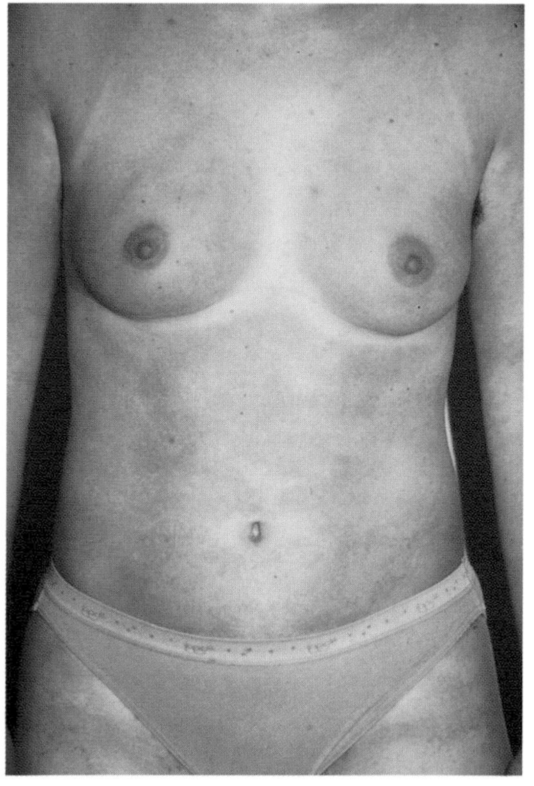

(**a**)

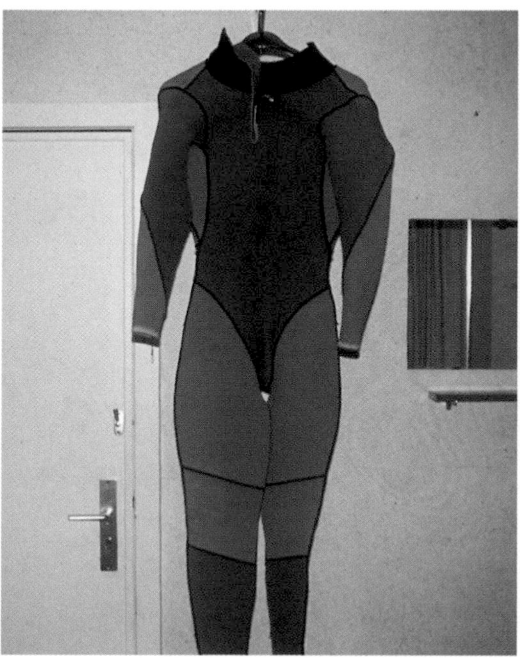

(**b**)

Figure 6.88 (**a**) Contact allergy was caused by diethylthiourea in the purple, but not the pink, synthetic lining of a wetsuit (**b**).

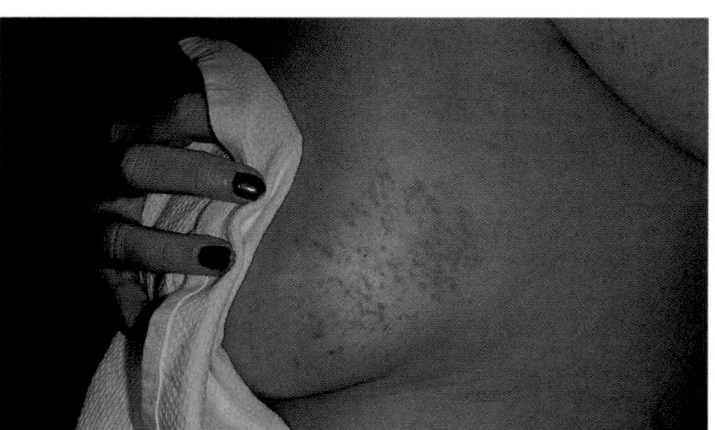

Figure 6.89 Dermatitis was present along the lateral thorax and spread over the breasts of this young woman who was patch-test positive to several permanent press textile finishes.

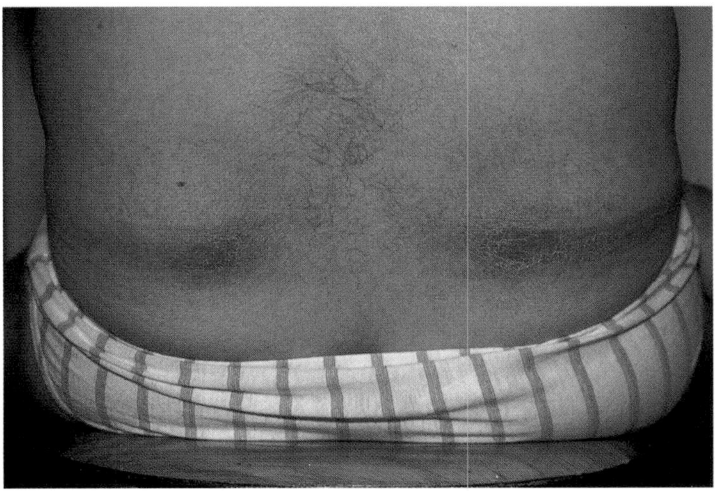

Figure 6.90 Clothing accessories can cause contact dermatitis, as seen on the waist of this patient who was allergic to *p-tert*-butylphenol–formaldehyde resin in a leather belt. This allergen is usually present in leather goods as an adhesive to bind the leather together.

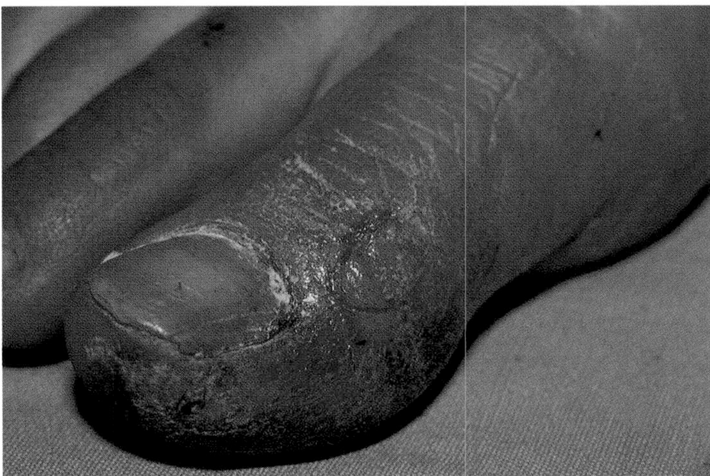

Figure 6.91 The same allergen identified in Figure 6.90 was present in the glue of the shoes of this patient, and caused the dermatitis seen here.

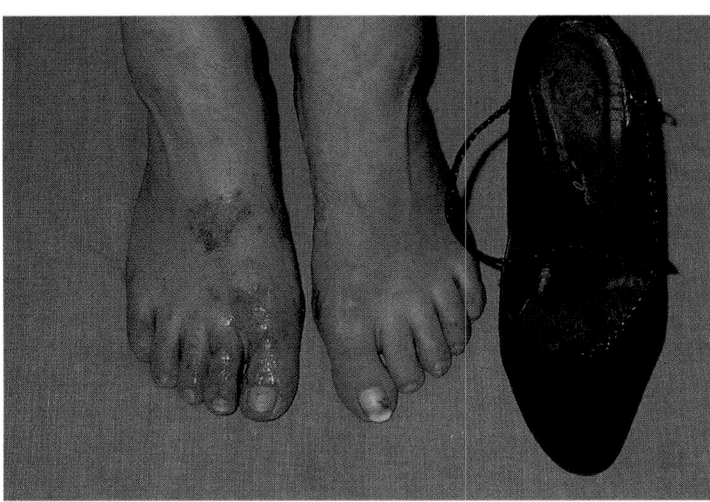

Figure 6.92 Shoe dermatitis was due to dyes present in the footwear of this patient. The unilateral localization is unusual. Sometimes unilateral presentations such as this can be explained by one shoe having stepped in a puddle of water or a similar circumstance, which could act to liberate materials from the outer or mid-portions of the shoe, allowing allergens to migrate to parts of the shoe that have more intimate contact with the skin surface.

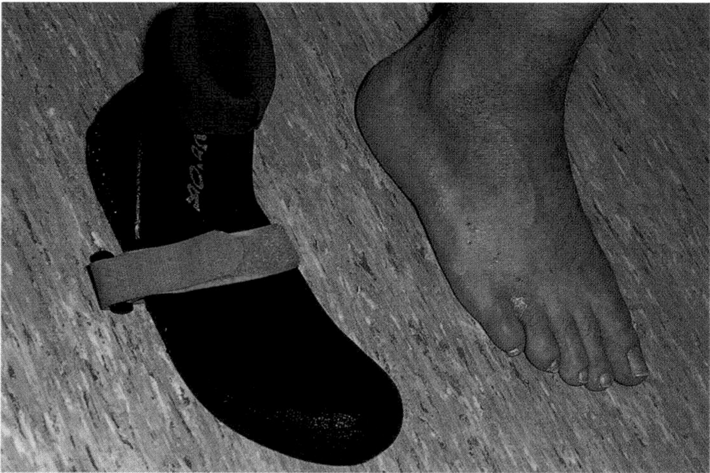

Figure 6.93 Contact dermatitis of the feet due to surfing shoes. The cause was allergy to diethylthiourea. Thioureas are associated with neoprene rubber products, such as these shoes and the wetsuit shown in Figure 6.88. It should be noted that this patient also has athlete's foot.

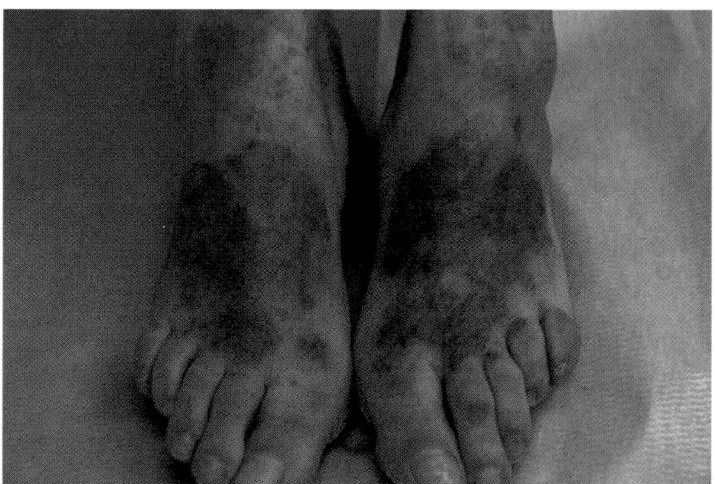

Figure 6.94 Patients who are allergic to chromates in leather components of shoes have dermatitis on the dorsal aspects of the feet, as seen in this case of chromate allergy. Potassium dichromate is the substance used to screen for this allergy.

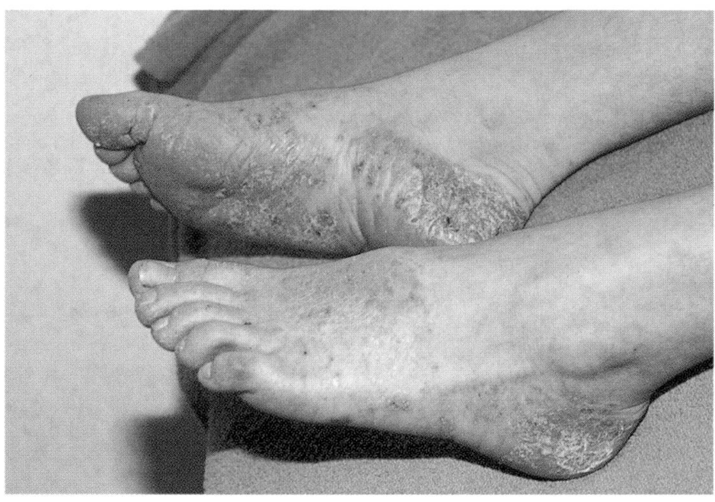

Figure 6.95 Rubber components of shoes and rubber cements used to bind shoes of various construction tend to cause dermatitis on the sides, heels and even the thick plantar surfaces of the feet, as seen in this case of mercaptobenzothiazole allergy.

REFERENCES

Adams RM, Maibach HI (1985) A five year study of cosmetic reactions. *J Am Acad Dermatol* **13**:1062–9.

Andersen KE, Hjorth N, Menné T (1984) The baboon syndrome: systemically-induced allergic contact dermatitis. *Contact Dermatitis* **10**:97–100.

Angelini G (1995) Topical drugs. In: *Textbook of Contact Dermatitis*, 2nd edn (Rycroft RJG, Menné T, Frosch PJ, eds). Berlin: Springer-Verlag: 477–503.

Benezra C, Ducombs G, Sell Y et al (1985) *Plant Contact Dermatitis*. Toronto: BC Becker/St Louis MO: CV Mosby.

Berne B, Lundin A, Enander Almros P (1994) Side effects of cosmetics and toiletries in relation to use: a retrospective study in a Swedish population. *Eur J Dermatol* **4**:189–93.

Camarasa JG, Burrows D, Menné T et al (1991) Palladium contact sensitivity. *Contact Dermatitis* **24**:370–1.

Conde-Salazar L, Guimaraens D, Romero L et al (1985) Erythema mulitformae-like contact dermatitis from lincomycin. *Contact Dermatitis* **12**:59–61.

Conde-Salazar L, Llinas Volpe M, Guimaraens D, Romero L (1988) Allergic contact dermatitis from a suction socket prosthesis. *Contact Dermatitis* **19**:305–6.

Consumers' Association (1979) *Reactions of the Skin to Cosmetic and Toiletry Products*. London: Consumers' Association.

de Groot AC, Nater JP, van der Lende R et al (1987) Adverse effects of cosmetics: a retrospective study in the general population. *Int J Cosmet Sci* **9**:255–59.

Dooms-Goossens A (1993) Contact allergy to cosmetics. *Cosmetics Toiletries* **108**:43–6.

Fisher AA (1978) Dermatitis associated with transcutaneous electrical nerve stimulation. *Cutis* **21**:24.

Foussereau J (1995) Clothing. In: *Textbook of Contact Dermatitis*, 2nd edn (Rycroft RJG, Menné T, Frosch PJ, eds). Berlin: Springer-Verlag: 504–15.

Fowler JF Jr (1987) Selection of patch test materials for gold allergy. *Contact Dermatitis* **3**:280.

Hausen BM (1988) *Allergiepflanzen. Pflanzenallergene*. Munich: Verlagsgesellschaft.

Hjorth N, Fregert S, Schildknecht H (1969) Cross-sensitization between synthetic primin and related quinones. *Acta Derm Venereol (Stockh)* **49**:552.

Knight TE, Hausen BM (1994) Melaleuca oil (tea tree oil) dermatitis. *J Am Acad Dermatol* **30**:423–7.

Laine J, Kalimo K, Forssell H, Happonen RP (1992) Resolution of oral lichenoid lesions after replacement of amalgam restorations in patients allergic to mercury compounds. *Br J Dermatol* **126**:10–15.

Lee JY, Wang BJ (1995) Contact dermatitis caused by cetrimide in antiseptics. *Contact Dermatitis* **33**:168–71.

Lepoittevin JP, Drieghe J, Dooms-Goossens A (1995) Studies in patients with corticosteroid contact allergy. Understanding cross-reactivity among different steroids. *Arch Dermatol* **131**:31–7.

McGeorge BC, Steele MC (1991) Allergic contact dermatitis of the nipple from Roman chamomile ointment. *Contact Dermatitis* **24**:139–40.

Maibach HI (1987) Oral substitution in patients sensitized by transdermal clonidine treatment. *Contact Dermatitis* **16**:1–8.

Mallory SB, Miller OF III, Tyler WB (1982) *Toxicodendron radicans* dermatitis with black lacquer deposit on the skin. *J Am Acad Dermatol* **6**:363.

Meijer C, Bredberg M, Fischer T et al (1995) Ear piercing, and nickel and cobalt sensitization in 520 young Swedish men doing compulsory military service. *Contact Dermatitis* **32**:147–9.

Mitchell JC, Rook AJ (1979) *Botanical Dermatology*. Vancouver, BC: Greengrass.

Oliwiecki S, Beck MH, Hausen BM (1991) Compositae dermatitis aggravated by eating lettuce. *Contact Dermatitis* **24**:318–19.

Podmore P (1995) Shoes. In: *Practical Contact Dermatitis: A Handbook for the Practitioner* (Guin JD, ed). New York: McGraw-Hill, 325–32.

Rietschel RL, Fowler JF Jr (1995) *Fisher's Contact Dermatitis*. Baltimore, MD: Williams and Wilkins.

Romaguera C, Grimalt F, Villaplana J (1988) Contact dermatitis from nickel: an investigation of its source. *Contact Dermatitis* **19**:52–7.

Schorr WF, Keran E, Plotka E (1974) Formaldehyde allergy. The quantitative analysis of American clothing for free formaldehyde and its relevance in clinical practice. *Arch Dermatol* **110**:73–6.

Storrs FJ (1984) Permanent wave contact dermatitis: contact allergy to glyceryl monothioglycolate. *J Am Acad Dermatol* **11**:74–85.

Thune P, Solberg Y, McFadden N et al (1982) Perfume allergy due to oak moss and other lichens. *Contact Dermatitis* **8**:396–400.

Veien NK, Hattel T, Justesen O, Nørholm A (1986) Aluminium allergy. *Contact Dermatitis* **15**:295–7.

Westat Inc (1975) *An Investigation of Consumers' Perception of Adverse Reactions to Cosmetic Products*. National Technical Information Service, US Department of Commerce.

Whitmore SE (1992) The importance of proper vehicle selection in the detection of minoxidil sensitivity. *Arch Dermatol* **128**:653–6.

7

Occupational Contact Dermatitis

OCCUPATIONAL DERMATOSES

In the 1930s, the American Medical Association defined occupational dermatoses as 'ailments of the skin in which it can be shown that work was the fundamental cause or a factor which contributed to them' (Noojin, 1954), but with the passage of time and the appearance of new technologies, that definition has had to be enlarged, and so today we can define occupational dermatoses as 'all ailments of the skin or mucous or associated membranes, which are directly or indirectly caused, conditioned, maintained or aggravated by all those things that are used in occupational activity or exist in the working environment' (Ortiz de Frutos and Conde-Salazar, 1996).

Epidemiology and prognosis

The study of the epidemiology of occupational dermatology is complicated by the need to define the various tasks carried out, and, even with such definitions, the results can appear contradictory and can be difficult to evaluate (Conde-Salazar, 1993). Nevertheless, several authors have shown that 90–95% of occupational dermatoses are contact dermatitis (Mathias, 1988; Lushniak, 1995). In the latter study, extensive reference is made to the difficulties of obtaining data on this subject and also to the sources of information available in the USA. Data obtained from a nationwide survey in the USA on the incidence of occupational contact dermatitis from 1973 to 1991 showed that the populations most at risk worked in agriculture, forestry and fishing. People employed in these fields had an incidence of 345 cases per 100 000 persons, while those employed in industry had an incidence of 179 cases per 100 000.

Tacke et al (1995) provided data indicating that, over a period of three years, the incidence of occupational dermatoses among workers in the food industry in northern Bavaria was 67 cases per 100 000. The incidence for bakers was 84 cases per 100 000 and for cooks 34 cases per 100 000. The most common occupational dermatosis seen was irritant contact eczema. Atopic bakers were shown to have a relative risk of developing irritant contact dermatitis of 9.7, while cooks had a relative risk of developing this form of dermatitis of 5.2. Murer et al (1995) studied the occupational dermatoses on the hands of 192 Danish dental technicians, and found a cumulative prevalence of 53% and a one-year prevalence of 43%.

It is believed that between 40% and 65% of occupational diseases are occupational dermatoses (40.6% in California in 1973 and 65% in England in 1976 (Rycroft and Calnan, 1976)).

Lobel (1995) has commented on the prognosis and development of occupational eczemas among workers with chronic dermatitis. He concluded that although there are occupations that do not have a negative influence on the dermatoses of such workers, many have difficulty in finding jobs and in securing pensions – a situation that is particularly trying for young people.

According to a study of 230 persons with occupational dermatoses by Holness and Nethercott (1995), 78% continued to hold jobs two years after receiving a diagnosis of occupational dermatitis, 57% had changed jobs (67% of these because of their dermatitis) and 35% had been out of work for at least one month; 43% had applied for economic compensation because of their dermatitis.

Agriculture

The dermatological risks in agriculture are numerous and varied, and are generally not as familiar as the risks in industry. This is, in part, because many of those employed in agriculture work on small farms where they are self-employed, i.e. are both worker and employer. In large countries, such farms may be some distance from specialist clinics. Some farmers have two occupations, since they both till the soil and raise livestock, and, in general, there is less scientific interest in their problems.

The occupational skin diseases seen in an agricultural environment can be caused by both chemical and physical agents, and include exposure to sunlight and various plants and woods, stings, infections transmitted by animals, animal secretions, and veterinary medications.

With regard to chemicals, the chief risks arise from the use of pesticides as well as products used in the operation and maintenance of machinery.

The most common irritants and allergens are listed in the box.

Irritants	Allergens
Animal secretions:	Animal feed additives:
amniotic fluid	vitamin K3
Cement	cobalt
Diesel oil	Animal secretions:
Fertilizers	amniotic fluid
Fungicides	Cement:
Herbicides	chromium salts
Milk containers	cobalt
Paraffin oil	Pesticide components
Pesticides	carbamates
Plants	thiourea
Rat poisons	thiurams
Soaps and products used	Plants
to clean cowsheds, stables etc.	Rubber components or
Wood	additives:
Wood preservatives	boots
	gloves
	Veterinary medications:
	spiramycin
	tylosin
	etc.
	Wood

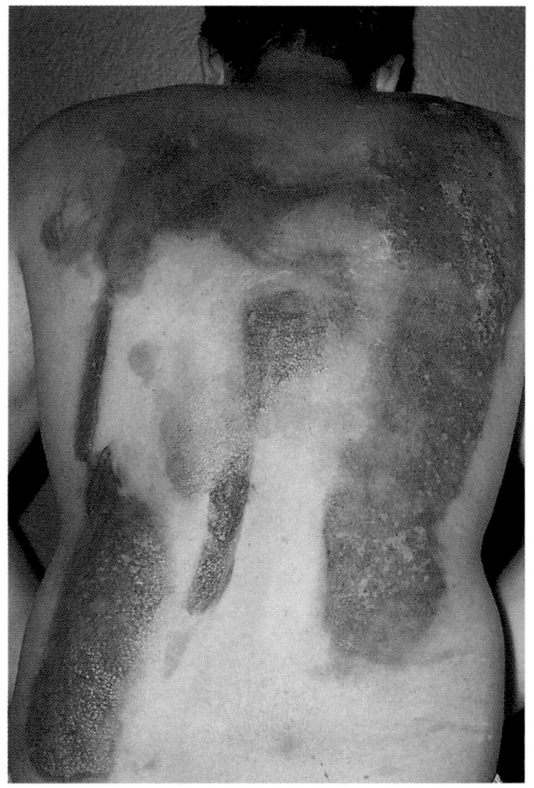

Figure 7.1 A severe toxic skin reaction occurred on the back of an agricultural worker. A pesticide was the source of the reaction. This is a form of irritant contact dermatitis.

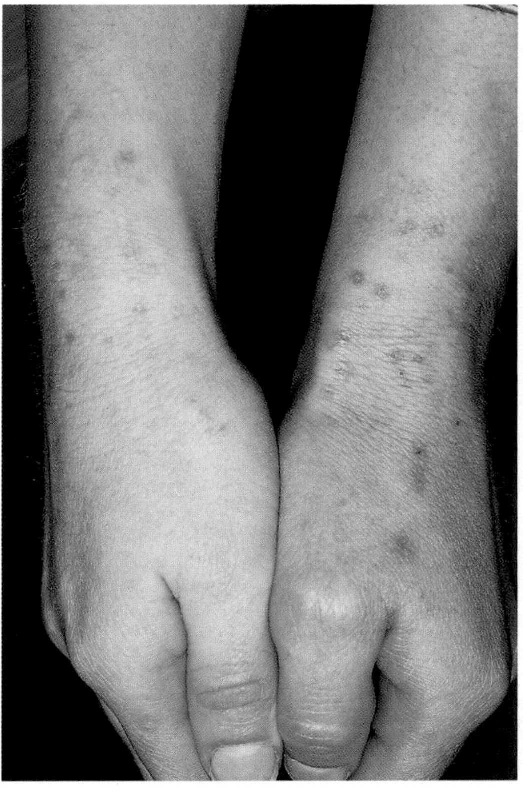

Figure 7.2 This 38-year-old farmer had mechanical irritant contact dermatitis from straw.

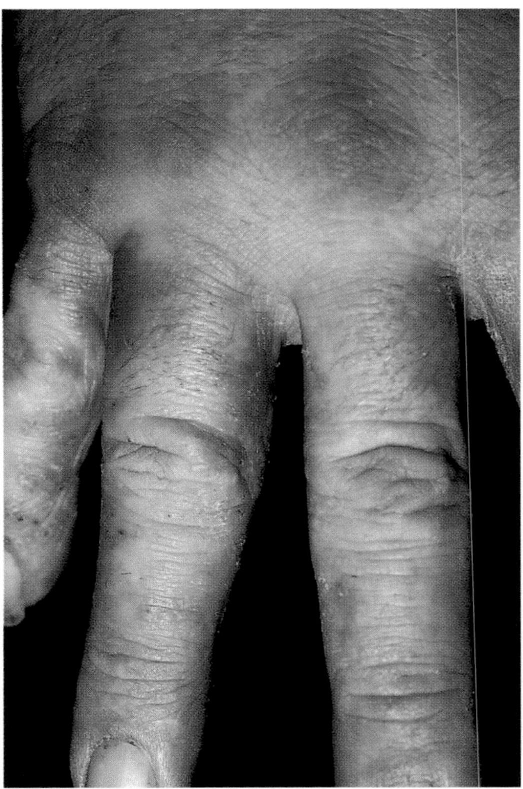

Figure 7.3 This 62-year-old dairy farmer developed acute irritant contact dermatitis of the sides of the fingers after contact with sodium hydroxide used to clean milking equipment.

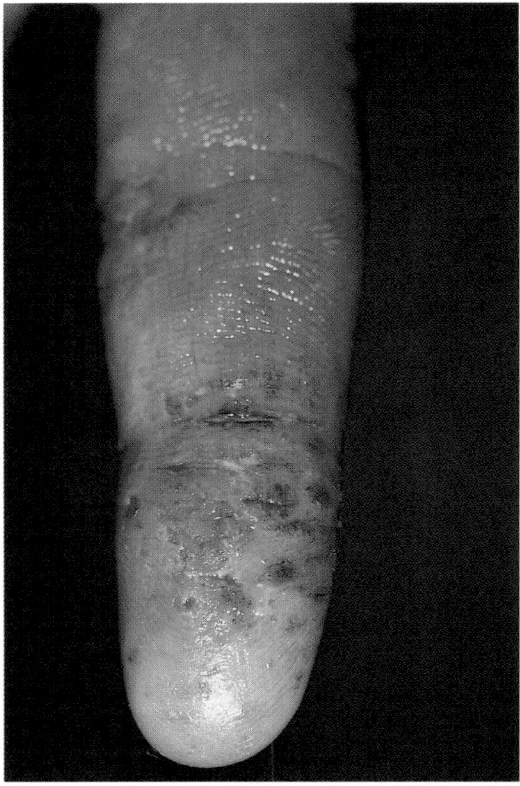

Figure 7.4 A 36-year-old pig farmer injected his pigs to combat diarrhoea. He used tylosin. His dermatitis occurred only on those fingers that touched the vials containing the drug and the syringes. He was patch-test positive to 5% tylosin tartrate (Neldner, 1972; Veien et al, 1980; Veien, 1987).

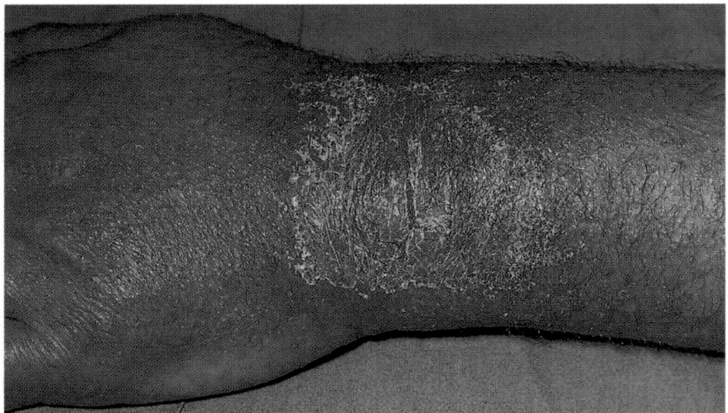
(a)

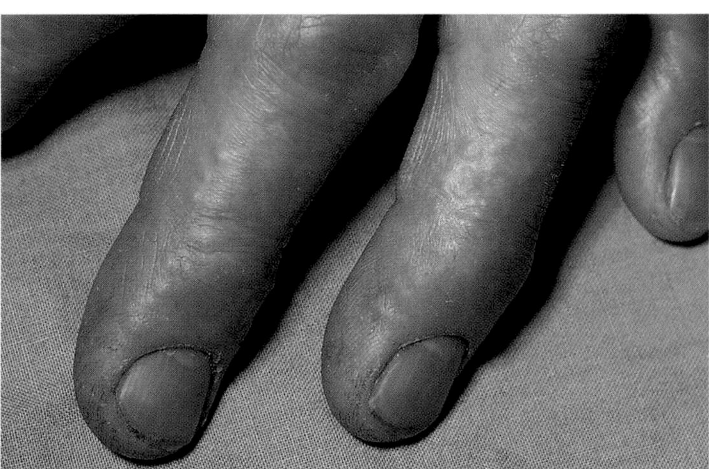
(b)

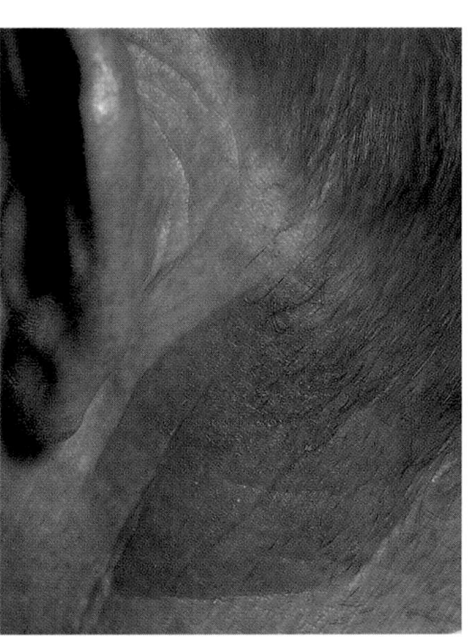
(c)

Figure 7.5 Allergic contact dermatitis can occur as a result of farmers treating themselves with veterinary products. In this case, the animal antifungal agent etisazole was applied to the wrist (**a**), and dermatitis developed in other areas due to transfer from the original site. Vesicular dermatitis was seen on the fingers (**b**), the neck showed a plaque-like lesion (**c**), and the upper lip and subnasal areas were also affected (**d**). The positive patch test to 2% etisazole in petrolatum is seen in (**e**).

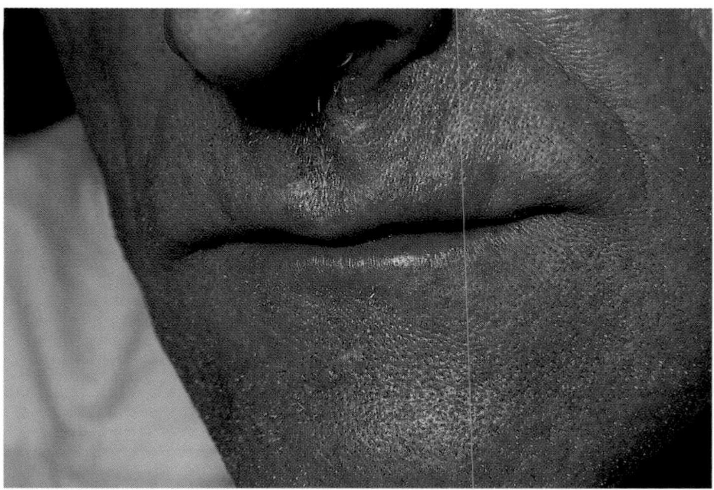

(**d**)

Figure 7.5 *continued*

(**e**)

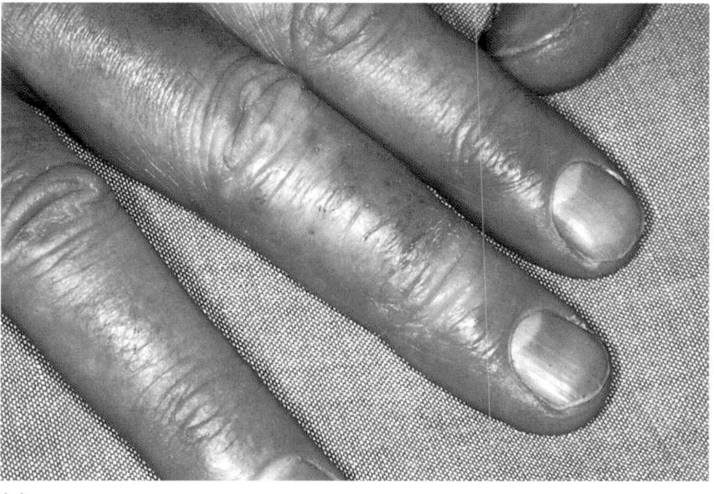

(**a**)

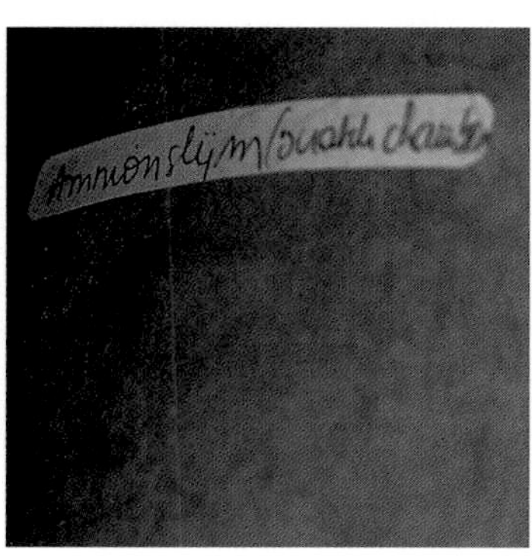

(**b**)

Figure 7.6 Protein from animals can cause contact urticaria, and if persistent contact occurs, the urticarial features are lost and chronic dermatitis occurs (protein contact dermatitis). (**a**) The hand of a veterinarian in whom specific IgE to bovine amniotic fluid was detected and found to be the source of his hand dermatitis. (**b**) The positive scratch test to bovine amniotic fluid in this patient.

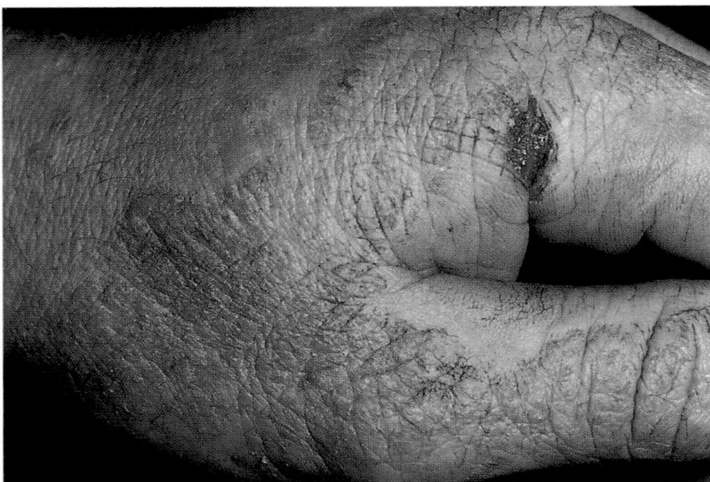

Figure 7.7 A 31-year-old dairy farmer had severely pruritic dermatitis, especially on the left hand and forearm, after contact with cows. He touched the cow with his left hand and arm, while the right hand was used to attach the milking equipment. The dermatitis was contact urticaria/protein contact dermatitis from cow dander, and he had a positive prick test to cow dander (Susitaival et al, 1995).

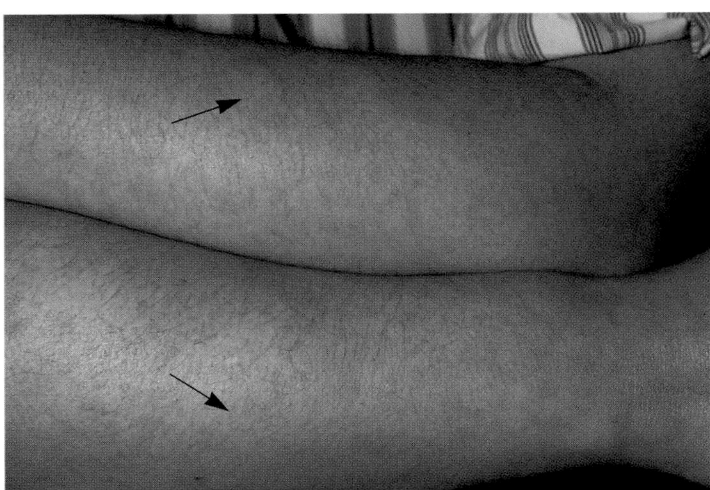

Figure 7.8 A 29-year-old female veterinary surgeon developed pruritic dermatitis on the forearms immediately after delivering calves. Protection with long plastic gloves and sleeves did not solve the problem, since the sharp teeth of the calves made holes in the gloves. A prick test with amniotic fluid was positive, and the dermatitis was diagnosed as contact urticaria/protein contact dermatitis from bovine amniotic fluid. The dermatitis faded after she stopped working with cattle (Schmidt, 1978).

Construction Industry

More than 200 occupations can be included within the scope of the construction industry (bricklayers, tilers, plasterers, concrete workers, carpenters, joiners, etc.). To various extents, all of the above persons use products commonly called 'cements' or 'hydraulic aggregates'. Such products, when mixed with water, set and harden to become solid. These cements are composed primarily of three raw materials: lime, clay and plaster. According to the proportions of these three components, the resultant finished product will have different properties. The main sensitizers found in clay are chromates, cobalt and nickel. These are found in small quantities (ppm), and the amounts vary depending on the geographical origin of the clay. These allergens are also found in items that contain them, i.e. machinery that contains oil, etc. In order to manufacture cements with specific properties, certain additives (sodium lignosulfonate, canitite, calcium nitrate and calcium chloride), in concentrations of up to 5%, may be added to, for example, speed up or slow down the setting process or to allow the cement to set in water (for the building of dykes or bridge foundations) (Turk and Rietschel, 1993). Epoxy or epoxy–acrylic resins are used with cements for laying floors.

In addition to the chemicals used in the construction industry, various kinds of wood are also used for the building of scaffolds, windows, doors, floors, etc., and woods can also cause occupational dermatitis. Tropical woods, also referred to as 'exotic' woods, and pine are more likely to cause skin reactions than other types of wood.

Other sources of occupational dermatitis are the use, maintenance and cleaning of machinery, when workers come in contact with oil, petrol and other substances.

The indiscriminate use of topical medications from the first-aid boxes found on construction sites can cause iatrogenic sensitization to neomycin, sulfonamides and preparations containing mercury.

Construction workers may also develop occupational dermatoses if they work in conditions where protective measures are not easily taken. Many construction workers are employed for only short periods at various building sites and may experience frequent changes of job and employer, adding to the difficulty of taking precautionary measures.

The most common irritants and allergens are listed in the box.

Irritants	Allergens
Cement	Acrylic resins
Cement additives	Chromates
Lime	Cobalt
Machine oil	Epoxy resins
Plaster	Exotic woods
Rubber gloves and boots	Latex
Wood	Nickel (in cement and many tools)
Wood preservatives	Rubber components and additives:
	carbamates
	mercaptobenzothiazoles
	thiourea
	thiurams
	Topical medications:
	neomycin
	sulfonamides
	thiomerosal
	Turpentine

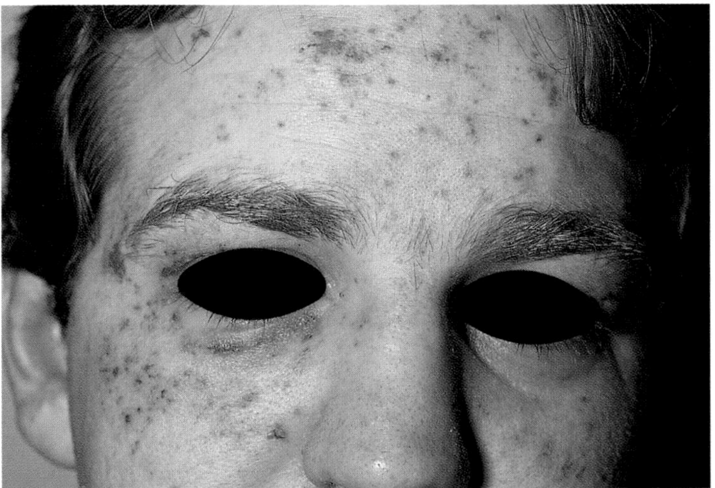

Figure 7.9 This is the face of a 28-year-old man who was employed at a cement manufacturing plant and was accidentally exposed to cement dust. He developed acute irritant dermatitis due to the alkaline reaction of the cement.

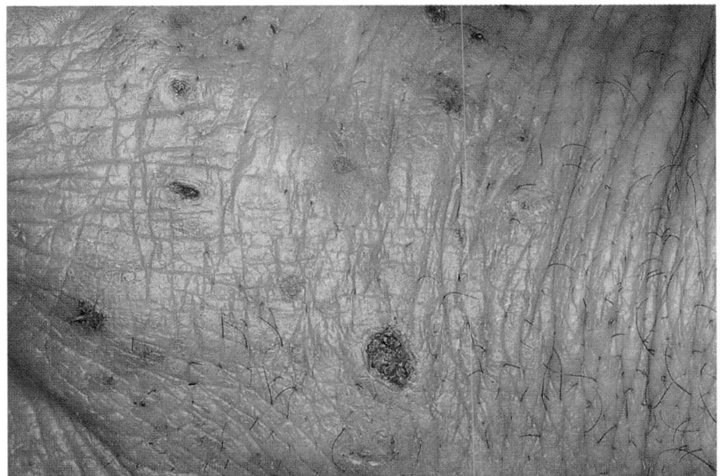

Figure 7.10 Irritant contact dermatitis due to cement may be caused by components of cement other than chromate. The small ulcerated lesions seen in this worker were believed to be due to silica particles found in cement. Chromium salts have also been associated with ulceration. Patch testing with potassium dichromate was also negative (Conde-Salazar et al, 1995a).

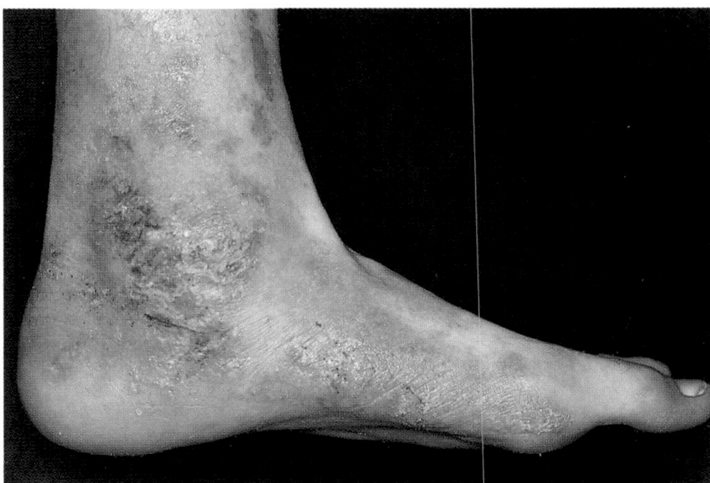

Figure 7.11 A 24-year-old man developed irritant contact dermatitis on the lower legs and feet at sites of contact with wet cement used to make repairs in his home. Wet cement is highly alkaline, usually with a pH of more than 12. Patch testing with potassium dichromate was negative.

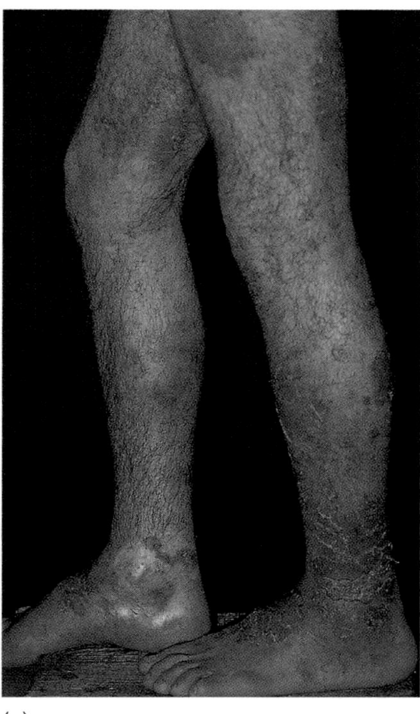

(a)

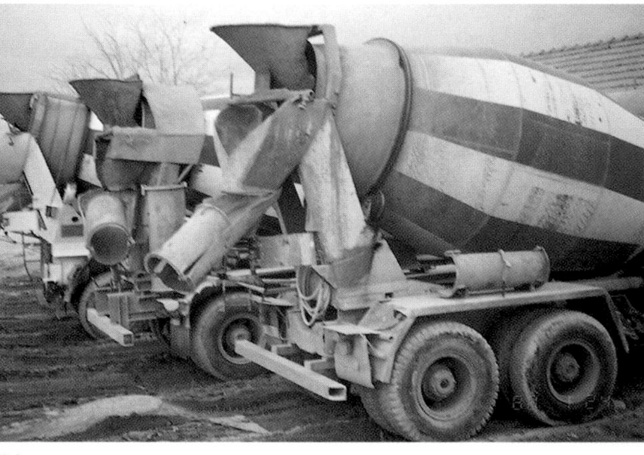

(b)

Figure 7.12 (**a**) An acute irritant reaction to cement in a construction worker who unloaded cement trucks – these reactions are referred to as 'burns'. (**b**) The high alkalinity of cement has already been mentioned, but the heat generated during its mixing gives added meaning to the concept of cement 'burns': the temperature of the cement in these trucks exceeds 80°C (Conde-Salazar et al, 1995a).

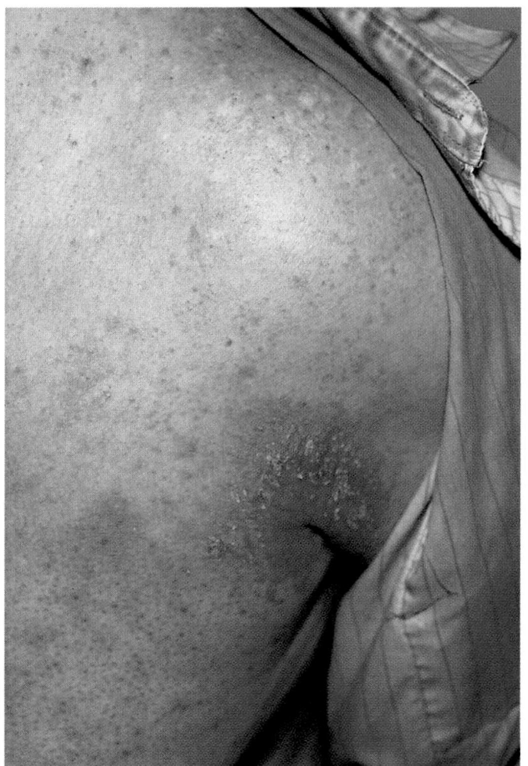

Figure 7.13 Inadequate protection of a worker can result from poor decisions on his or her part. This 39-year-old man worked at a cement manufacturing plant and developed intertriginous dermatitis of the neck, axillary folds and chest. He was overweight, and the working environment was hot. He felt it was too hot to wear the dustproof overalls he had been provided with, so he opened the zippered front and was thus exposed to cement dust. The dust turned his originally white shirt grey, as seen here. His eruption was irritant contact dermatitis from the alkaline cement dissolved in his sweat.

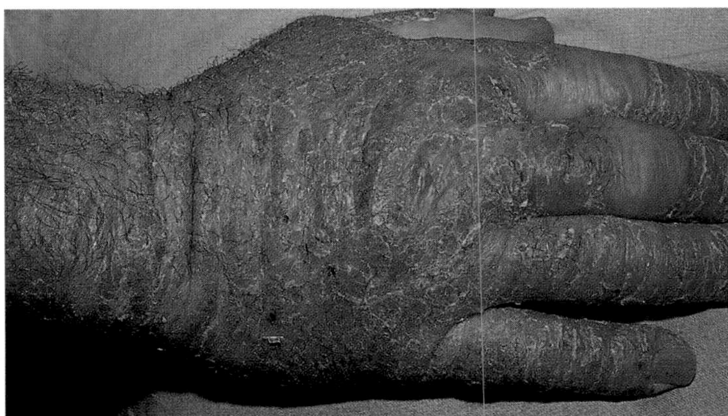

Figure 7.14 These lesions on the back of the hand are typical of chromate allergic contact dermatitis in the construction trades. This worker was sensitive to both chromate and cobalt.

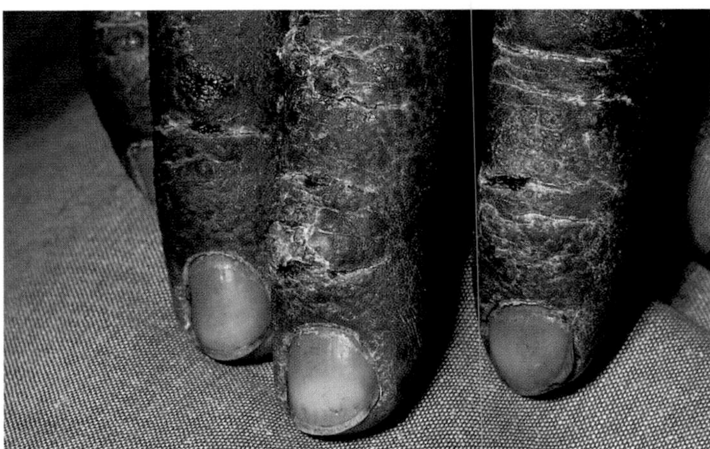

Figure 7.15 Chronic exposure to chromates in cement can be associated with hyperkeratotic and crusted changes, as seen here (Conde-Salazar et al, 1995a).

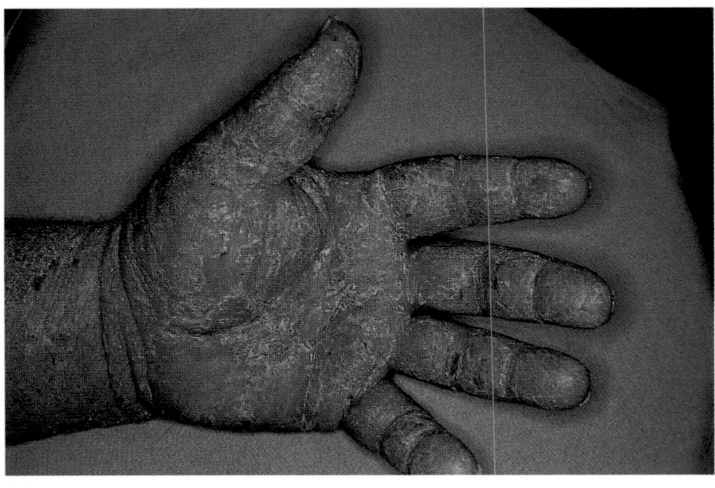

(**a**)

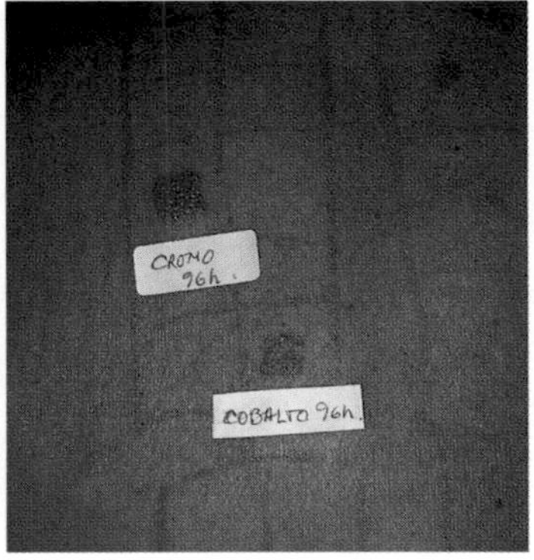

(**b**)

Figure 7.16 (**a**) The palm may also be involved in allergic contact dermatitis due to chromate in cement. (**b**) These are the patch tests of the patient: he was allergic to cobalt and chromate, both of which are found in cement.

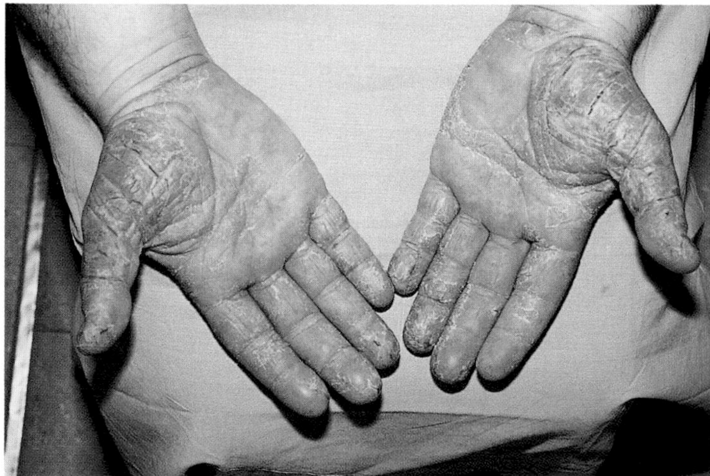

Figure 7.17 This is another example of the hyperkeratotic features that can develop into allergic contact dermatitis to chromate.

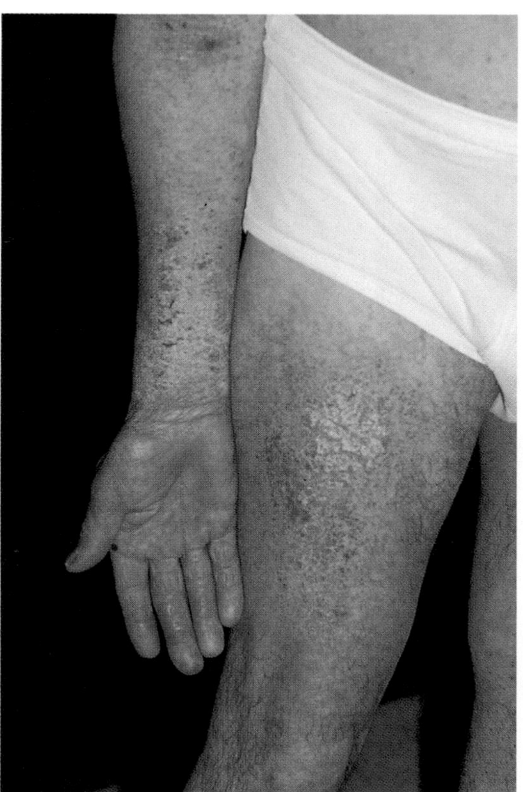

Figure 7.18 Occupational contact dermatitis to chromate from cement is not confined to the hands. It can spread to other areas, as seen here, and can be made worse by other factors. This patient was allergic to chromate, cobalt and nickel. Metal objects carried in his pockets contributed to the eruption on his thighs.

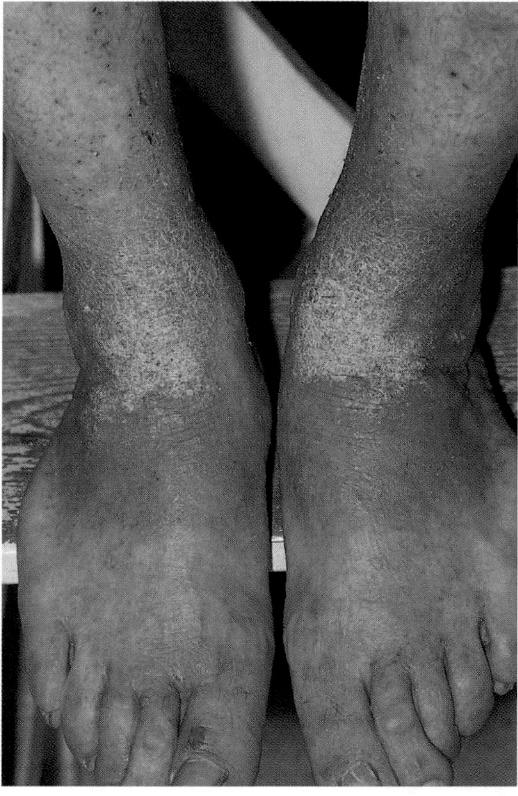

Figure 7.19 This construction worker experienced a similar problem to that seen in Figure 7.11. The use of inappropriate footware (i.e. sandals) provided inadequate protection. In this case, he was actually found to be allergic to chromate.

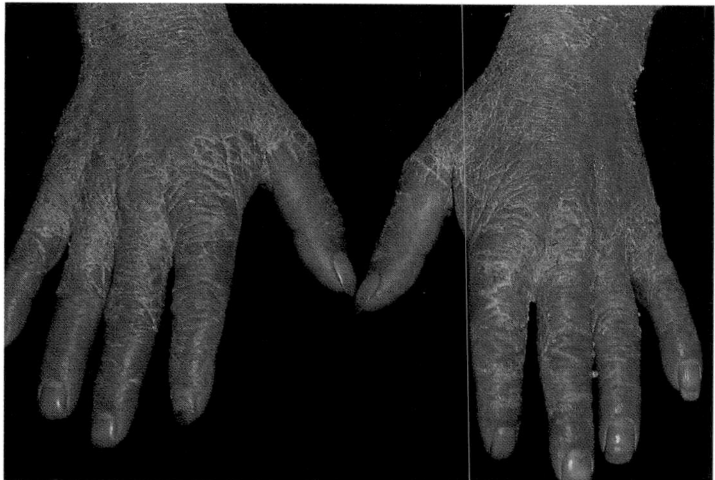

Figure 7.20 Efforts to protect this worker who was allergic to chromate in cement were not helpful. He was told to wear rubber gloves, but proved to be allergic to the rubber allergens thiuram and mercapto mix (Hogan et al, 1990).

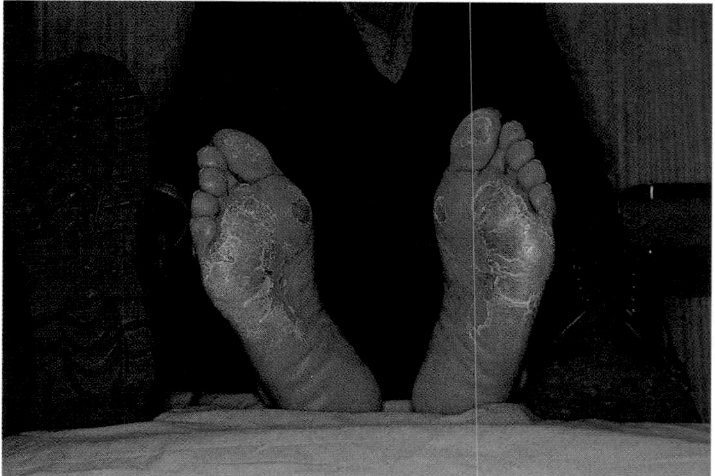

Figure 7.21 This is another example of persistent dermatitis caused by protective clothing. Rubber boots were to be worn for protection. However, the worker was allergic to the rubber antioxidants found in his boots, which were detected with the black rubber mix patch test chemicals.

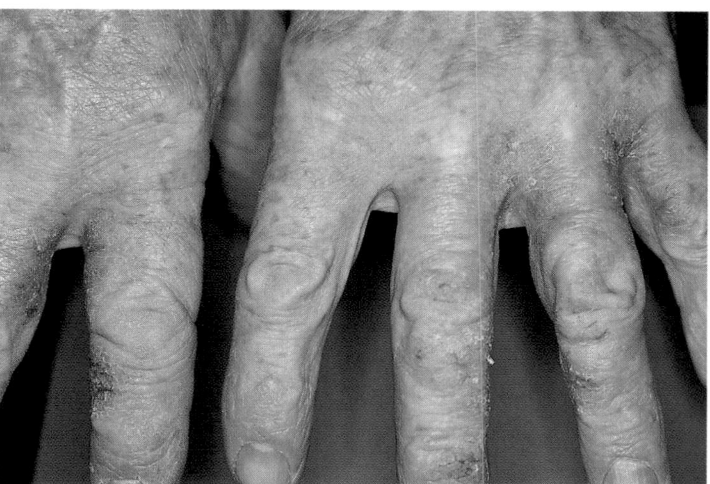

Figure 7.22 This 61-year-old man developed pruritic interdigital dermatitis after using fibre insulating material. The dermatitis was mechanical irritant contact dermatitis from the fibres. Allergic sensitization to fibreglass is rare (Fisher, 1982).

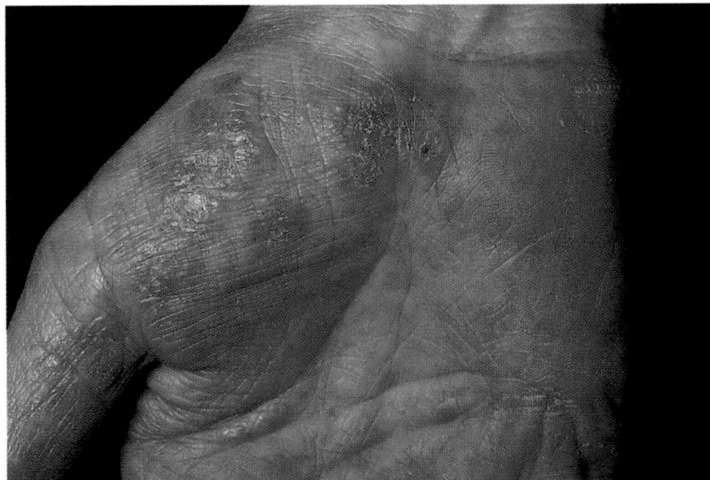

Figure 7.23 A 58-year-old male builder developed dermatitis of the right palm. The dermatitis appeared after he began working with plywood. Patch testing was negative. This proved to be a mechanical irritant contact dermatitis caused by constant testing of the surface of the plywood with his right palm.

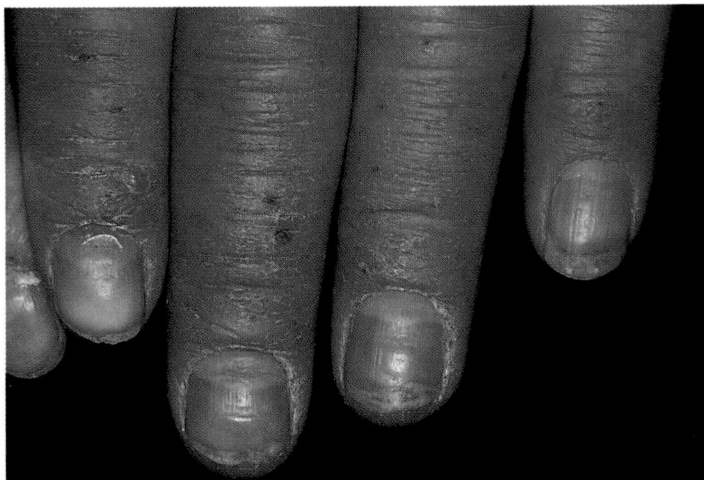

Figure 7.24 This is a 45-year-old house painter who was seen for hand dermatitis suspected to have an occupational cause. He had used a water-based paint that contained methylchloroisothiazolinone–methylisothiazolinone (Kathon CG) as a preservative. He was allergic to this preservative.

Health Care

Health professionals can be defined as 'all workers who have the common mission of promoting or preserving health'. This group of professionals includes those directly associated with health (doctors, nurses, auxiliaries, etc.) and those employed in health services (food, housekeeping, maintenance, etc.) as well as workers in the pharmaceutical industry. In many countries, health personnel (including those involved in the manufacture of pharmaceutical products) make up one of the largest occupational groups.

In the United Kingdom, the National Health Service is the largest employer in the country, with a staff of more than a million, while in the USSR during the 1980s, there were more than one million doctors.

In Eastern Europe there are, on average, 100–200 physicians per 100 000 inhabitants, the nurse–physician ratio being about 4:1.

Occupational dermatoses in health workers are difficult to classify because there are so many professions, in which the risks are very different (radiologists, surgeons, biochemists, pharmacists, nurses, dentists, etc.), and one can find dermatoses not only of chemical origin (irritant and allergic), but also of infectious and physical origin (radiodermitis).

In general, contact dermatitis of health workers is due to the handling of different chemical products – sometimes used as work materials, sometimes for hygiene and disinfection. In particular, dentists and dental technicians, because of their use of various (mainly acrylic) resins, show a fairly high level of sensitization. Similarly, orthopaedic surgeons have a high level of sensitization due to the use of acrylic cements.

The incidence of irritant dermatitis can be high among nurses and operating theatre staff, because of the use of many antimicrobial products and the frequent washing of hands. In addition, sensitization to latex, particularly allergic contact urticaria from contact with latex, is frequent, resulting in serious repercussions among this group of personnel.

Most cases of contact dermatitis in the health professions involve the hands. The variety of insults to the hands include frequent exposure to detergents and disinfectants, medications, gloves, and chemicals unique to the profession. Among the more allergenic chemicals are antimicrobials and acrylates.

The common irritants and allergens are shown in the box.

Irritants	Allergens
Antimicrobial products	Acrylic resins
Disinfectant soaps	Components of rubber gloves:
Formaldehyde solution	carbamates
Laboratory materials	mercaptobenzothiazoles
Solvents	thiurams
	Epoxy resins
	Formaldehyde solution
	Glutaraldehyde
	Latex
	Medications:
	analgesics (e.g. propacetamol; see Barbaud et al, 1995)
	antibiotics
	sulfonamides
	Photographic developers (radiologists)

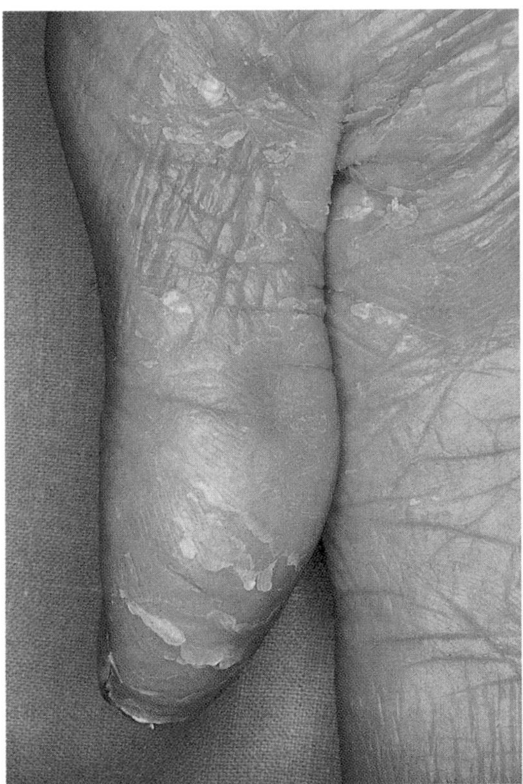

Figure 7.25 A case of irritant contact dermatitis in a surgical nurse.

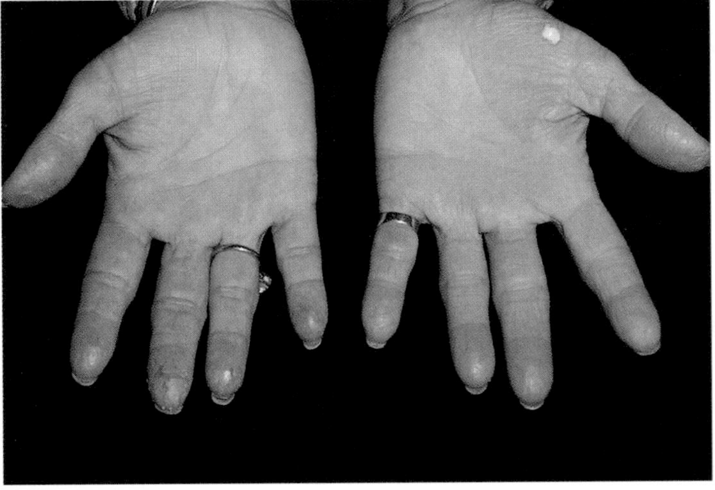

Figure 7.26 This member of a surgical staff had irritant contact dermatitis. She washed her hands many times a day, but had no positive patch test reactions (Camarasa and Conde-Salazar, 1987).

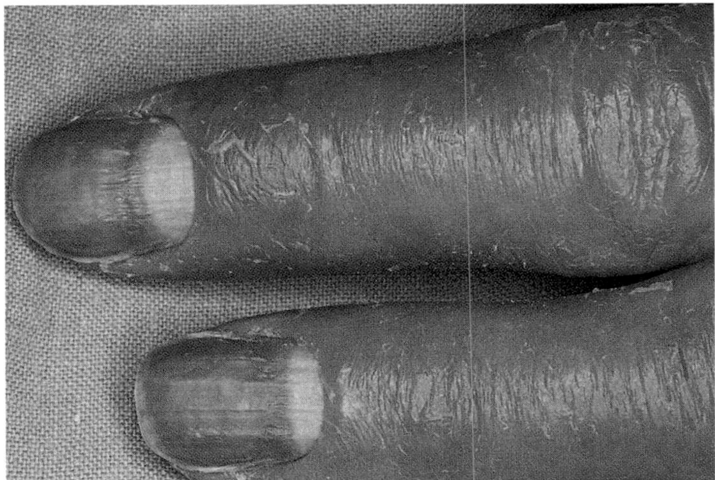

Figure 7.27 This intensive care unit nurse had irritant contact dermatitis. Patch tests were negative, and repeated washing of the hands with disinfectant products was believed to be the source of this dermatitis. Irritant contact dermatitis is more common than allergic contact dermatitis in most studies (Camarasa and Conde-Salazar, 1987; Meding and Swanbeck, 1990).

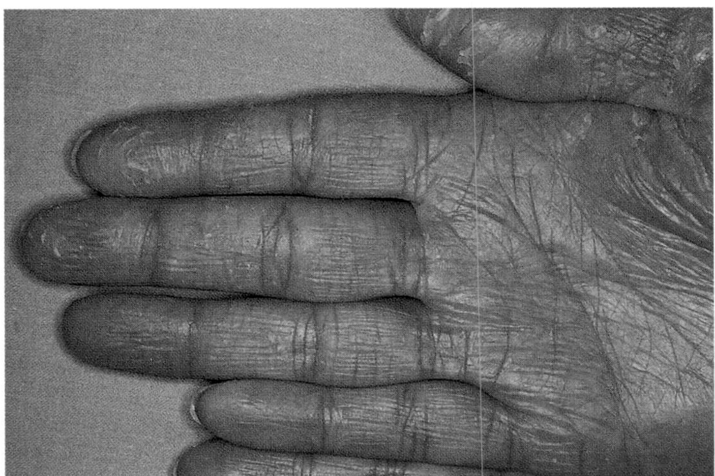

(**a**)

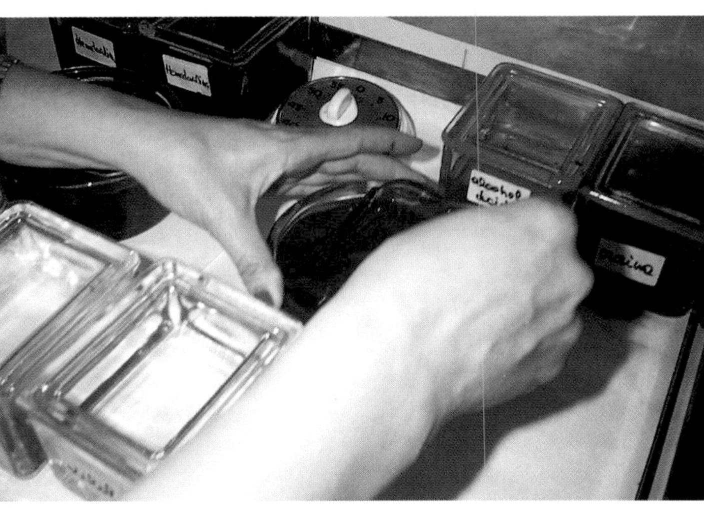

(**b**)

Figure 7.28 It is not unusual for a worker to suspect the chemicals that they handle in their work to be responsible for their dermatitis. (**a**) A laboratory technician worked with the materials seen in (**b**), and believed these to be the cause of the eruption. The correct diagnosis was irritant contact dermatitis, and patch tests were negative (Camarasa and Conde-Salazar, 1987).

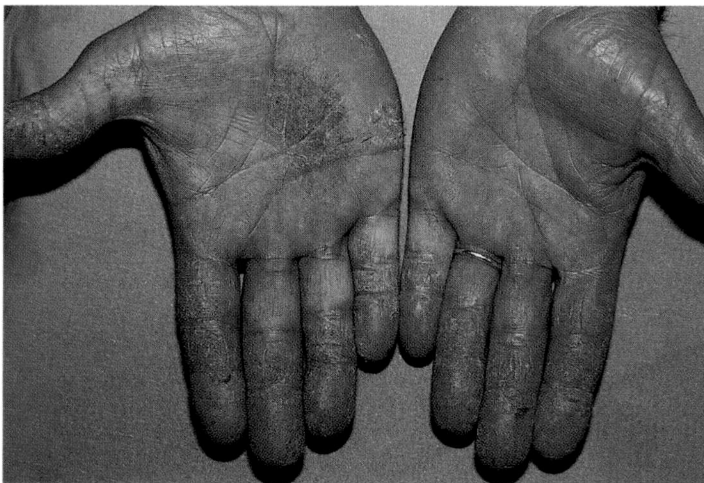

Figure 7.29 This laboratory technician was frequently exposed to formaldehyde, and patch testing revealed allergy to formaldehyde. The morphologies of irritant and allergic contact dermatitis can be very similar, and patch tests are required to clarify the source of the problem.

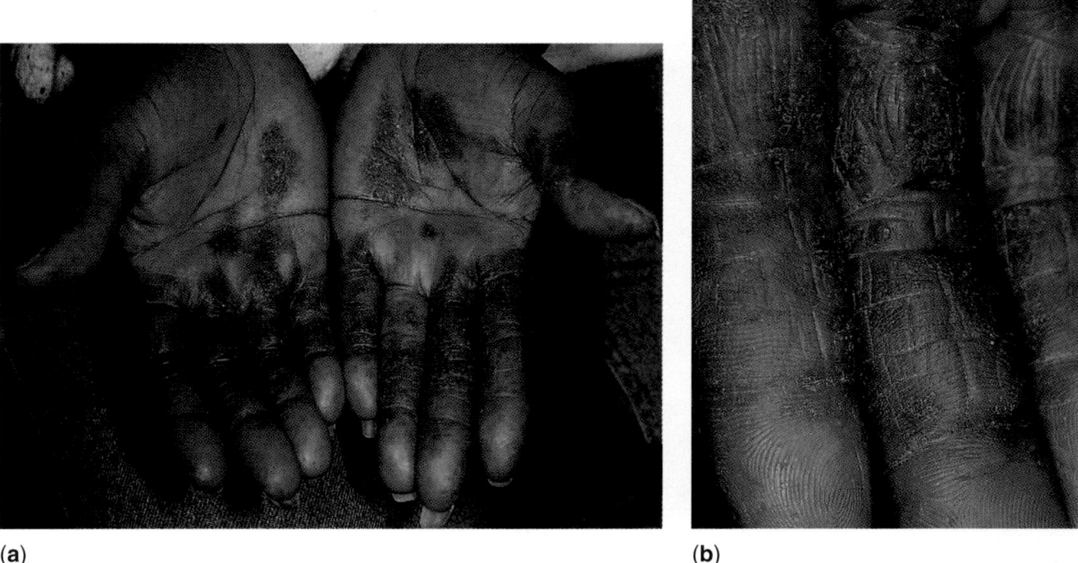

(**a**) (**b**)

Figure 7.30 (**a**, **b**) This darkly-pigmented African–American housekeeper worked at a nursing home and had had hand dermatitis for 15 years. Hyperpigmentation was prominent in this case. Patch testing revealed allergy to nickel and thiuram derivatives, the latter being present in the gloves she wore at work and home.

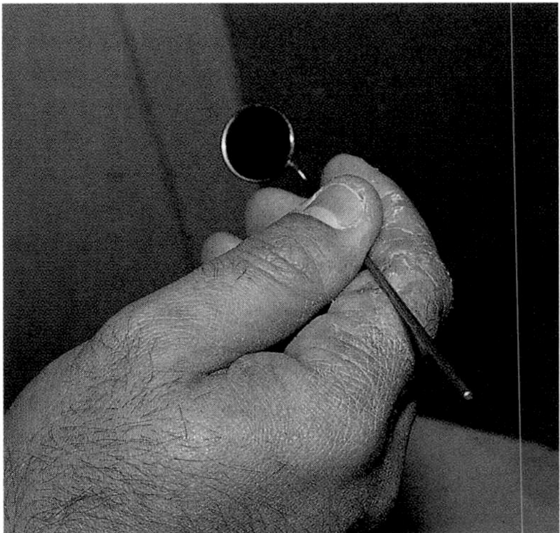

Figure 7.31 Nickel is the most commonly identified allergen detected by screening patch test series, and can be a problem in the health professions if metal instruments release nickel – as was the case for this individual. Stainless steel instruments are usually safe and do not release enough nickel to cause dermatitis.

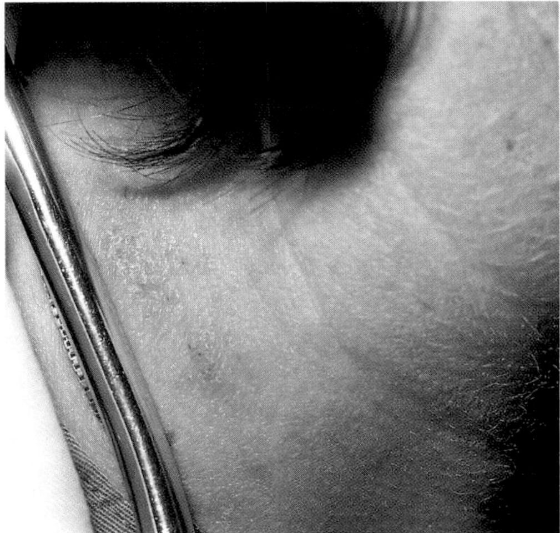

Figure 7.32 Nickel released from the metal components of this stethoscope led to dermatitis of the neck. This patient had previously been sensitized by costume jewellery.

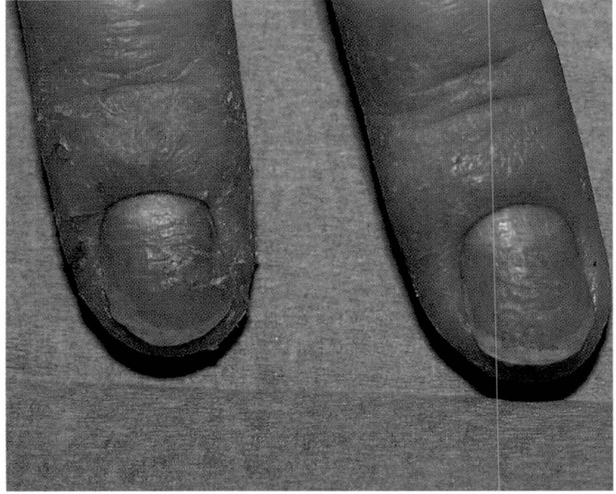

(**a**)

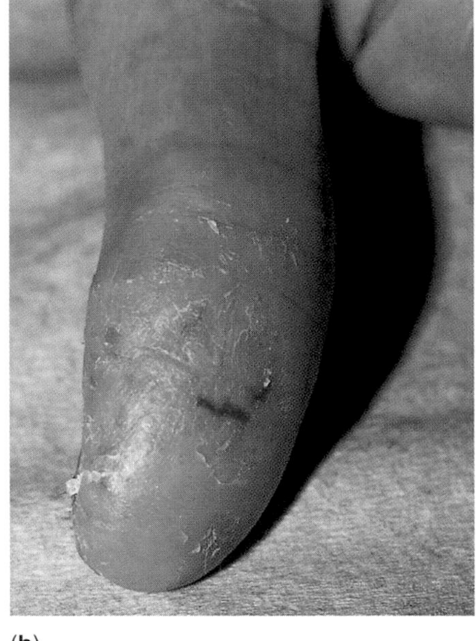

(**b**)

Figure 7.33 (**a**, **b**) Allergic contact dermatitis of the fingertips developed in a nurse who was exposed to cephalosporins and semisynthetic penicillins, which were the source of this reaction.

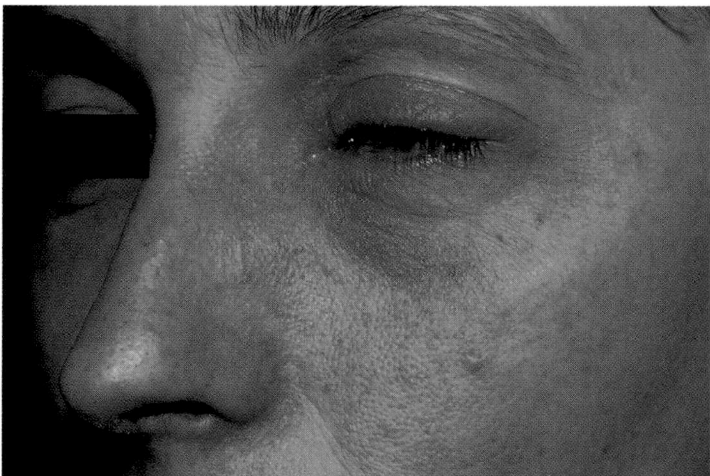

Figure 7.34 Allergic contact urticaria on the eyelids of a nurse due partially to airborne and partially to hand transfer of latex proteins present in natural rubber gloves. Immediate hypersensitvity to latex protein has been a new development over the past decade, and is most commonly manifested as itching and swelling of the hands within minutes of wearing latex gloves. It has been estimated that 5–10% of hospital-based doctors and nurses have this immediate-type hypersensitivity (Hamman, 1993).

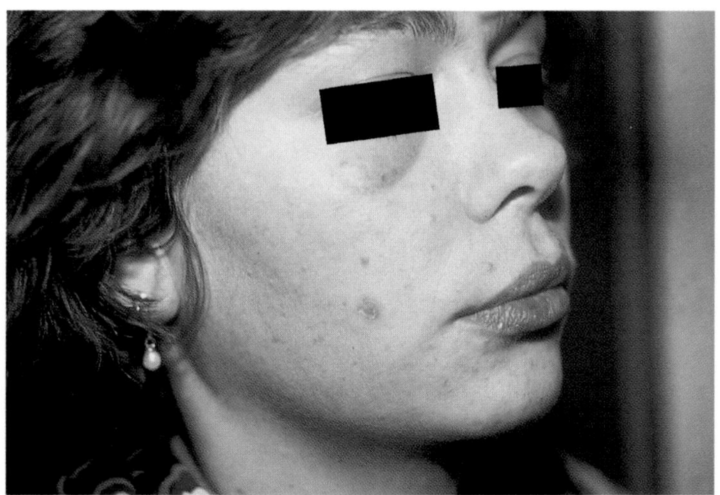

Figure 7.35 Powder in gloves can absorb natural latex protein, and the powder can become an airborne source of this allergen when gloves are removed. In this nurse, airborne latex caused dermatitis on areas of the face occluded by her surgical mask.

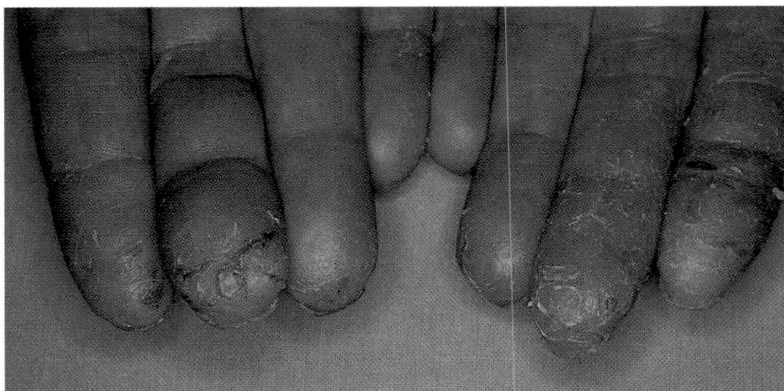

(a)

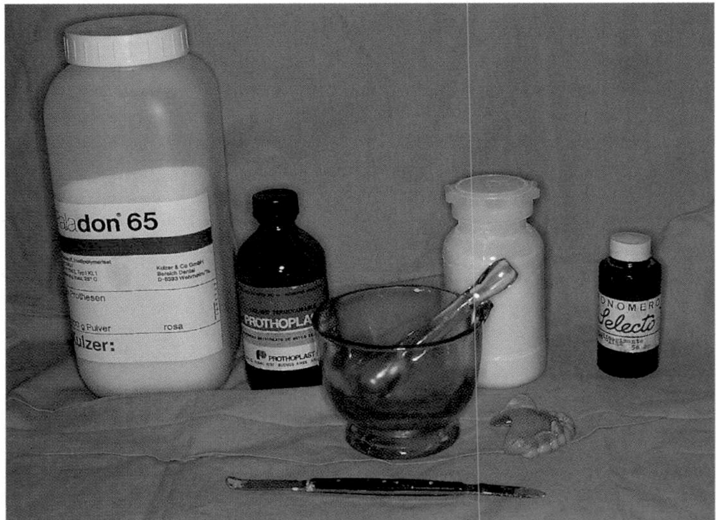

(b)

Figure 7.36 (**a**) Fingertip dermatitis is characteristic of acrylate allergy in the dental profession. Prostheses are made from acrylates, as seen in (**b**).

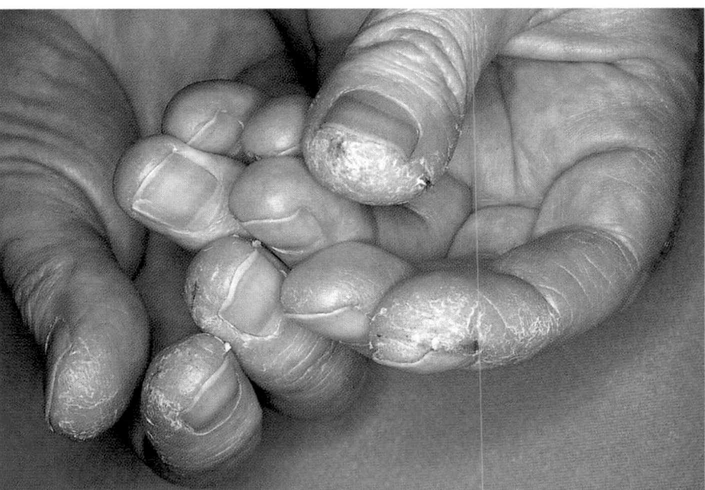

(a)

Figure 7.37 Acrylates were also responsible for the dermatitis seen here (**a**).

Cont.

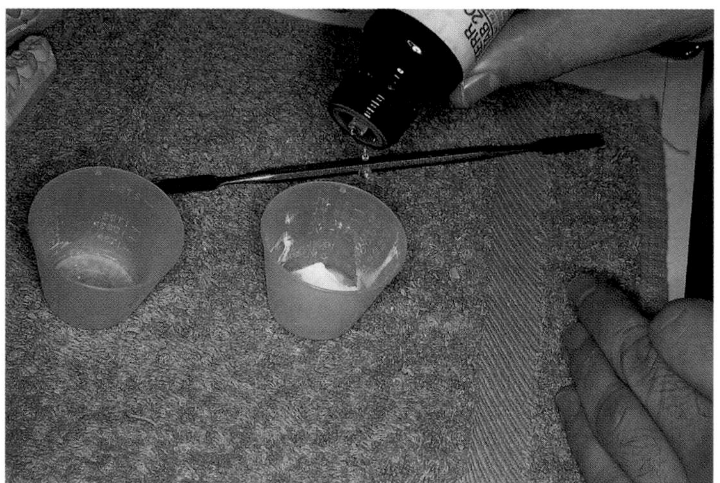
(**b**)

Figure 7.37 *continued* The method of handling these allergens is seen in (**b**). No protective measures were taken in the mixing of resin and hardener. The method of finishing the work is illustrated in (**c**), and (**d**) is the finished acrylate product.

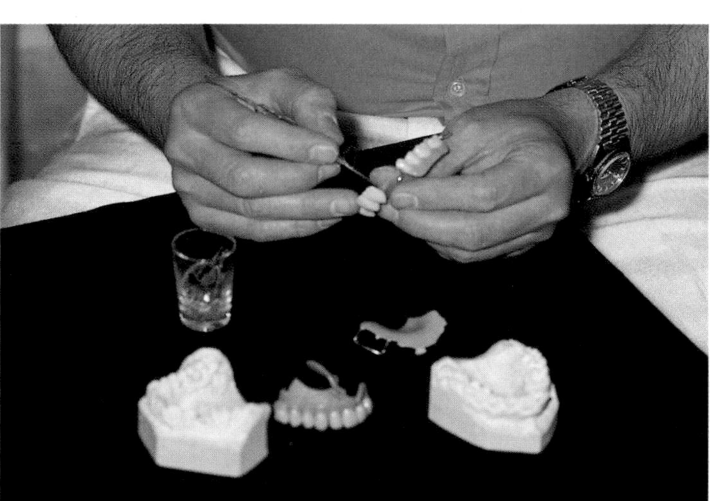
(**c**)

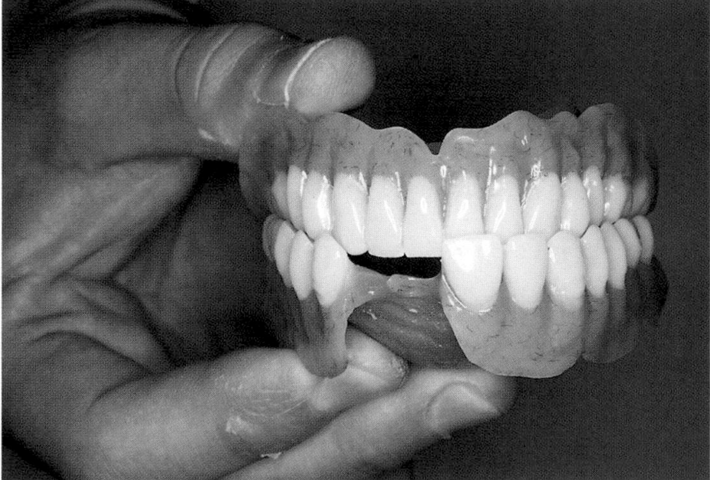
(**d**)

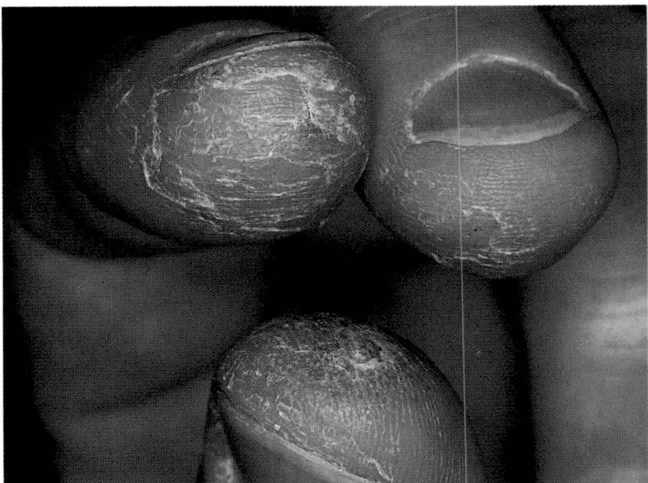

Figure 7.38 This 49-year-old dentist developed fissured dermatitis on the thumb, index and middle fingers of his left hand. These fingers were used in direct and indirect contact with acrylate dental fillings. Patch testing showed a strongly positive reaction to acrylates. He was able to continue to work as a dentist by protecting his hands with gloves whenever possible and by exchanging the offending acrylates with other types of plastic. Ordinary rubber gloves do not protect against acrylates, but some degree of protection is afforded by nitrile rubber (Rietschel et al, 1984; Conde-Salazar et al, 1988a).

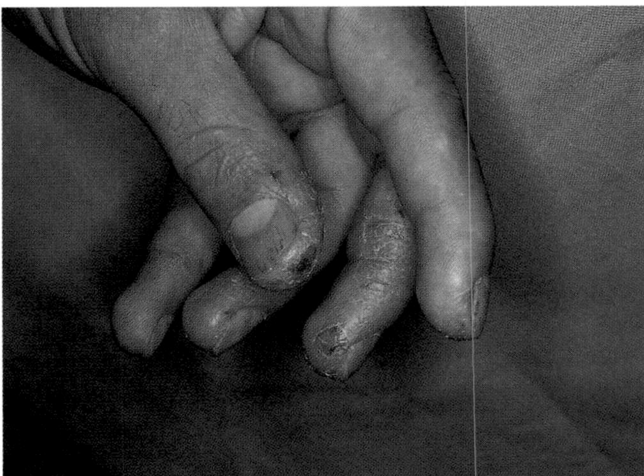

Figure 7.39 A pattern similar to acrylate sensitivity was seen in this dentist, who was allergic to mercury and was exposed to it in dental amalgam (Conde-Salazar et al, 1988a).

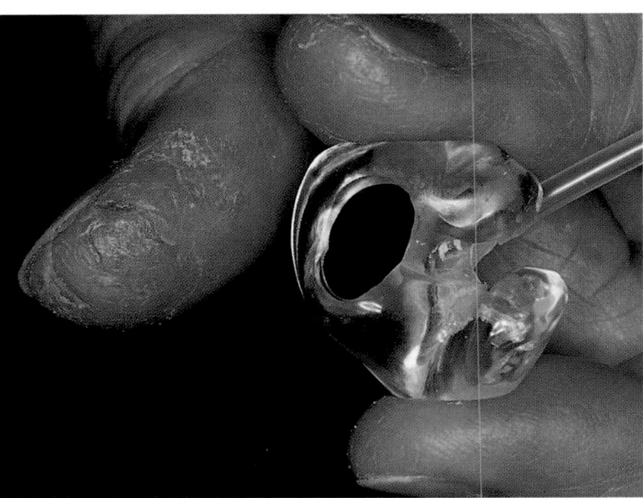

Figure 7.40 A 63-year-old woman developed fissured dermatitis on her right thumb. There was similar, but less extensive, dermatitis on the index and middle fingers of the right hand. Patch testing revealed a positive reaction to methyl methacrylate. The dermatitis persisted in spite of treatment with topical corticosteroids, because she did not want to give up her job and because it was not possible to protect the fingers against contact with acrylates. 4-H gloves, which effectively block the penetration of acrylates, are too coarse to wear when working with small objects. She achieved some degree of protection by cutting off the fingertips of the 4-H gloves and wearing them inside rubber gloves.

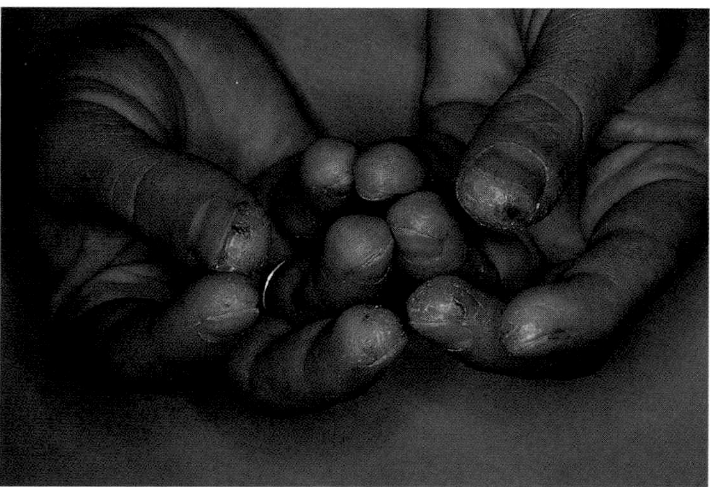

(**a**)

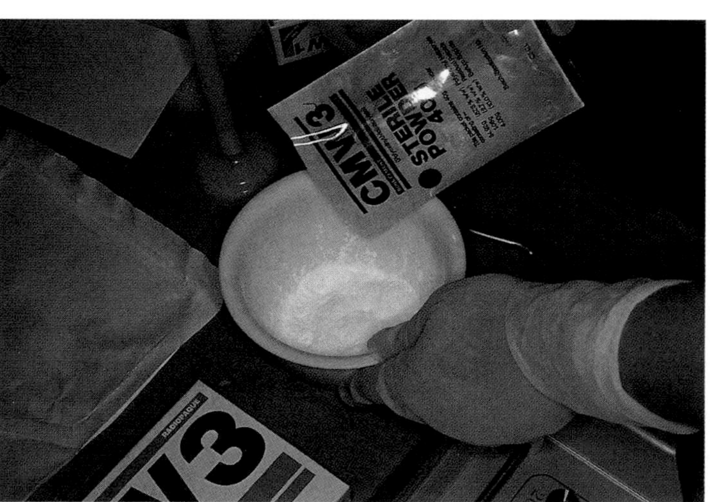

(**b**)

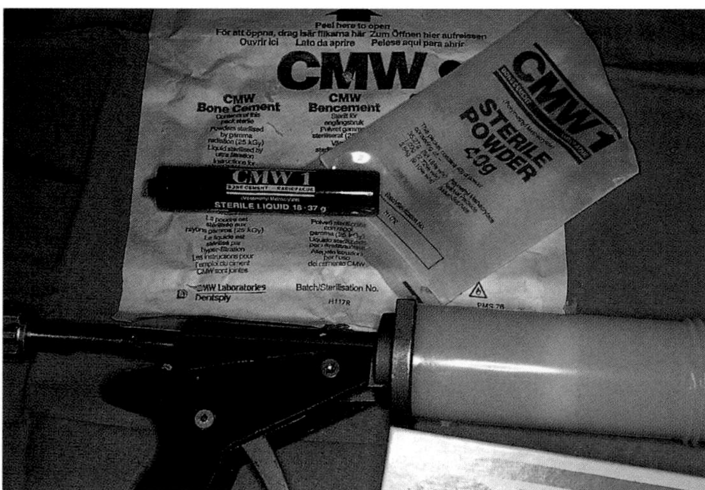

(**c**)

Figure 7.41 Orthopaedic surgeons use acrylate bone cement to attach hip prostheses, and may develop contact dermatitis to this material, which passes rapidly through gloves (Fisher, 1975). (**a**) The hands of such a surgeon, who was patch-test positive to multiple acrylates. (**b**) The method of making bond cement. (**c**) The components.

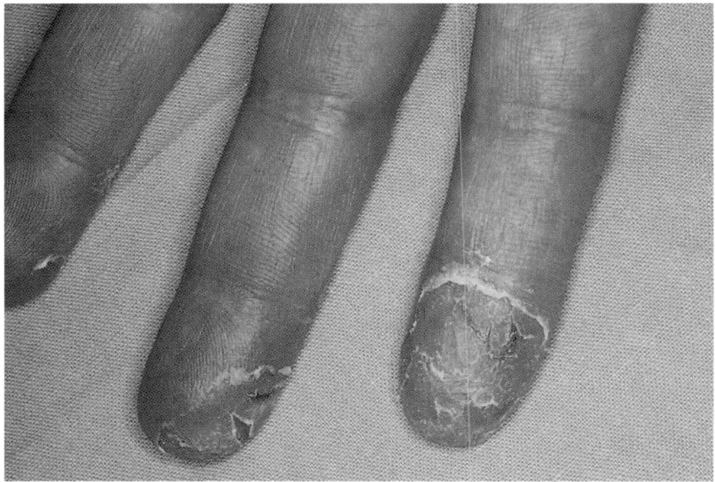

(**a**)

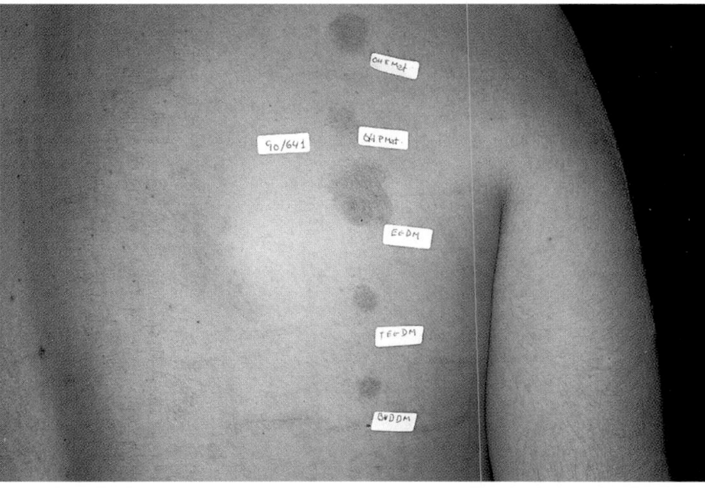

(**b**)

Figure 7.42 This is another example of an orthopaedic surgeon with the same problem, but to a lesser degree, as the surgeon in Figure 7.41. (**a**) The fingers typically involved – these are used to mould the embedding cement. (**b**) The multiple positive patch tests to acrylates in this surgeon.

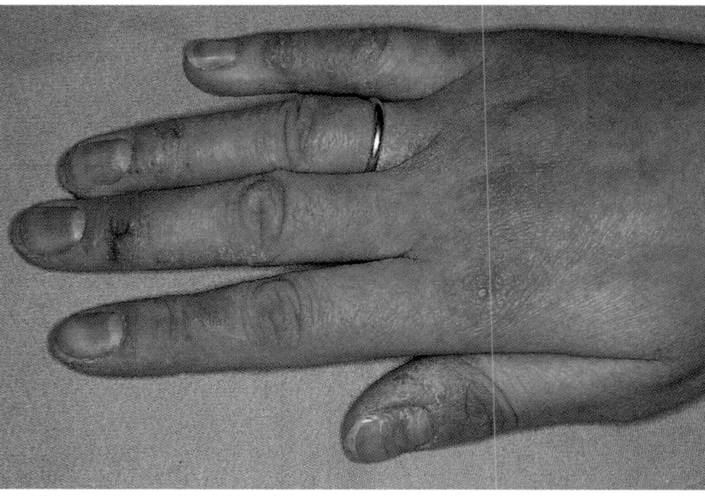

Figure 7.43 Another resin that can cause fingertip dermatitis in pathologists and technicians is epoxy resin, as in the case seen here. The exposure occurs during the embedding process for electron microscopy. Epoxy resin components are sometimes also used in immersion oils for microscopy (Le Coz and Goossens, 1998).

Acrylates, Epoxy and Other Resins

Epoxy resins are such common allergens that they are included in routine patch test series. About 75% of epoxy resins are based on the diglycidyl ether of bisphenol A (Kanerva et al, 1992). The lower-molecular-weight resins are the most allergenic. Resins with a molecular weight of around 340 are liquid and are the most versatile in industrial applications, while resins of higher molecular weight are solid. Testing for allergy to resins, particularly phenol–formaldehyde resins, may require use of the specific industrial material, since a standard patch test chemical may be sufficiently different from the industrial chemical to give a false-negative patch test reading (Bruze, 1986).

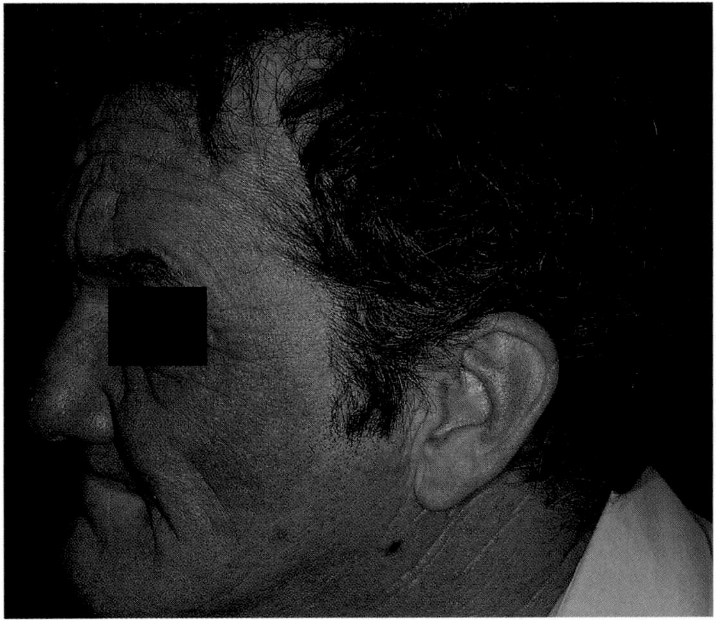

Figure 7.44 Facial dermatitis with involvement of the eyelids occurs with airborne exposure to epoxy resin vapours. This is especially a problem when the resin is heated. This man was sensitized when an industrial accident resulted in an explosion that covered him with epoxy resin. After the dermatitis from that accident cleared, he experienced the dermatitis seen here when working around areas where epoxy resins were being mixed and heated. No direct skin contact was necessary to produce this reaction.

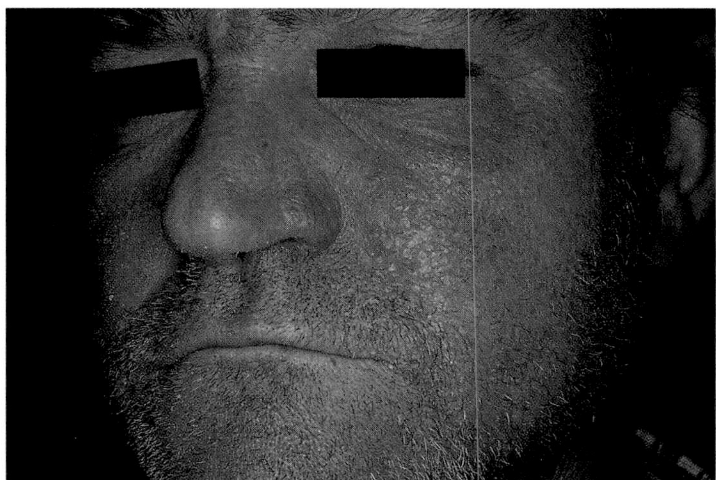
(**a**)

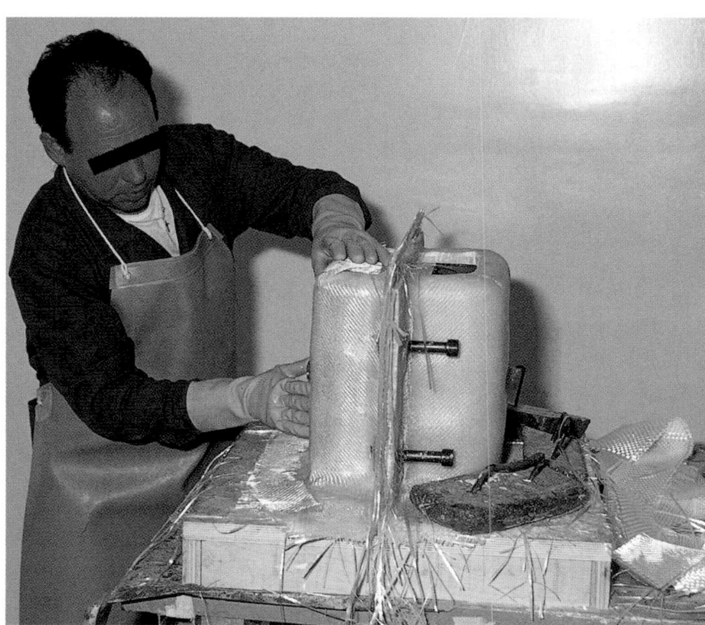
(**b**)

Figure 7.45 This man worked with epoxy resin in the aeronautical industry, and experienced the airborne pattern of dermatitis seen in (**a**). The nature of his exposure in the workplace is illustrated in (**b**).

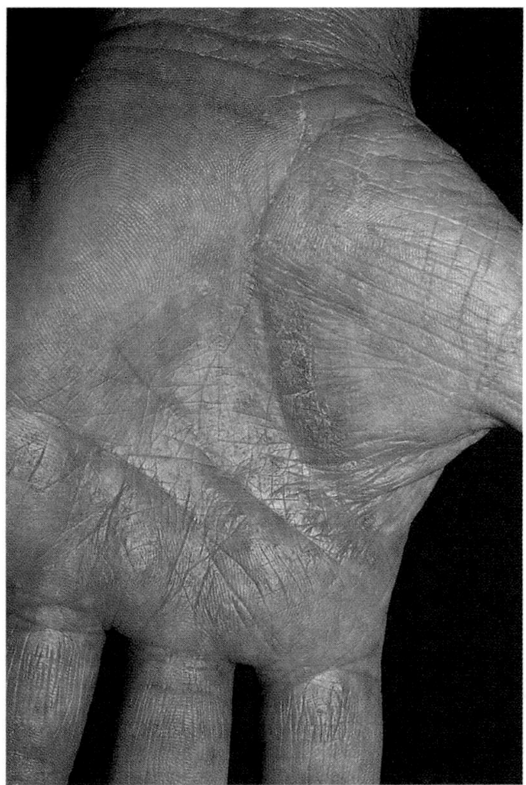

(**a**)

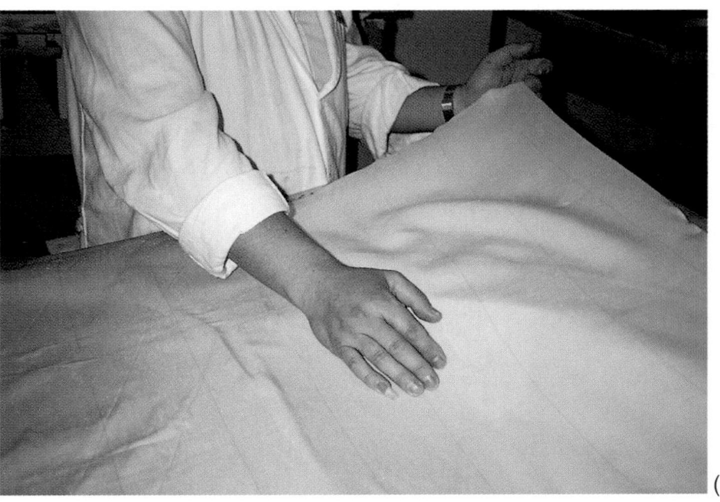

(**b**)

Figure 7.46 This man also worked in the aeronautical industry, and handled cloth coated with epoxy resin. He was patch-test positive to epoxy resin, and his hand dermatitis is seen in (**a**). The nature of his work exposure is seen in (**b**).

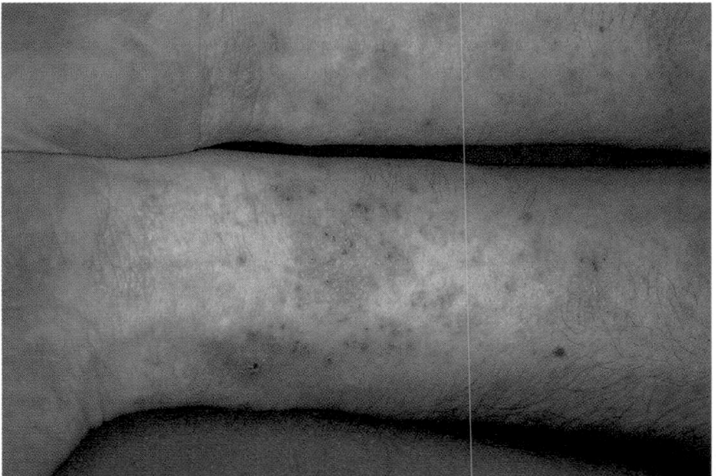

(a)

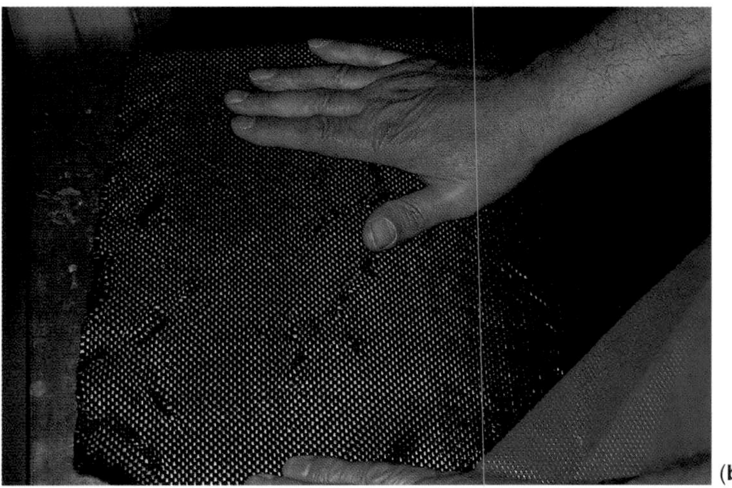

(b)

Figure 7.47 This man had dermatitis of the forearms from handling cloth treated with epoxy resin used in the manufacture of aircraft fuselages. (**a**) The allergic contact dermatitis. (**b**) The work exposure.

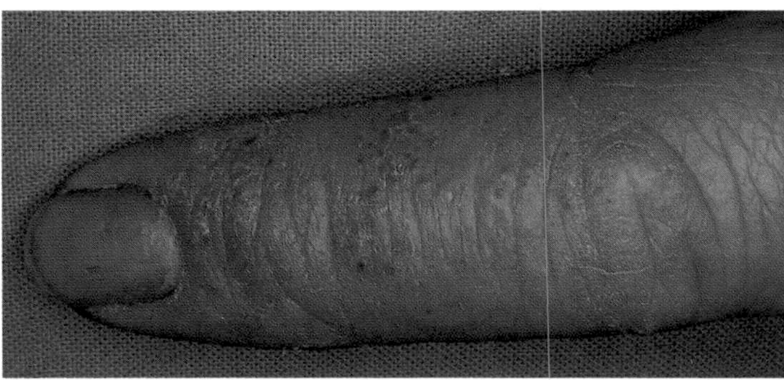

Figure 7.48 Finger dermatitis occurred in this plumber, who used epoxy resin for sealing cracks (Conde-Salazar et al, 1993a).

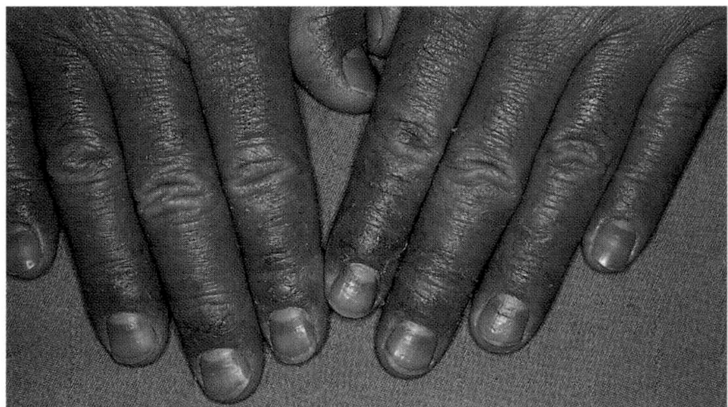

(**a**)

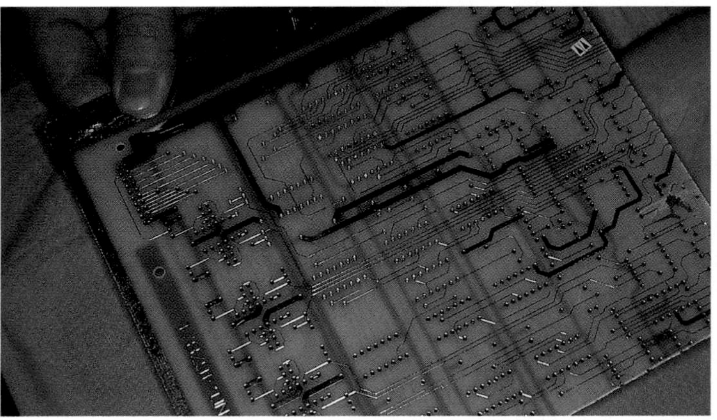

(**b**)

Figure 7.49 Epoxy resins are used as adhesives in the manufacture of electronic printed circuit boards and electronic chips. The hand dermatitis seen in (**a**) was caused by contact with objects such as those seen in (**b**). A patch test to epoxy resin was positive.

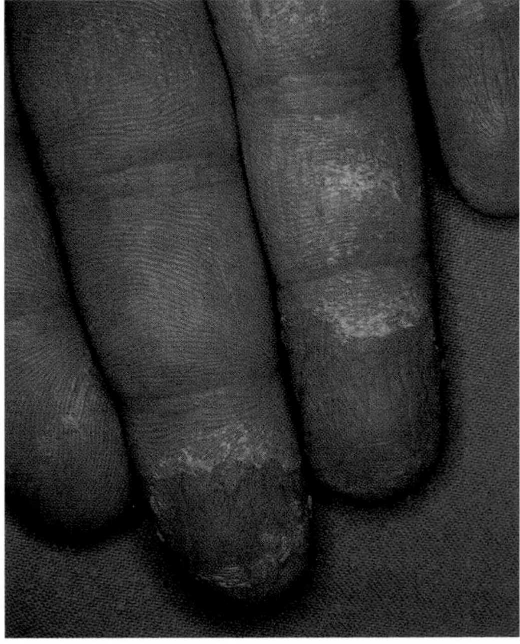

Figure 7.50 Costume jewellery was repaired with epoxy resin by the patient shown here: allergic contact dermatitis of the fingertips resulted from contact with the various objects.

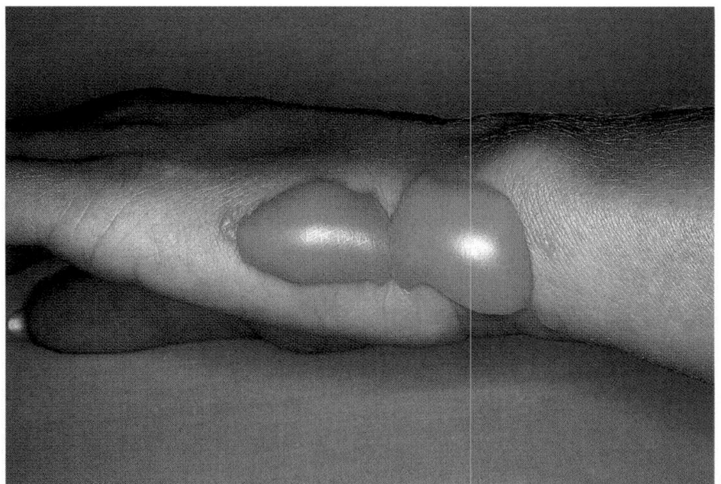
(**a**)

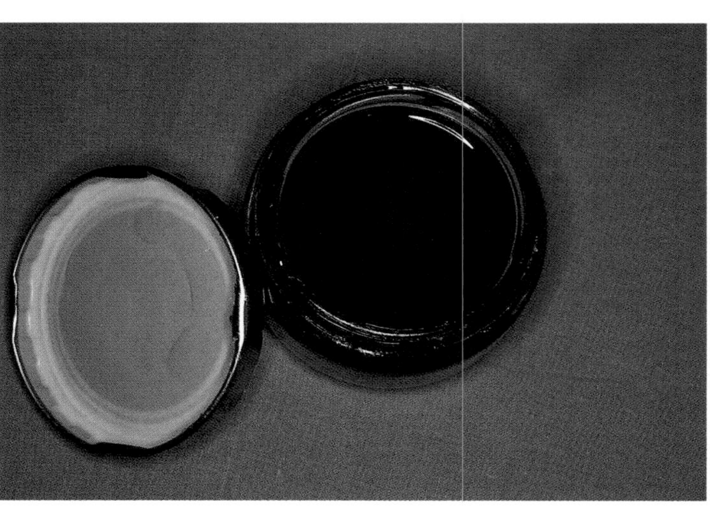
(**b**)

Figure 7.51 Acute dermatitis developed in this woman after she made leather handbags glued together with a *p-tert*-butylphenol–formaldehyde resin type of product. The dermatitis is seen in (**a**). The glue is seen in (**b**). Patch test to the *p-tert*-butylphenol–formaldehyde resin in the standard screening series was negative, but, as noted in the introduction to this section, the specific resin may be required to confirm the allergen.

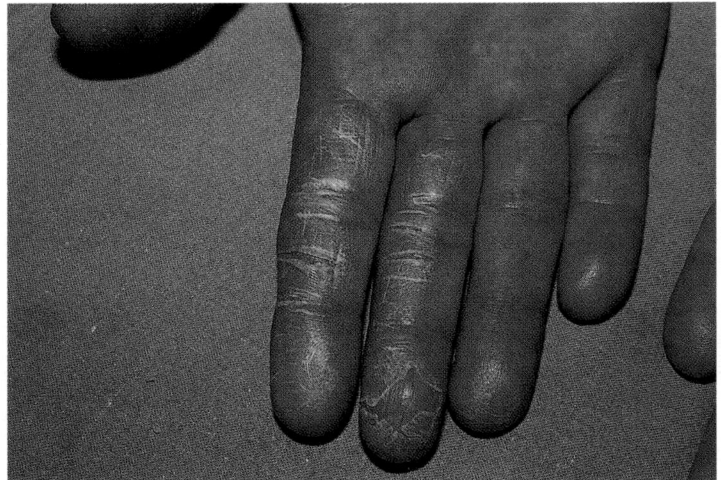

(**a**)

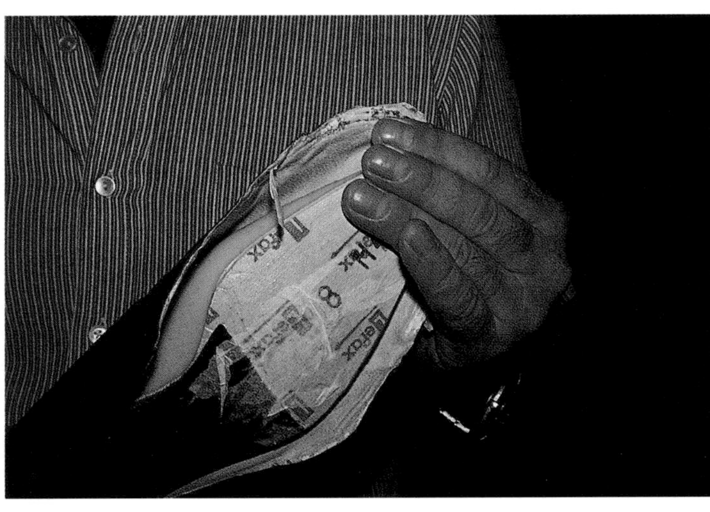

(**b**)

Figure 7.52 The most commonly used shoe repair glues contain *p-tert*-butylphenol–formaldehyde resins. This shoemaker developed a dry, hyperkeratotic palmar eruption seen in (**a**). He had a positive patch test to *p-tert*-butylphenol–formaldehyde resin, and the nature of his contact with the material is illustrated in (**b**) (Conde-Salazar et al, 1984).

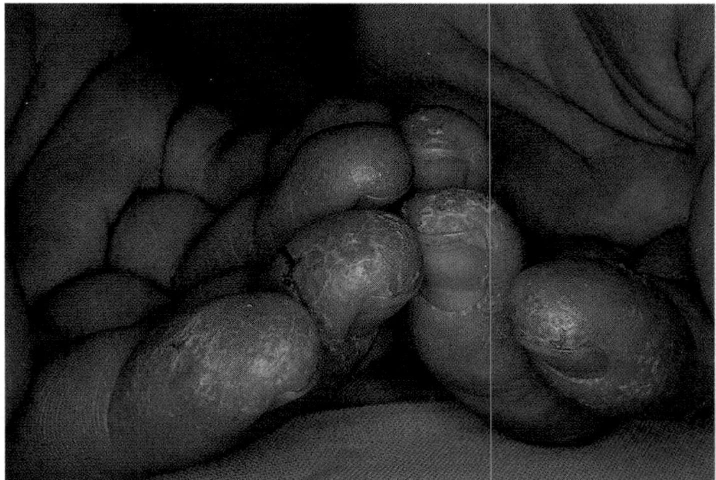

(**a**)

(**b**)

Figure 7.53 Dry, hyperkeratotic dermatitis of the distal one-third of the fingers occurred in this automobile worker from exposure to anaerobic sealants that contain acrylates, especially methyl methacrylate (Dempsey, 1982). The common usage of these sealants is illustrated in (**b**) (Conde-Salazar et al, 1988b).

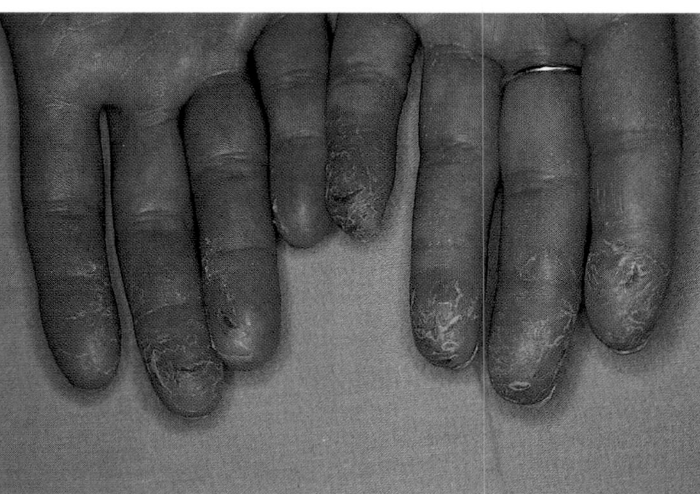

Figure 7.54 Acrylates can also be used to repair jewellery. Compare this case of allergic contact dermatitis due to methyl methacrylate with that in Figure 7.50, which was due to epoxy resin.

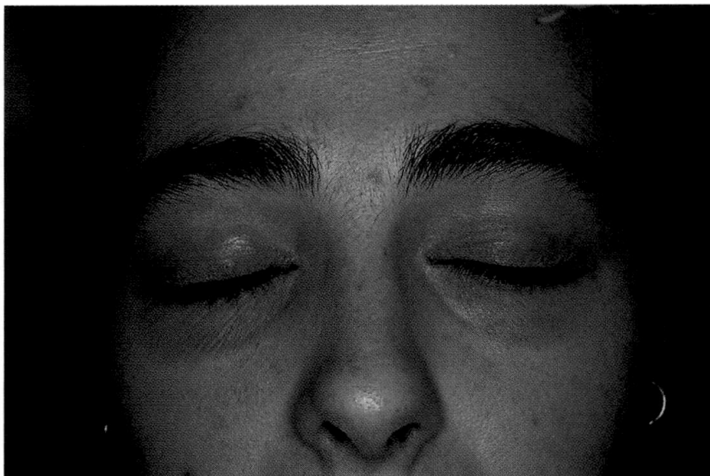

Figure 7.55 Acrylic nails were applied by this woman, who developed dermatitis of the eyelids, believed to be due to airborne exposure to the acrylates used to make artificial nails.

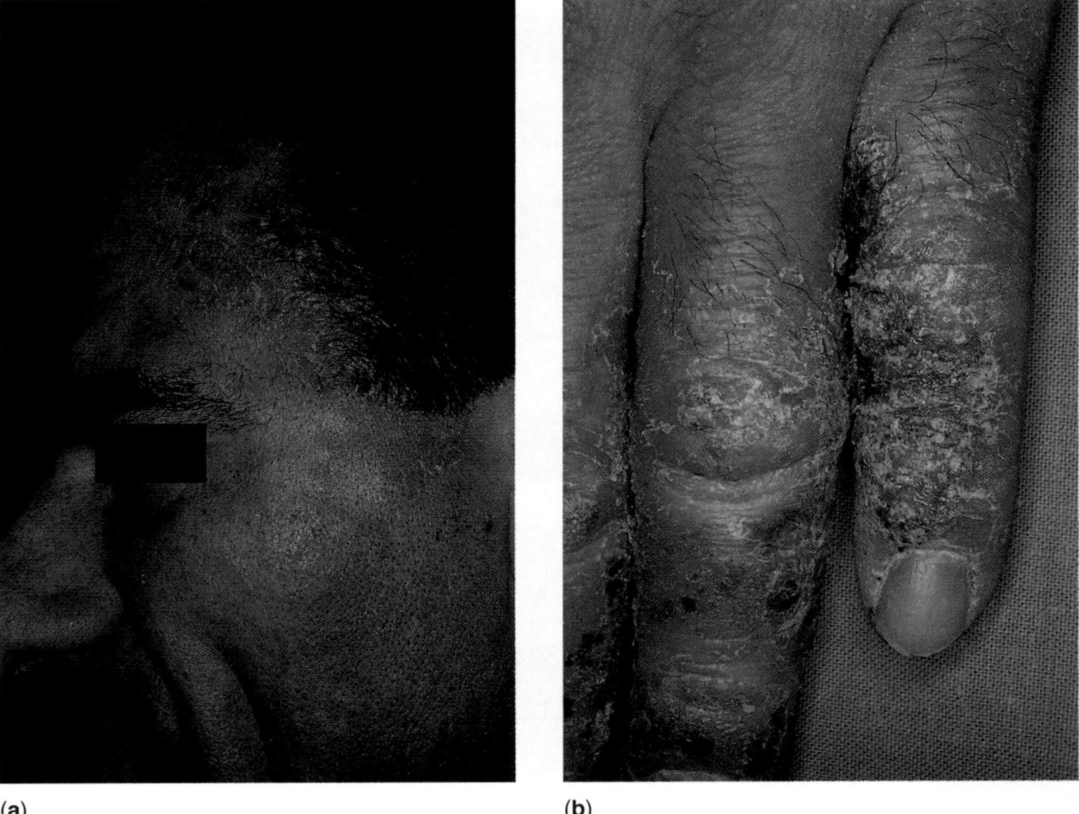

(**a**) (**b**)

Figure 7.56 This construction worker installed industrial flooring, and worked with various materials containing epoxy resin. He developed allergic contact dermatitis of the face (**a**), hands (**b**) and feet (**c**) (Conde-Salazar et al, 1994).

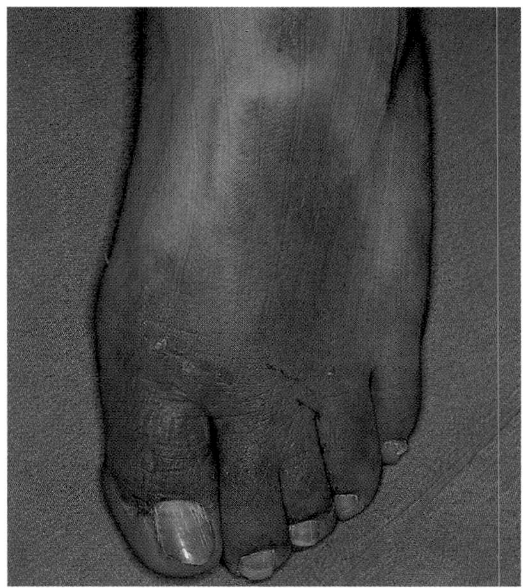

(c)

Figure 7.56 *continued*

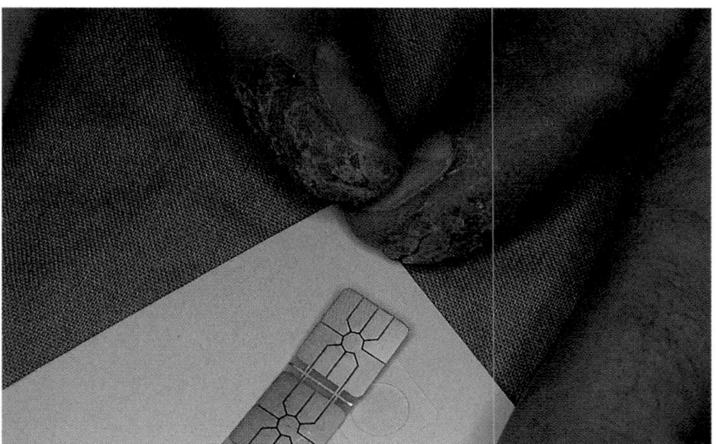

(a)

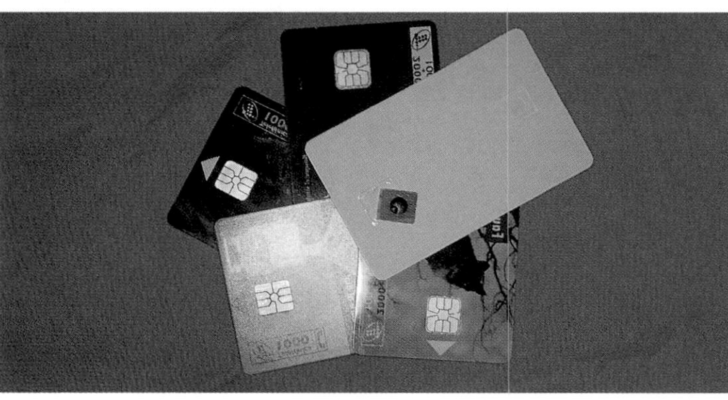

(b)

Figure 7.57 (**a**) The resin that caused this fingertip dermatitis was a cyanoacrylate. The patient manufactured telephone cards that required the gluing of a chip onto the card, as seen in (**b**). He was patch-test positive to cyanoacrylate (Conde-Salazar et al, 1998).

Rubber

Rubber allergens that cause contact dermatitis of the typical delayed hypersensitivity type are usually additives used to speed up the vulcanization process (rubber accelerators) or additives used to retard rubber oxidation (antioxidants) (Conde-Salazar, 1990). Immediate hypersensitivity to natural rubber latex is usually type 1 hypersensitivity with urticarial skin changes.

Contact urticaria is a common cutaneous reaction to natural rubber latex, and respiratory symptoms of type 1 hypersensitivity are sometimes seen in these patients. This immediate type of reaction will not be covered in this chapter.

Rubber screening patch test series contain the following chemicals or mixtures of chemicals:

- mercaptobenzothiazole;
- mercapto mix;
- thiuram mix;
- carba mix.

The mixture of paraphenylenediamine chemicals, commonly called the black rubber mix, is no longer available, and has been replaced in the standard series by *N*-isopropyl-*N'*-phenyl-*p*-phenylenediamine (IPPD). The latter is a rubber antioxidant, while the other components of the black rubber mix are rubber accelerators (Rietschel and Fowler, 1995, pp.24–7). Rubber antioxidants are a more common problem in industrial rubber products compared with accelerators, which are most commonly associated with consumer goods.

The typical distribution of rubber dermatitis is illustrated on the facing page. Common contact allergens are given in the box (Conde-Salazar, 1990).

Allergens
Carbamates
N-Isopropyl-*N'*-phenyl-*p*-phenylenediamine
Mercaptobenzothiazoles
Thiourea
Thiurams

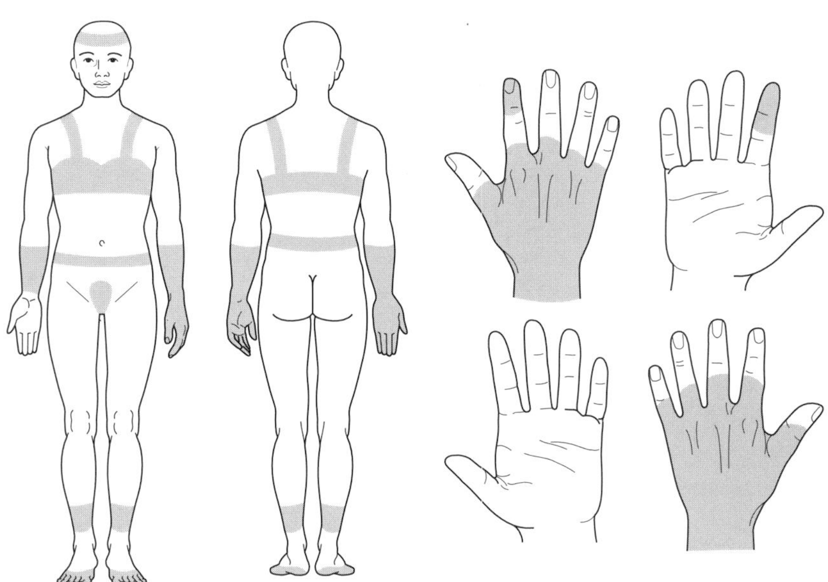

Typical distribution of rubber dermatitis

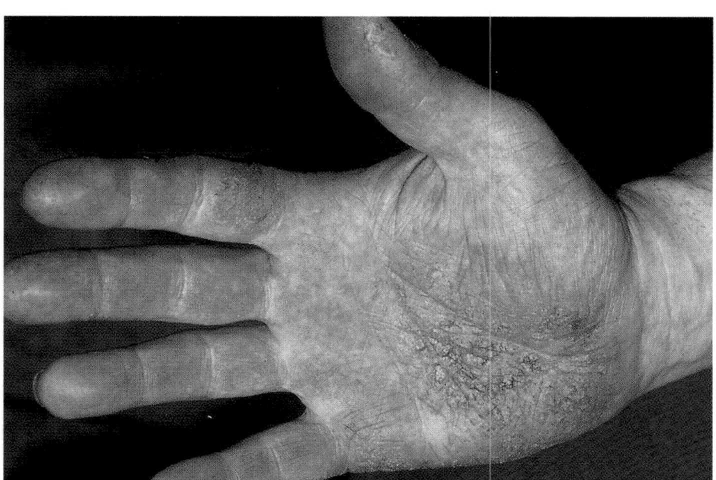

(a)

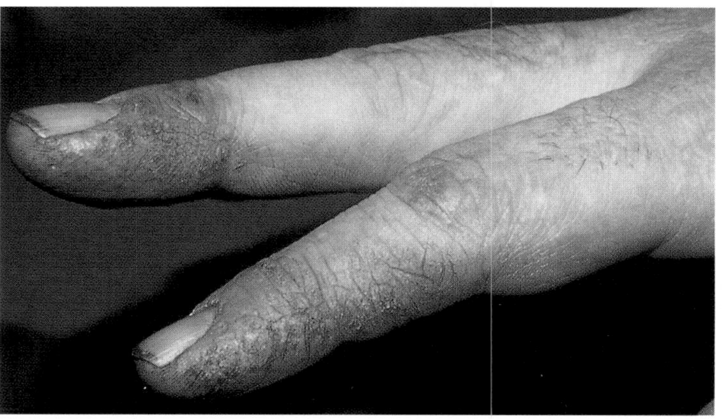

(b)

Figure 7.58 Hyperkeratotic eczema of the palms was due to mercaptobenzothiazole sensitivity in this mechanic, who was in daily contact with tyres, hoses and automobile belts. (**a**) Palmar side of the hand. (**b**) Detail of the fingers.

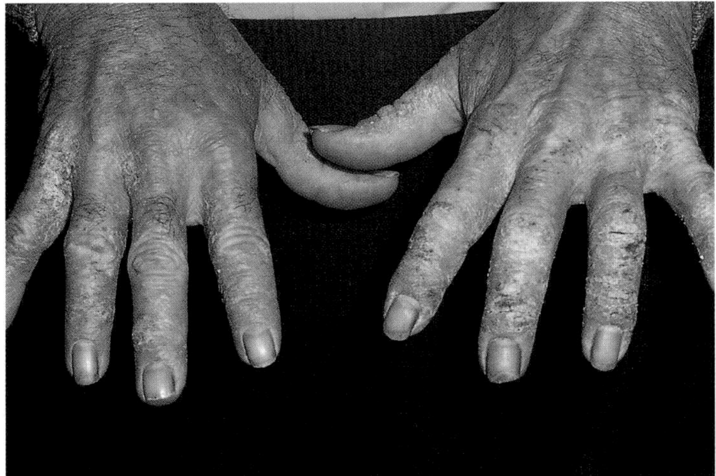

Figure 7.59 Rubber gloves were worn by this construction worker with allergic contact dermatitis. He was patch-test positive to a thiuram derivative present in his gloves (Conde-Salazar, 1990; Conde-Salazar et al, 1993b).

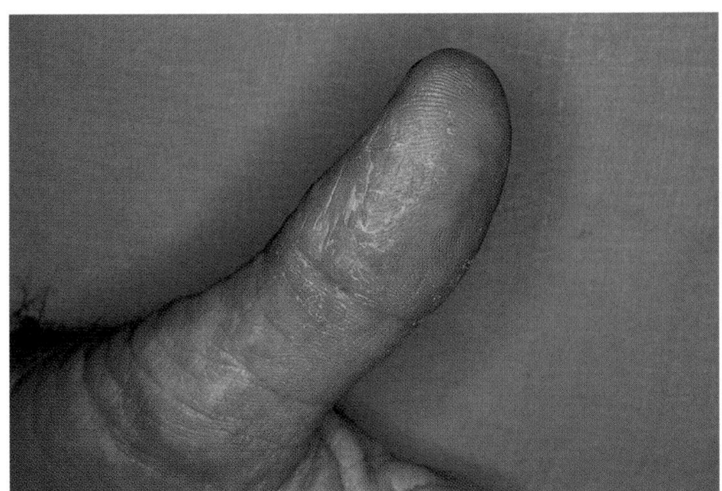

(**a**)

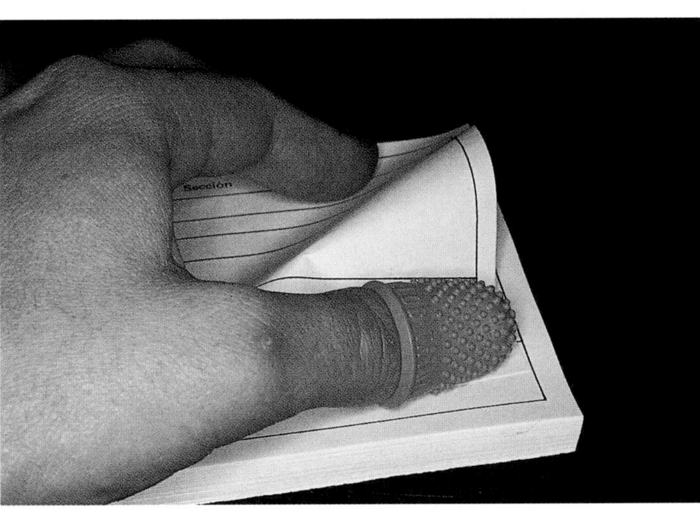

(**b**)

Figure 7.60 (**a**) The changes seen on the thumb of this office worker were allergic contact dermatitis due to a thiuram derivative. The cause of this dermatitis is seen in (**b**). A rubber thimble was worn on this digit (Conde-Salazar, 1990; Conde-Salazar et al, 1993b).

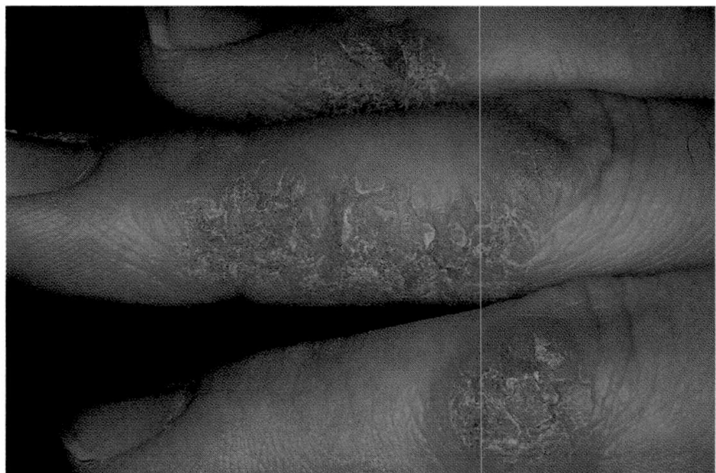
(**a**)

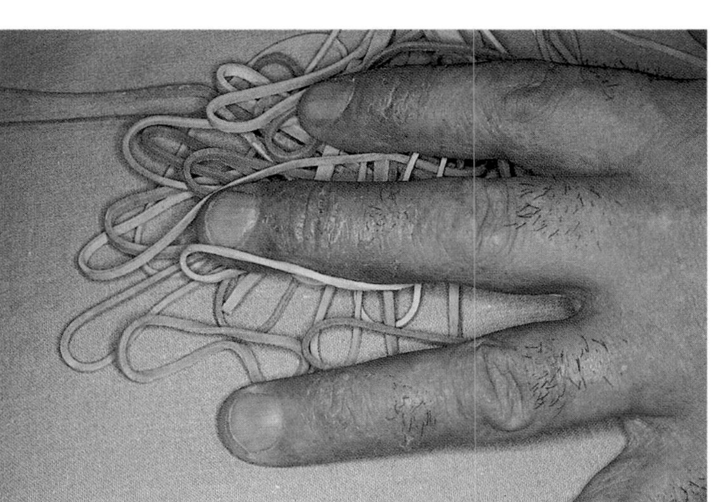
(**b**)

Figure 7.61 This bank worker developed vesicular hand dermatitis. Allergy to thiuram mix, and to a specific component of the thiuram mix known as tetramethylthiuram disulfide, was confirmed. Rubber bands were the cause of the dermatitis due to the handling seen in (**b**) (Conde-Salazar, 1990; Conde-Salazar et al, 1993b).

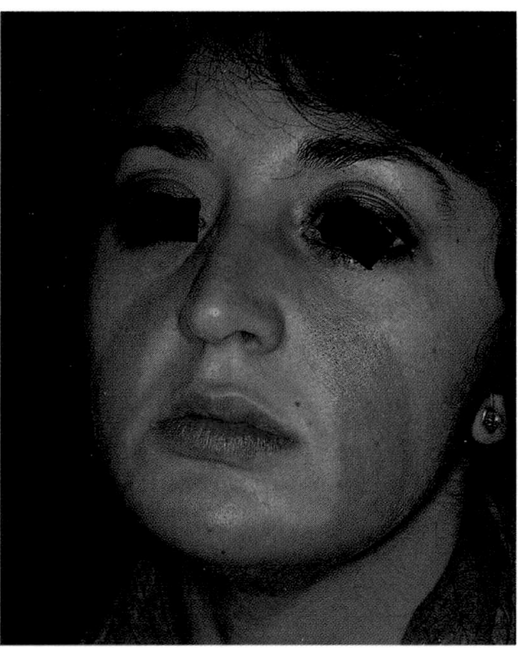

Figure 7.62 A safety mask caused this woman to develop facial dermatitis. Antioxidants were responsible, and were identified by the black rubber mix from the standard screening series of patch tests (Conde-Salazar, 1990; Conde-Salazar et al, 1993b).

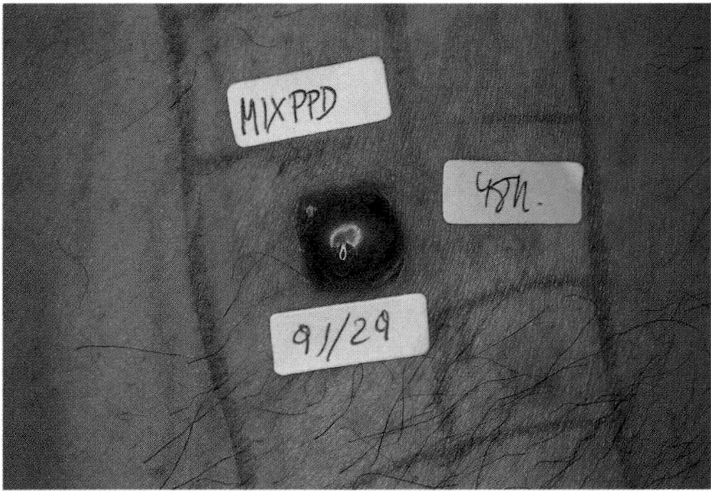

Figure 7.63 Black rubber mix is also known as paraphenylenediamine mix, and strong patch test reactions to this mix can occur, as seen here. The mix is composed of 0.1% *N*-isopropyl-*N'*-phenyl-*p*-phenylenediamine, 0.25% *N*-phenyl-*N'*-cyclohexyl-*p*-phenylenediamine 0.25% *N,N'*-diphenyl-*p*-phenylenediamine (Rietschel and Fowler, 1995, pp.24–7). Note that black rubber mix is no longer available, and has been replaced by *N*-isopropyl-*N'*-phenyl-*p*-phenylenediamine (IPPD).

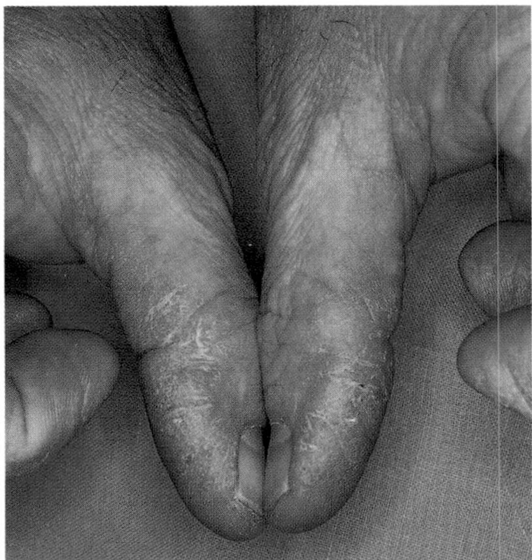

(**a**)

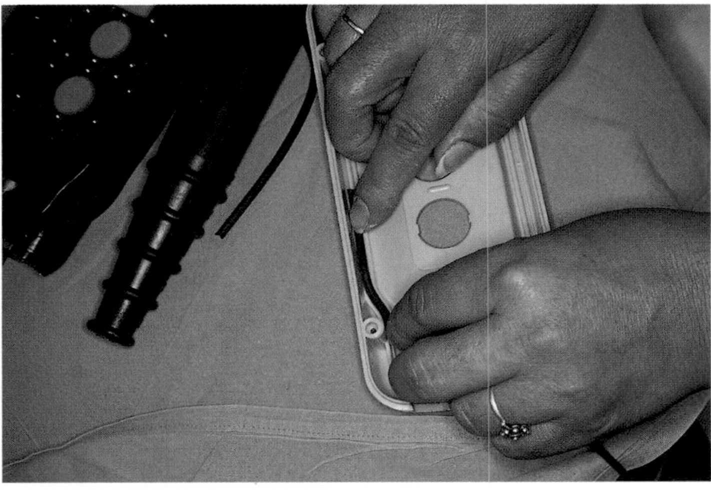

(**b**)

Figure 7.64 Black rubber mix allergy was responsible for the dry, hyperkeratotic dermatitis of the thumbs of this woman who worked in the automobile industry (**a**). The material she installed that led to the changes on her thumbs is seen in (**b**). The presence of black rubber mix chemicals was confirmed by thin-layer chromatography.

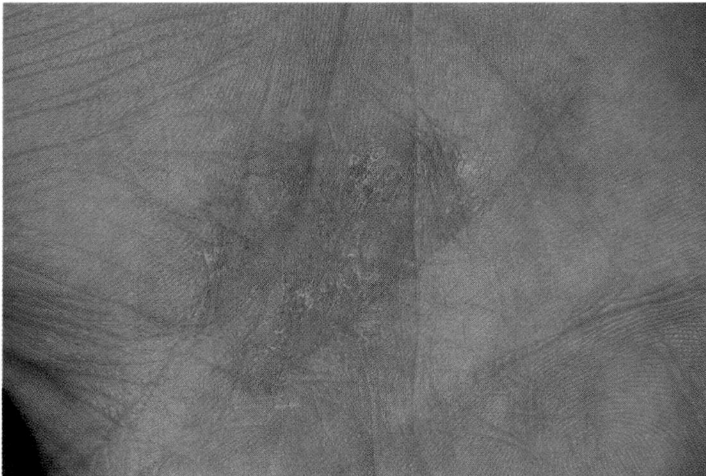
(**a**)

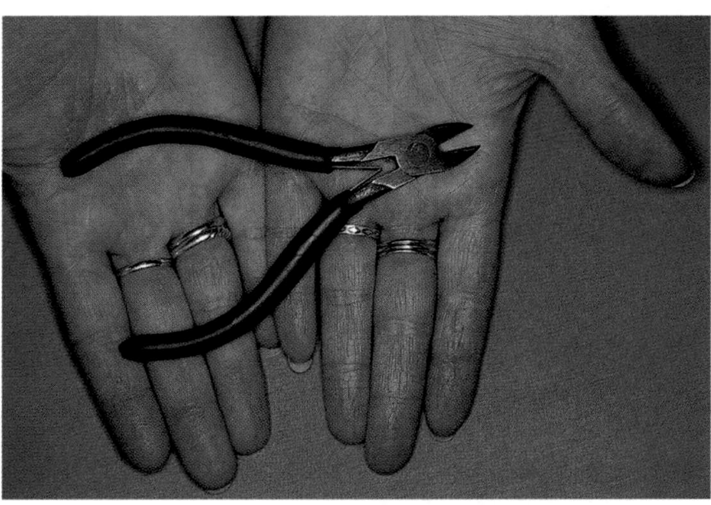
(**b**)

Figure 7.65 Dermatitis of the central area of the palm is usually of endogenous rather than exogenous origin. The palmar eruption in (**a**) is dry and hyperkeratotic, and was due to allergic contact dermatitis to black rubber mix chemicals. (**b**) The pliers that were covered by a material containing this allergen. The patient worked as an electrician.

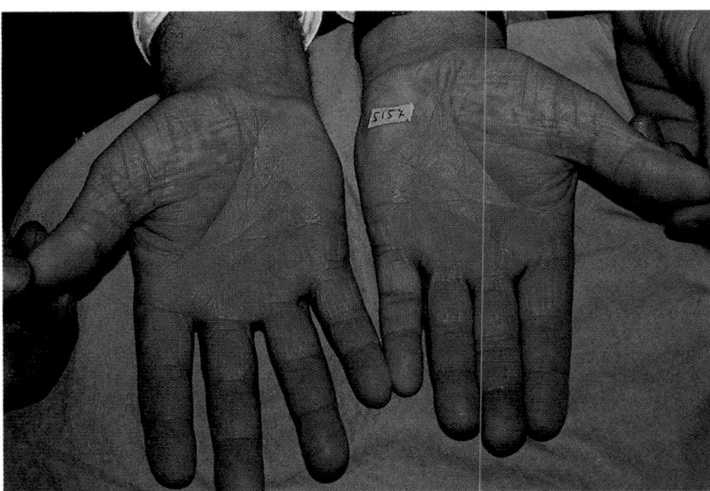

(a)

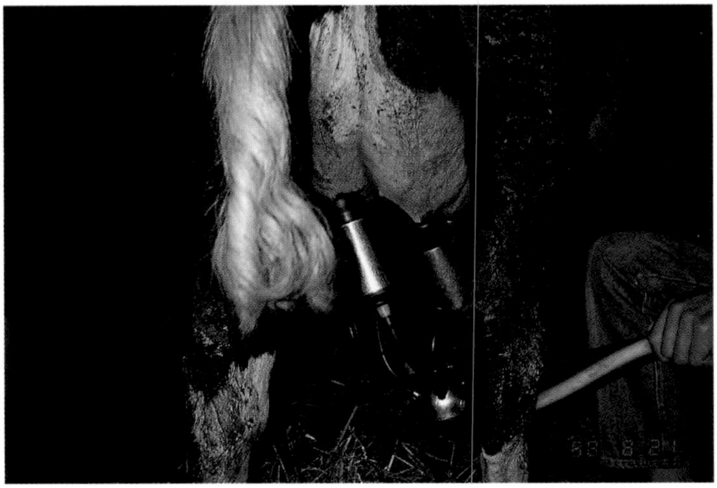

(b)

Figure 7.66 Dairymen use milking machines that contain rubber components and thiuram derivatives, and black rubber mix chemicals are commonly found in the milking machines. (**a**) The dry, hyperkeratotic dermatitis produced by the milking machine (**b**). The dairyman was allergic to the *N*-isopropyl-*N*'-phenyl-*p*-phenylenediamine (IPPD) component of the black rubber mix.

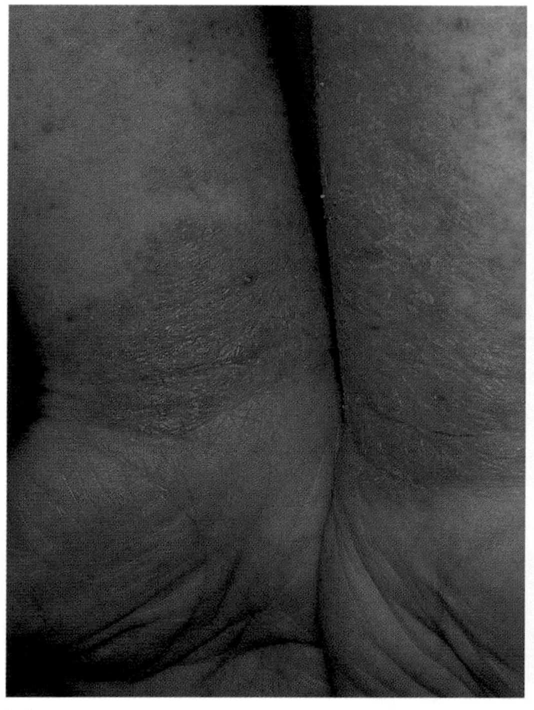

(**a**)

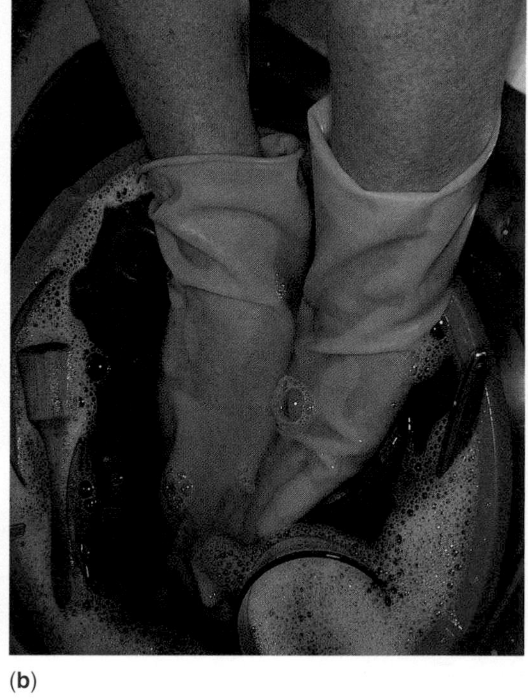

(**b**)

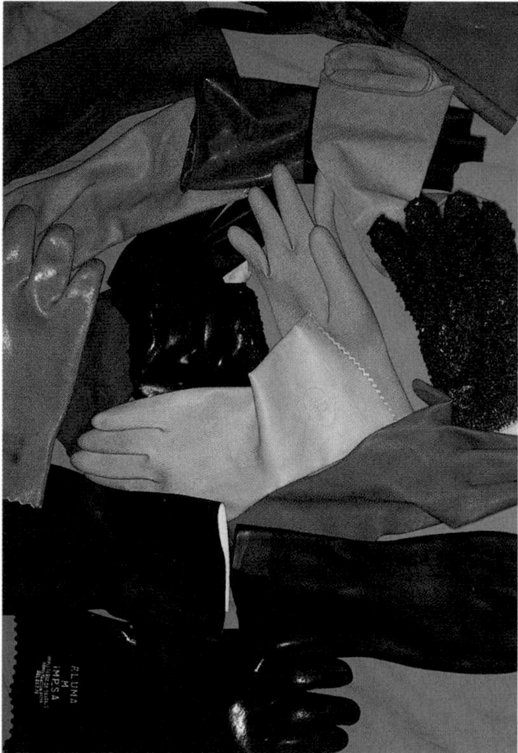

(**c**)

Figure 7.67 Rubber gloves commonly contain rubber accelerators. The hand and wrist dermatitis seen in (**a**) was found to be due to the presence of a thiuram derivative in the gloves that the patient wore at work (**b**). All the gloves pictured in (**c**) contained thiurams, carbamates and mercapto compounds.

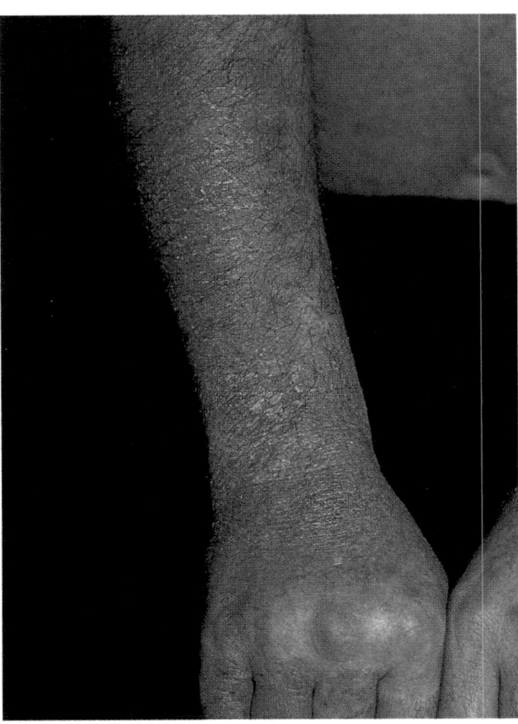

Figure 7.68 Severe chronic dermatitis of the hands and forearms occurred in this butcher due to thiuram derivatives in his rubber gloves.

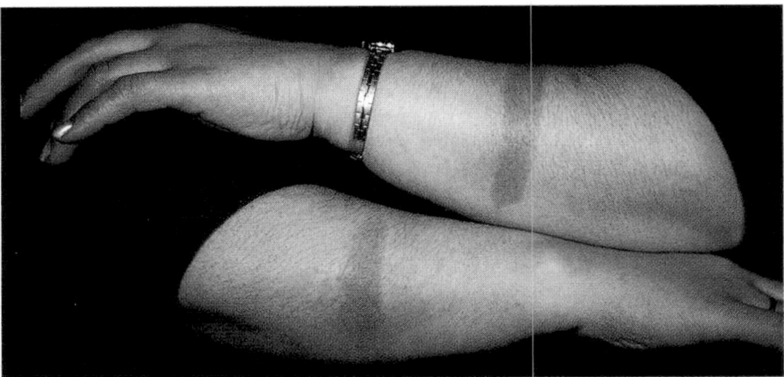

(a)

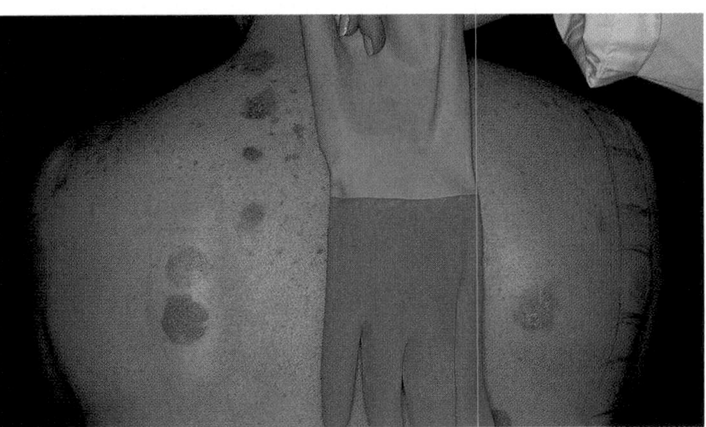

(b)

Figure 7.69 Liners are sometimes worn under gloves to prevent the accumulation of moisture. These are usually made of cotton. In (**a**), an unusual pattern of dermatitis occurred from wearing gloves with a liner that afforded protection, but not to the very top of the glove. It should be remembered that cotton is absorbent and will hold rubber allergens such as mercapto-benzothiazole even after washing and boiling (Rietschel, 1984). Pieces cut from rubber gloves can be used for patch testing, as seen in (**b**).

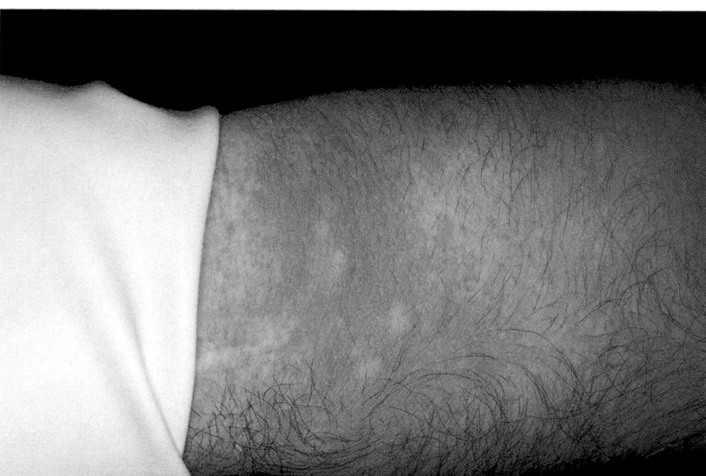

Figure 7.70 Contact urticaria to natural rubber latex was previously discussed in the section on health-care workers, but the problem can occur in other settings, as seen here. This is a dairy worker who wore a glove that caused IgE-mediated contact urticaria. Individuals with this type of allergy are at risk of anaphylaxis upon mucosal exposure to natural rubber latex (FDA, 1991; Conde-Salazar et al, 1997). (See also Figures 5.58–5.64.)

Metals and Metal Lubricants

The most common metal allergens are nickel, cobalt and chromates, and sensitization to these metals may be due to occupational or non-occupational exposure.

Metal lubricants are chemical substances used to reduce the coefficient of friction between two, usually metal, surfaces. The principal functions of metal lubricants are to lubricate the cutting surface between a tool and the metal item to be cut, to reduce heat, to remove metal filings (swarf) and to protect machine parts.

Metal lubricants differ according to their function, and contain a number of additives to maintain and increase lubrication, to reduce corrosion and to improve machinery performance. The most commonly used additives are biocides, antioxidants, colouring agents, fragrances and antifoaming agents. Biocides and antioxidants are the additives most likely to sensitize. These products can cause both allergic and irritant contact dermatitis, the irritant form being the most common. They can also cause changes in pigmentation (leucodermas and melanodermas), skin cancer and folliculitis (oil acne). The oil acne phenomenon is often seen in small 'epidemics' in companies where low-quality metal lubricants are used or in settings where appropriate precautions (the use of clean clothing, showering after work, etc.) have not been taken.

The most common irritants and allergens are listed in the box.

Irritants	Allergens
Aromatic hydrocarbons	Chromates
Formaldehyde solution	Cobalt
Laboratory materials	Components of metalworking fluids:
Metalworking fluids	benzothiazoles
Soaps and products used for cleaning hands and machines	colophony
Solvents	formaldehyde solution
	fragrances
	isothiazolinones
	mercaptobenzothiazole
	triazines
	Nickel

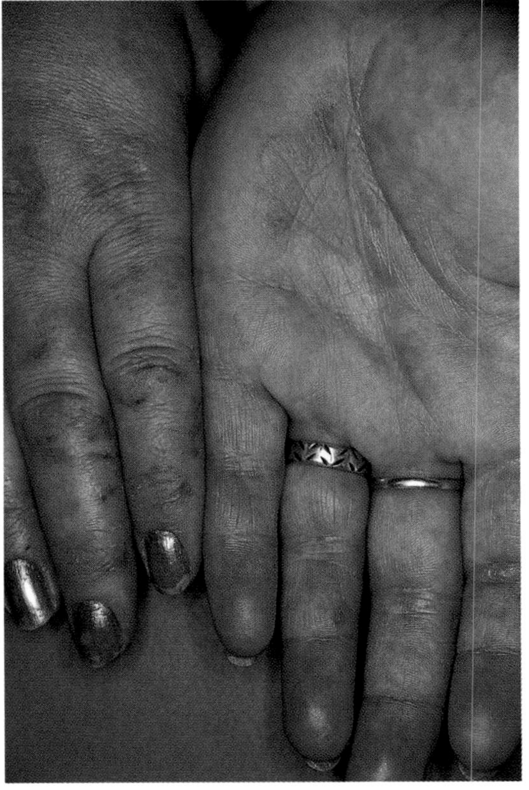

Figure 7.71 A 30-year-old nickel-sensitive woman worked at a newspaper stand, and handled a large number of coins every day. She developed the dermatitis seen here on the fingers of the right hand, used to take coins from the cash register, and in the left palm, in which coins were received from customers.

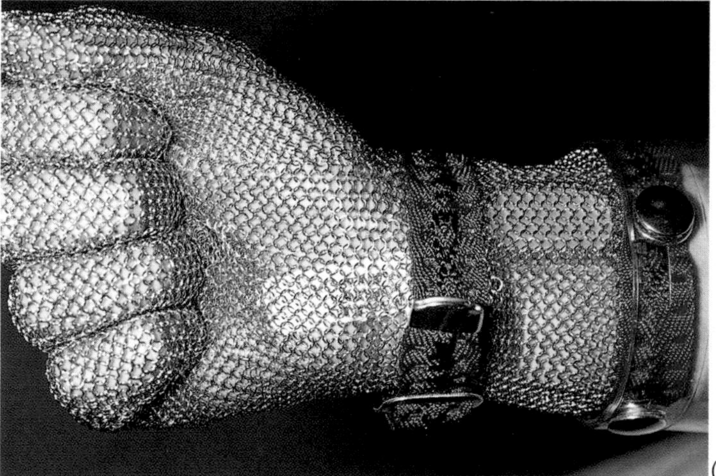

(**a**)

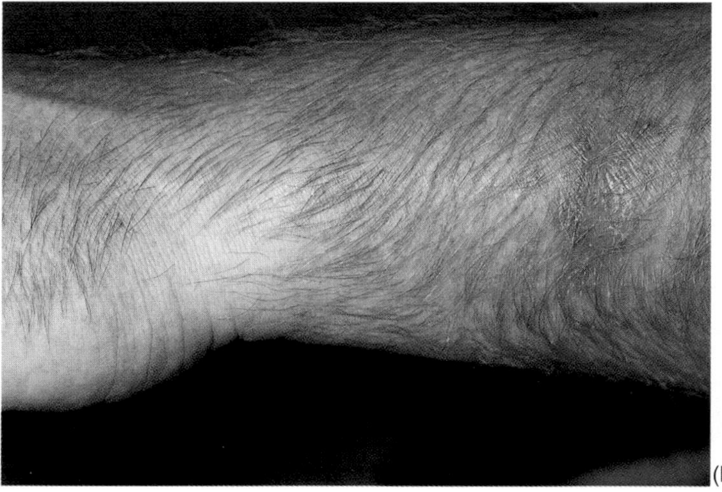

(**b**)

Figure 7.72 This 25-year-old man with no previous skin disease worked in a slaughterhouse. On his left hand, he wore a cotton glove and a protective steel mesh glove (**a**). He developed pruritic dermatitis on the ulnar aspect of his left forearm, just above the wrist (**b**). He was patch-tested with the European Standard Patch Test Series, and showed a strongly positive reaction to nickel. A button on the steel glove tested positive for nickel with the dimethylglyoxime test (see Figure 6.65).

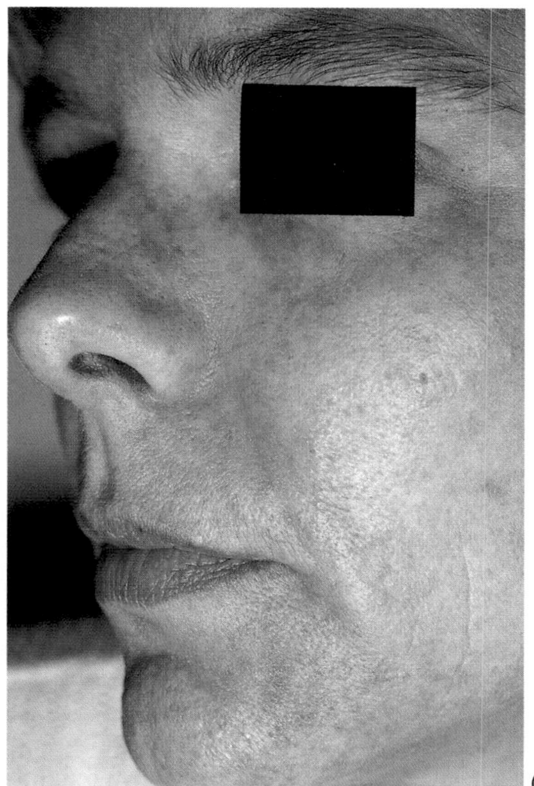

(**a**)

Figure 7.73 (**a**) This 26-year-old woman experienced pruritus and facial dermatitis while working in an electronics factory, where she drilled holes in dark-grey plastic cabinets and assembled electrical wires. The pruritus disappeared when she was off work for approximately a week, and reappeared after a few days back at work. Patch testing showed nickel allergy, and it was discovered that a nickel salt was used to colour the plastic cabinets (**b**). The pruritus and dermatitis disappeared after she was moved to another type of work within the same factory.

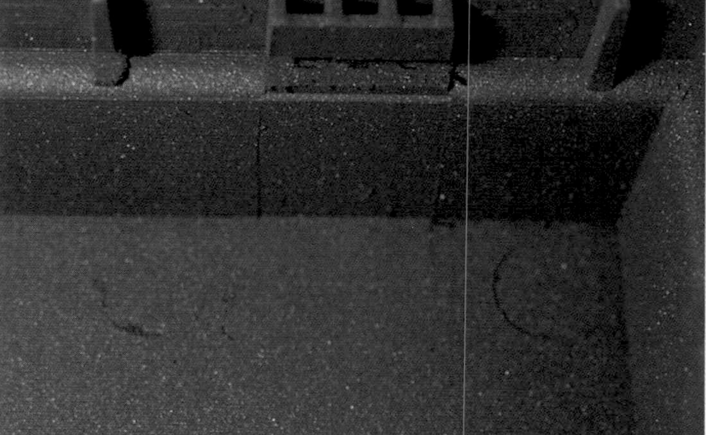

(**b**)

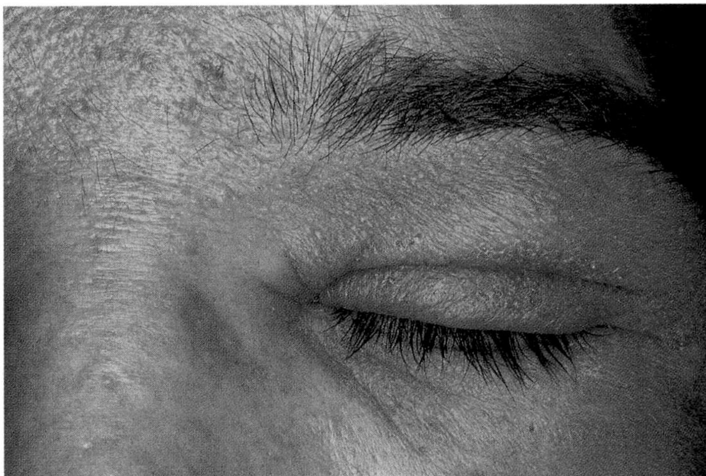

Figure 7.74 Dermatitis of the eyelids and face occurred in this electroplating worker, who was shown to be allergic to chromates. Electroplating is a notorious occupation for exposure to chromates. An airborne mechanism was suspected.

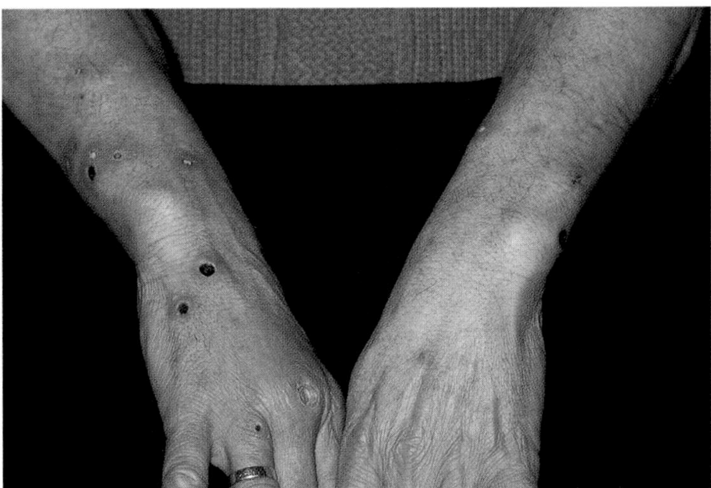

Figure 7.75 Skin ulceration is also associated with chromate exposure. This electroplating worker was not allergic to chromate. Ulceration was not thought to be due to sensitization. These are sometimes called 'chrome holes' (Samitz and Epstein, 1962; Conde-Salazar and Zambrano Zambrano, 1979).

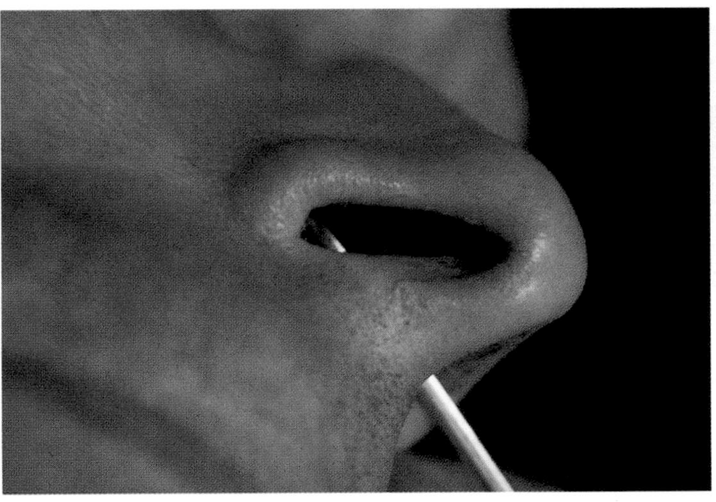

Figure 7.76 Perforation of the nasal septum by chromate occurred in this electroplating worker (Conde-Salazar and Zambrano Zambrano, 1979).

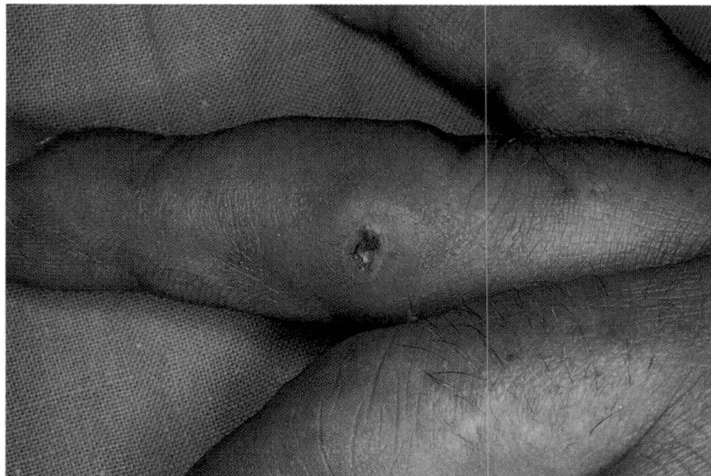

Figure 7.77 This ulceration occurred owing to nickel exposure in a worker manufacturing nickel catalysts.

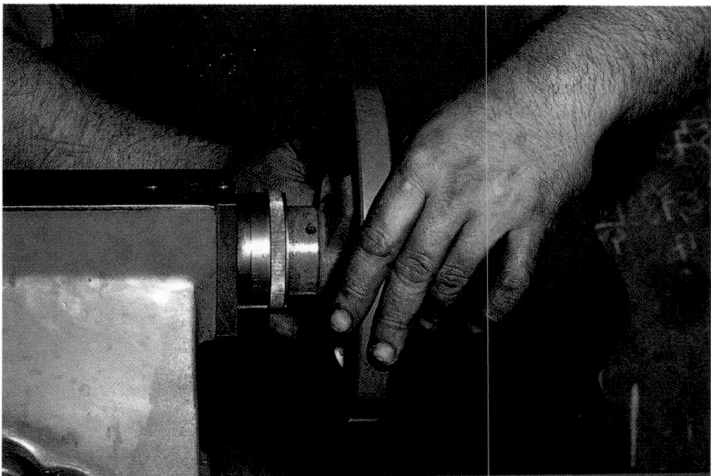

(**a**)

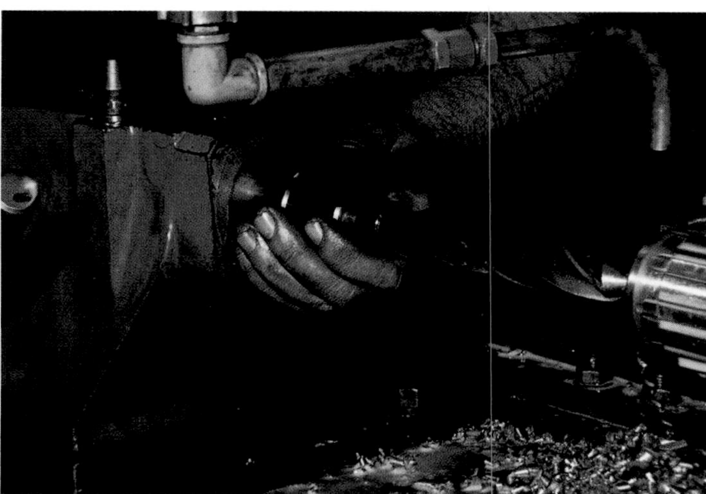

(**b**)

Figure 7.78 (**a**, **b**) These are examples of the types of machines that require coolants in the manufacture of various hard metal devices. The nature of the skin contact helps to explain the location of irritant and allergic reactions.

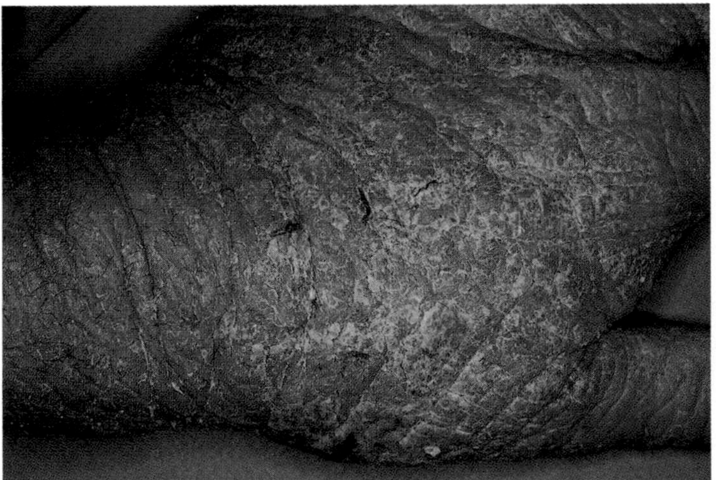
(a)

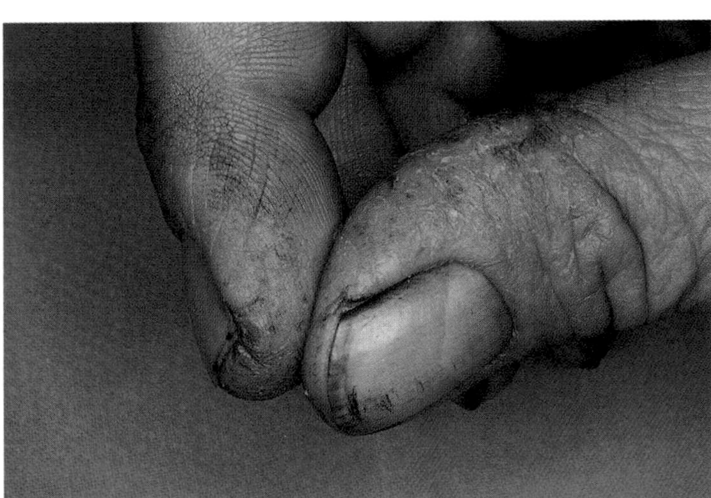
(b)

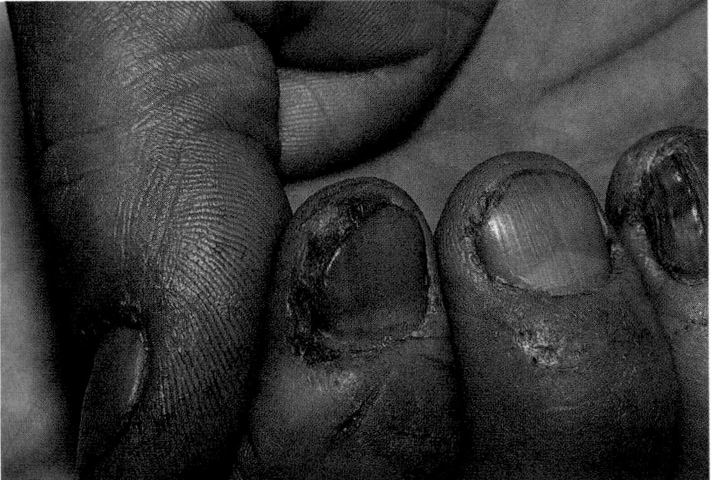
(c)

Figure 7.79 (**a**) This irritant dermatitis of the back of the hand is due to the repeated wet-to-dry nature of exposure to water-soluble machine-cooling lubricants. Irritation can also arise from small particles of metal, which result in the type of changes seen in (**b**) and (**c**) (Conde-Salazar et al, 1993c).

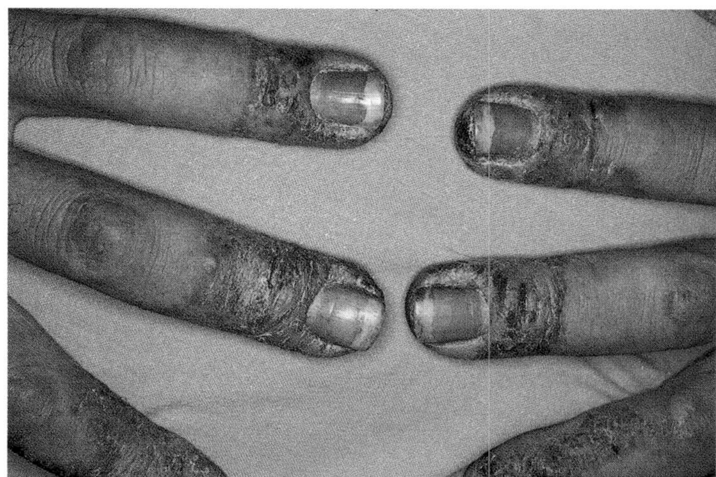
(a)

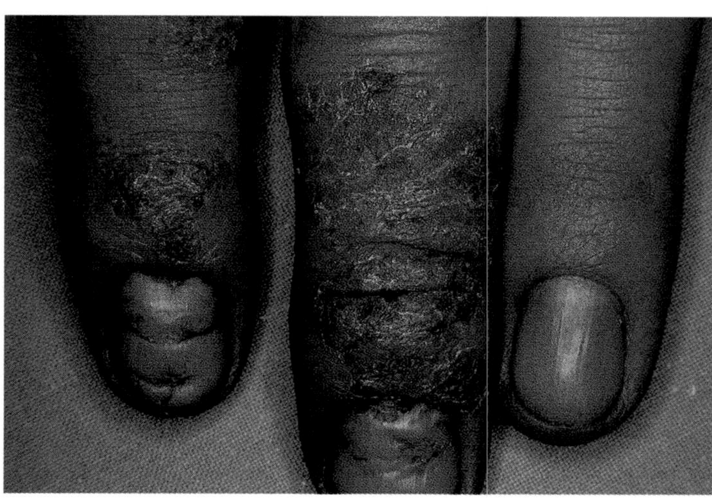
(b)

Figure 7.80 Allergic contact dermatitis to coolants can be similar in presentation to the irritant reactions seen in Figure 7.79. The machinist seen in (**a**) was allergic to formaldehyde present in a coolant. The machinist in (**b**) was allergic to paraphenylenediamine, formaldehyde and the biocide in his coolant, Bioban CS-1246. Note the secondary infection and the nail damage (Conde-Salazar et al, 1991a).

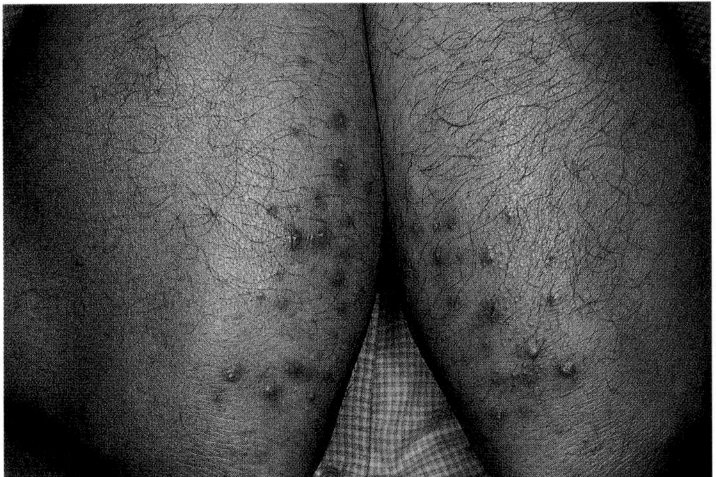

(a)

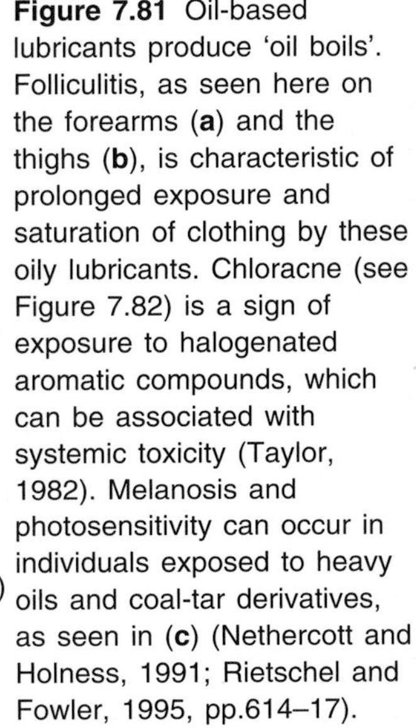

Figure 7.81 Oil-based lubricants produce 'oil boils'. Folliculitis, as seen here on the forearms (**a**) and the thighs (**b**), is characteristic of prolonged exposure and saturation of clothing by these oily lubricants. Chloracne (see Figure 7.82) is a sign of exposure to halogenated aromatic compounds, which can be associated with systemic toxicity (Taylor, 1982). Melanosis and photosensitivity can occur in individuals exposed to heavy oils and coal-tar derivatives, as seen in (**c**) (Nethercott and Holness, 1991; Rietschel and Fowler, 1995, pp.614–17).

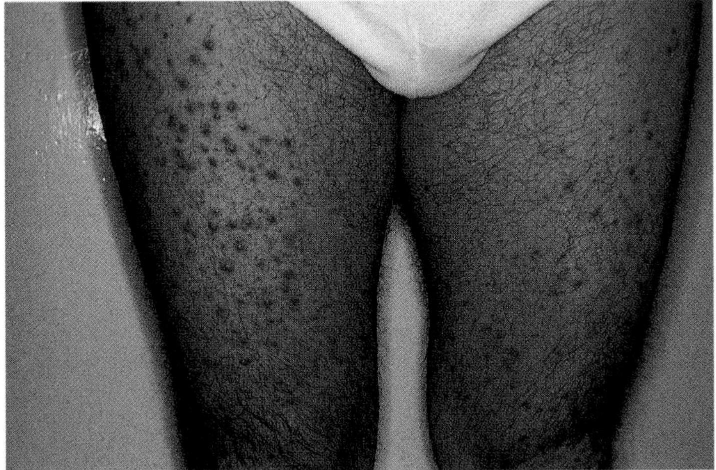

(**b**)

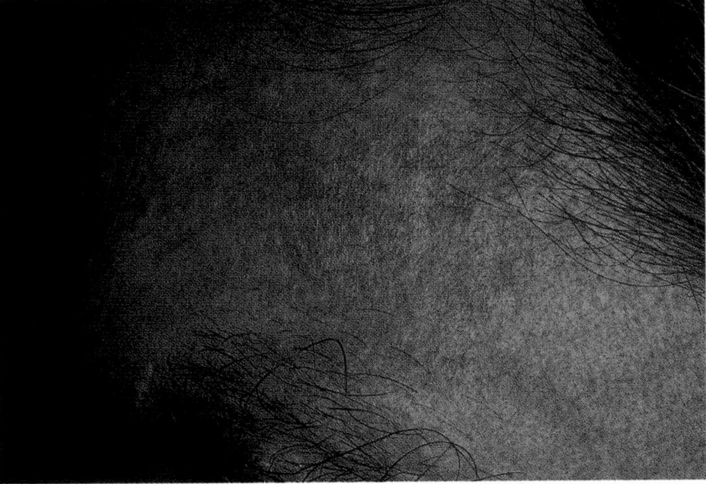

(**c**)

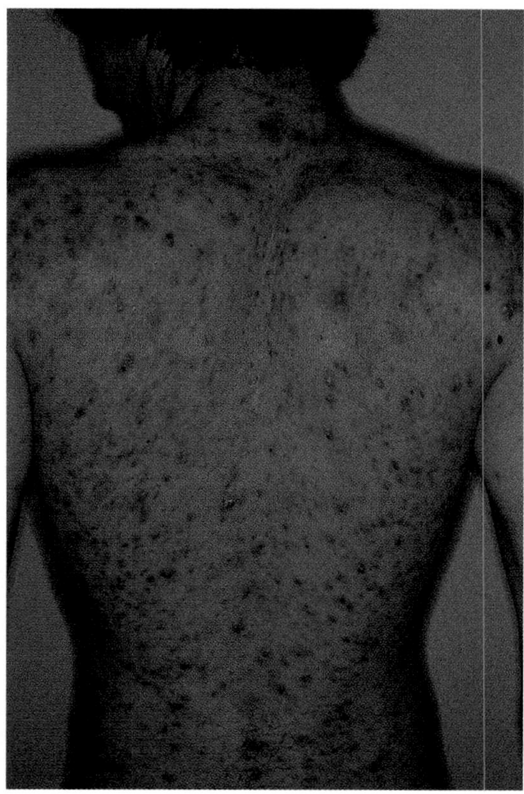

Figure 7.82 Chloracne in a patient who worked in a chemical products industry (pesticides), and was exposed to halogenated compounds (chloronaphthalenes).

Hair Care

There are two common hair-care treatments that can cause dermatitis on the hands of hairdressers and on the scalps of clients; this section will focus on hairdressers. Hair dyes based on paraphenylenediamine are those most commonly used in salons and provide the longest-lasting colour. Allergy to these dyes is sufficiently common that the instructions accompanying these products advise consumers to patch test themselves prior to use. Another procedure with moderate sensitizing potential commonly carried out by hairdressers is the permanent waving of hair. Some permanent-wave solutions are based on glyceryl thioglycolate (formerly called glyceryl monothioglycolate) (Storrs, 1988). Permanent waves in which such solutions are used are also known as 'acid' perms. An additional hazard to the hairdresser is ammonium persulfate, which can cause not only contact dermatitis and contact urticaria, but also anaphylactic reactions (Fisher and Dooms-Goossens, 1976). This product is found in bleaching solutions used to create a platinum-blonde colour.

The common irritants and allergens are shown in the box on the following page.

Irritants	Allergens
Dyes Permanent-wave solutions Shampoos Soaps	Ammonium persulfate Dyes and derivatives of paraphenylenediamine Formaldehyde solution Fragrances Nickel (utensils) Resorcinol Thioglycolates

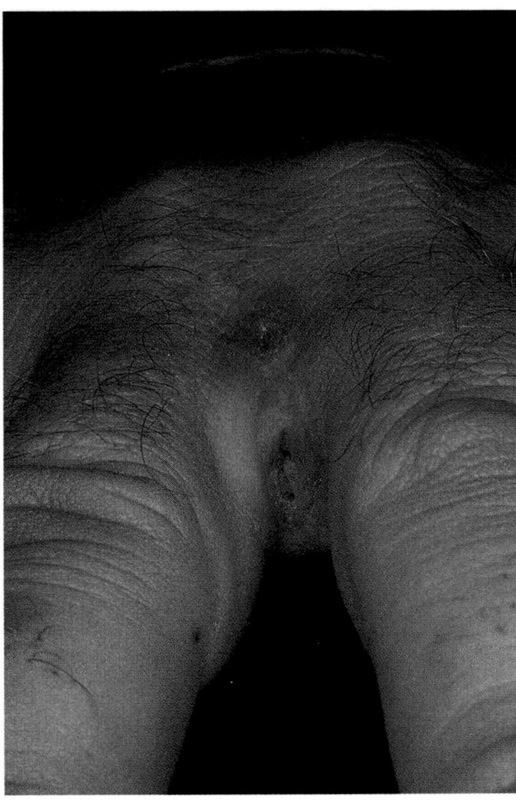

Figure 7.83 Hair cutting can lead to small fragments of hair becoming imbedded in the skin between the fingers of barbers. A sinus, as seen here, can result, and is known as 'barbers' hair sinus' (Price and Popkin, 1976). This is a mechanical rather than an allergic phenomenon (Conde-Salazar et al, 1995b).

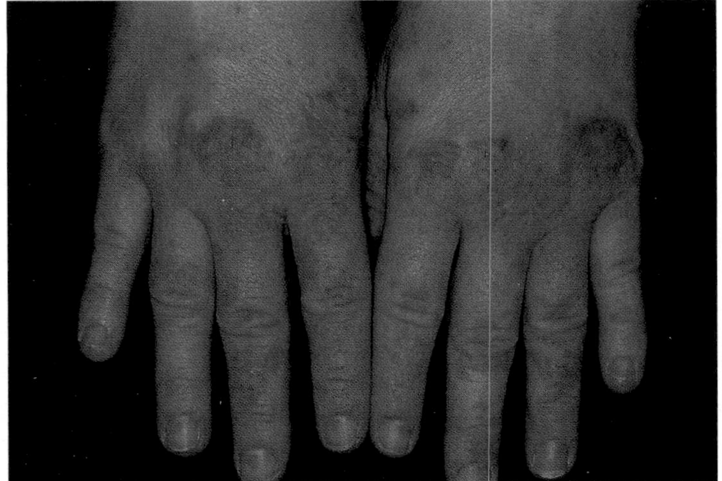

Figure 7.84 Dermatitis of the back of the hands can result from cumulative irritation due to shampooing clients' hair, as occurred in this hairdresser's apprentice. Her work consisted solely in washing hair (Conde-Salazar et al, 1995b).

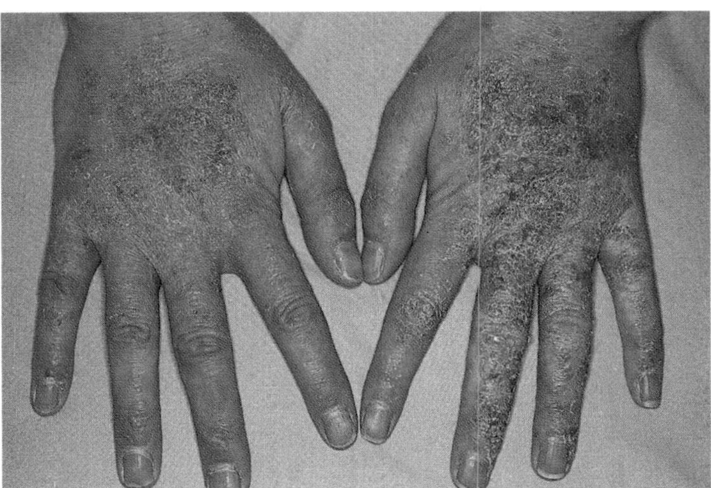

(**a**)

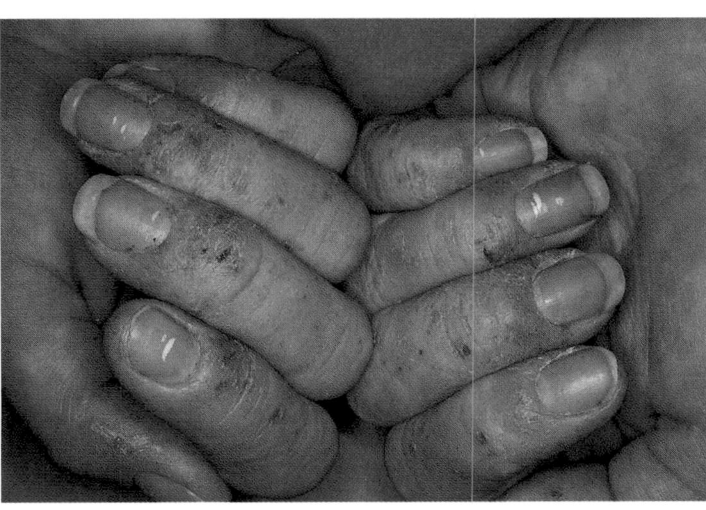

(**b**)

Figures 7.85 (**a**, **b**) Allergic contact dermatitis of the hands occurred in these hairdressers due to sensitization to paraphenylenediamine. The nails can take on a yellowish colour due to the use of these dyes (Conde-Salazar et al, 1995b).

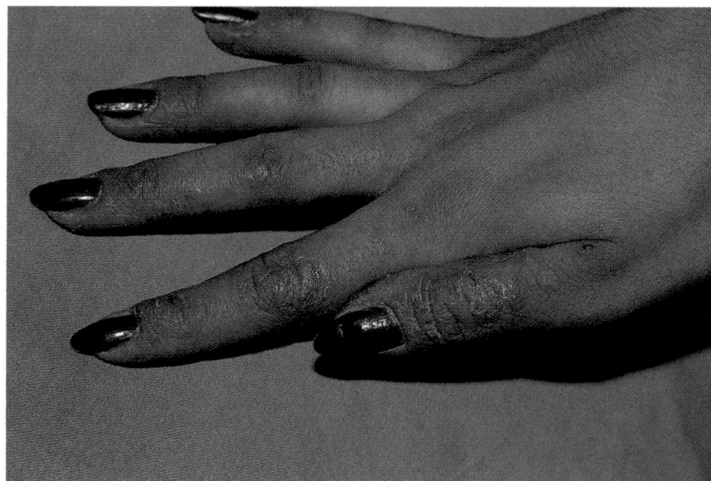
(**a**)

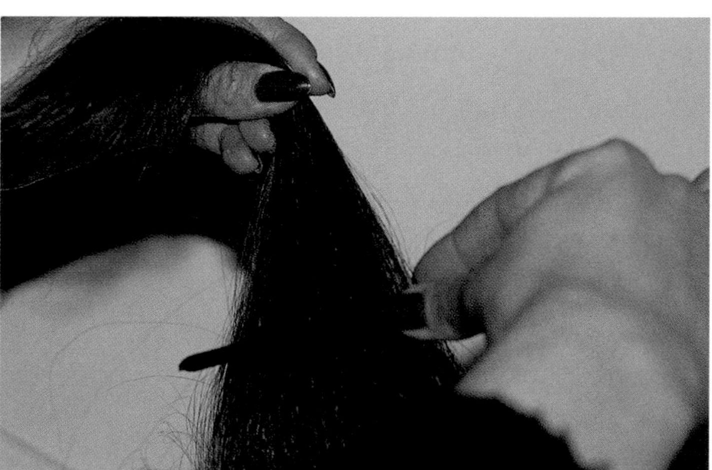
(**b**)

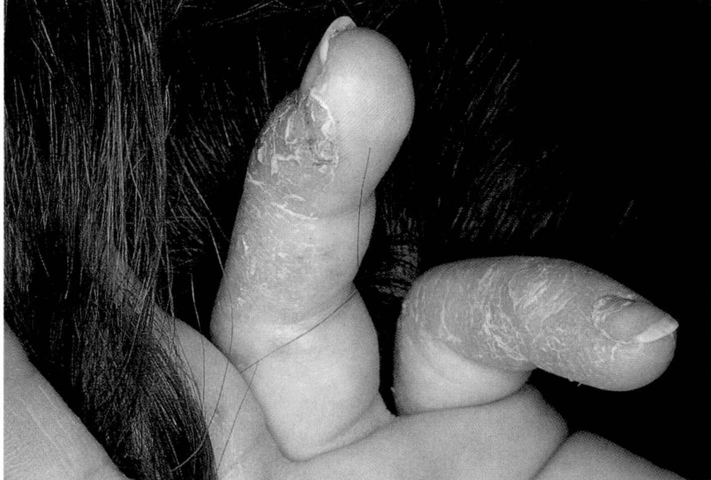
(**c**)

Figure 7.86 This hairdresser was allergic to paraphenylenediamine, but her dermatitis was very localized (**a**). The explanation for the localization is demonstrated in (**b**) and (**c**). The lesions were all located where there was greatest contact with hair (Conde-Salazar et al, 1995b).

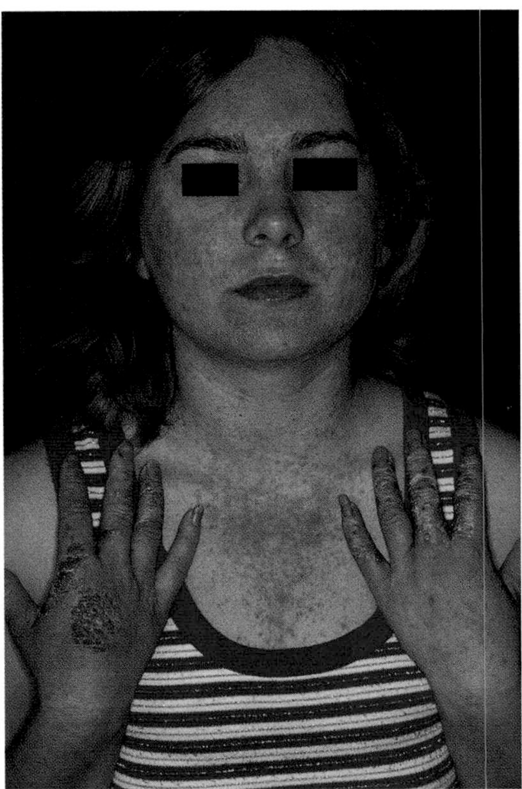

Figure 7.87 The dermatitis of this hairdresser spread from the hands to the face and trunk. She was sensitive to paraphenylenediamine (Conde-Salazar et al, 1995b).

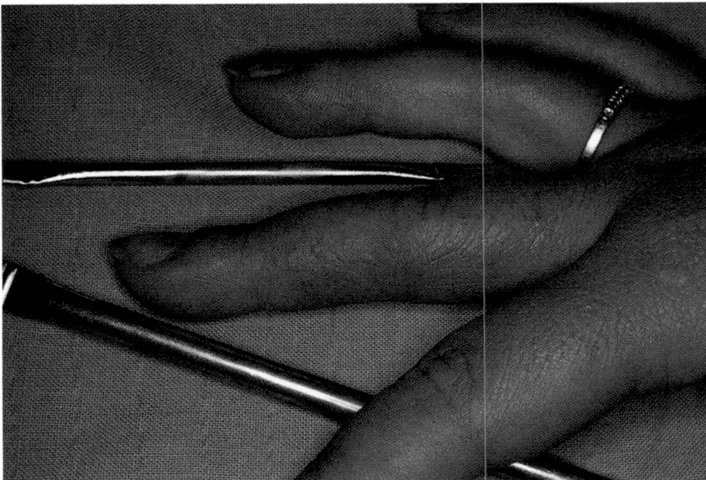

Figure 7.88 Implements containing nickel can be another source of allergic contact dermatitis for hairdressers, as was the case for this woman who had pre-existing nickel allergy from costume jewellery.

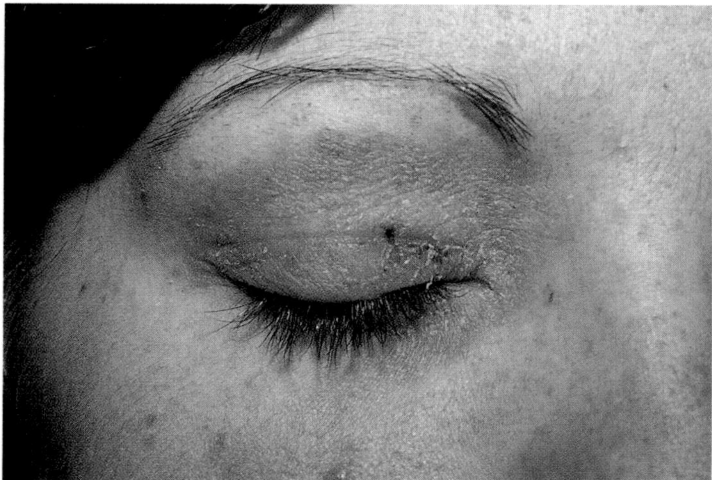

Figure 7.89 The eyelid dermatitis of this hairdresser was due to airborne exposure to ammonium persulfate, to which she was allergic.

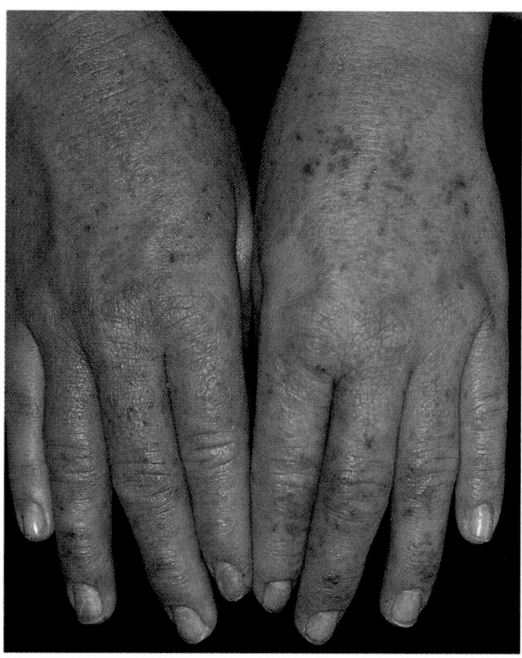

Figure 7.90 A 20-year-old apprentice hairdresser developed hand dermatitis one year into her apprenticeship, as seen here. Patch testing showed a strongly positive reaction to ammonium persulfate, which is used to bleach hair. She had severe flare-ups of dermatitis when she worked with ammonium persulfate, and, over time, just being in the room where it was used caused her dermatitis to flare. She had to give up her apprenticeship.

Figure 7.91 A positive prick test to ammonium persulfate. Ammonium persulfate can also cause immediate-type reactions such as rhinitis, asthma, and even anaphylactic reactions. Prick testing with ammonium persulfate should be undertaken with care, since anaphylactic reactions caused by this test procedure have been described.

Floristry, Horticulture and Woodwork

Many plants and various woods can cause both allergic and irritant contact dermatitis, and it is not possible to mention all of these here. The virtually worldwide popularity of house plants means that consumers as well as the growers and sellers of the plants in question may become sensitized.

The occupations most affected by sensitization to plants and woods are gardening, floristry, horticulture and woodworking, and persons who care for plants in hotels, restaurants, hospitals, etc. may also be affected. Chemical products used in the care of plants (insecticides, fertilizers and disinfectants) can cause dermatitis, and the use of rubber gloves to protect the hands may also result in sensitization.

The plants that most frequently cause sensitization are the Frullaniaceae, lichens, the Alliaceae, the Compositae, the Pinaceae, *Primula obconica,* the Anacardiaceae (poison ivy, poison oak) and the Tulipae.

The woods of major interest include the so-called tropical or exotic woods, and the most frequent sensitizers are pao ferro (*Machaerium scleroxylum*), Mansonia (*Mansonia altisima*), iroko (*Clorophora excelsa*) and Sucupira (*Bowdichia nitida*). The commercial name of a particular wood differs from country to country, and it is therefore necessary to be familiar with the botanical name.

Care should be taken in testing patients suspected to be sensitized to plants or woods, since the use of the plants themselves or sawdust may cause sensitization. For this reason, commercial allergens should be used where possible. If a particular allergen is not available, tests should be carried out using aqueous or alcoholic extracts of the plants or of the sawdust of the woods. For additional information regarding botanical dermatology, the reader is referred to Mitchell and Rook (1979) and Benezra et al (1985).

The most common irritants and allergens are listed in the box.

Irritants	Allergens
Fertilizers	Colophony
Herbicides	Diallyl disulfide (garlic)
Insecticides	Fertilizers
Plants	Gum components
Sawdust	Herbicides
Wood preservatives	Pesticides (carbamates)
Woods	Primin (primula)
	Quinones
	Tulipalin
	Tuliposide
	Turpentine
	Urushiol (poison ivy, poison oak)
	Usnic acid

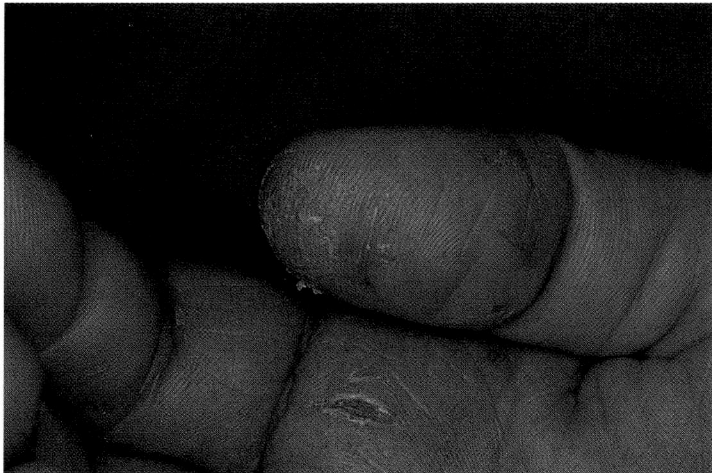

Figure 7.92 Florists may be exposed to primula (*Primula obconica*), as was this florist, who developed the dermatitis seen here (see also Figures 6.69–6.71).

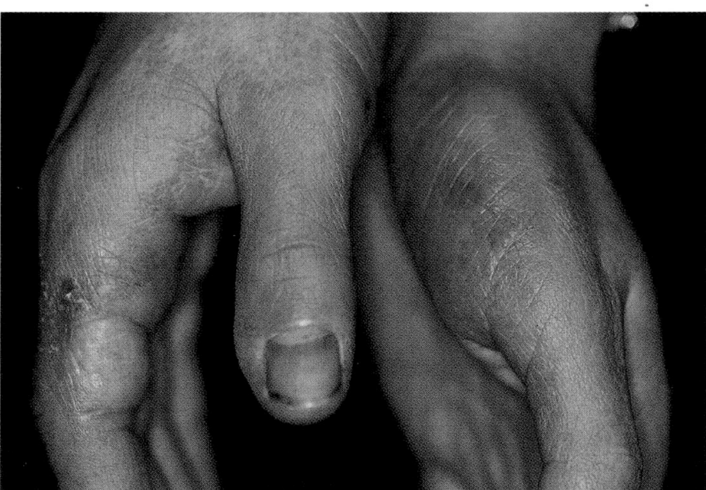

Figure 7.93 A 21-year-old man was employed in a plant nursery, where his job was to separate the stems of tulips from the bulbs. After a few weeks, he developed bullous dermatitis on the index finger of his right hand and on the left thumb, the areas of skin in closest contact with the bulbs, as seen here. He had a strongly positive patch test to the tulip bulb. The dermatitis cleared when he stopped working at the nursery.

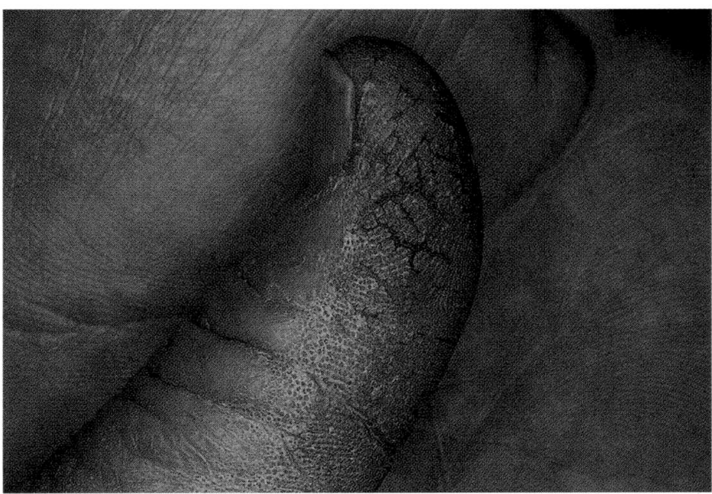

Figure 7.94 'Tulip finger' is the common name for the pulpitis seen in this gardener, which was due to handling tulips and hyacinths.

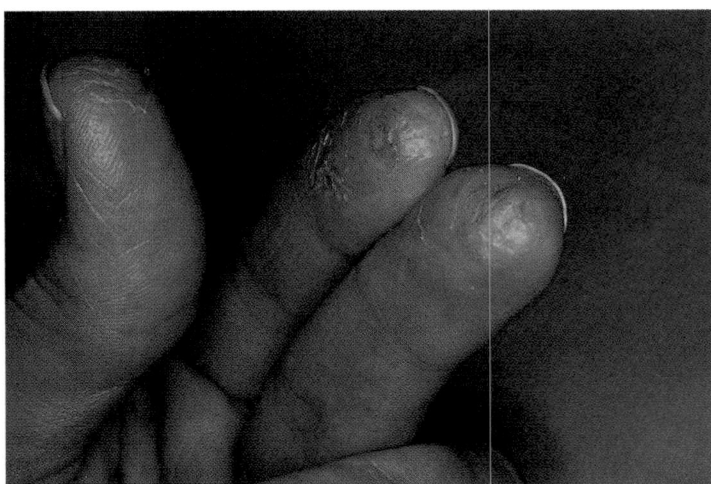
(a)

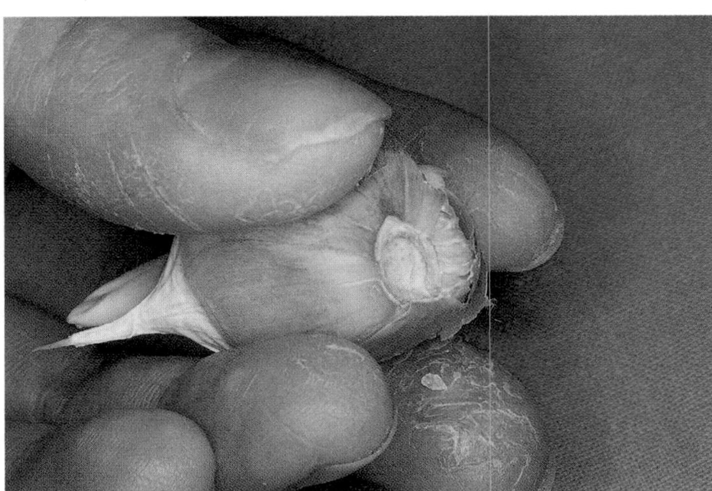
(b)

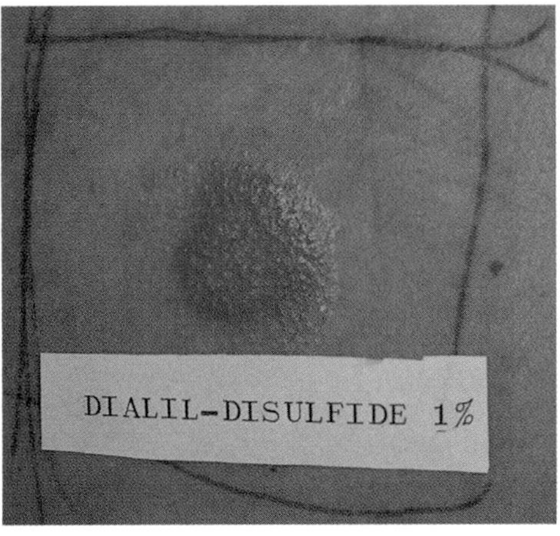

(c)

Figures 7.95 (**a**) A strong similarity exists between the pulpitis caused by *Alstroemeria*, tulip finger, and contact dermatitis to garlic, which is seen here. (**b**) This restaurant cook demonstrates the manner in which garlic is held for cutting, and why the dermatitis is so localized. (**c**) The allergen in garlic is diallyl disulfide, while the allergen in *Alstroemeria* is a tuliposide (Christensen and Kristiansen, 1995). (See also Figures 6.82–6.85.)

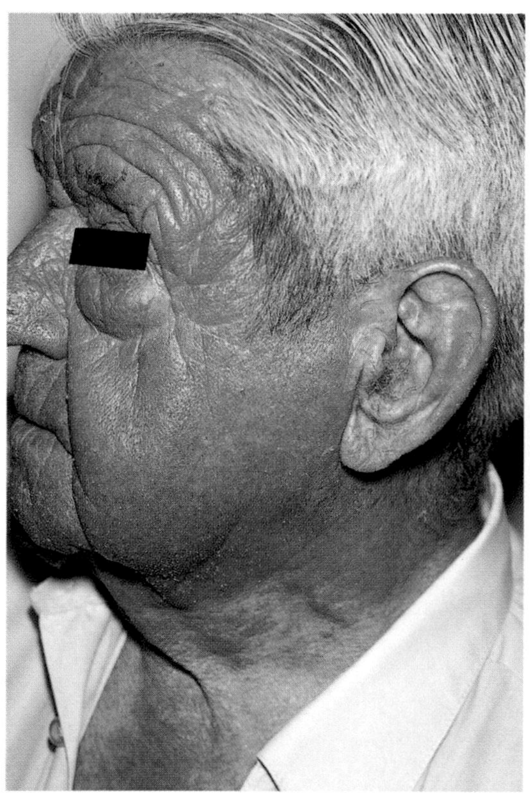

Figure 7.96 A 74-year-old retired florist helped make funeral decorations. He developed severe dermatitis of the exposed areas of his face, neck, hands and forearms, which improved when he was not working, and recurred both when he returned to work and when he worked in his own garden. Patch testing showed a strongly positive reaction to sesquiterpene lactones. He was unwilling to give up his job, and the dermatitis proved very persistent and refractory to treatment (Lamminpaa et al, 1996). Another hazard for florists is the leatherleaf fern (Hausen and Schulz, 1978).

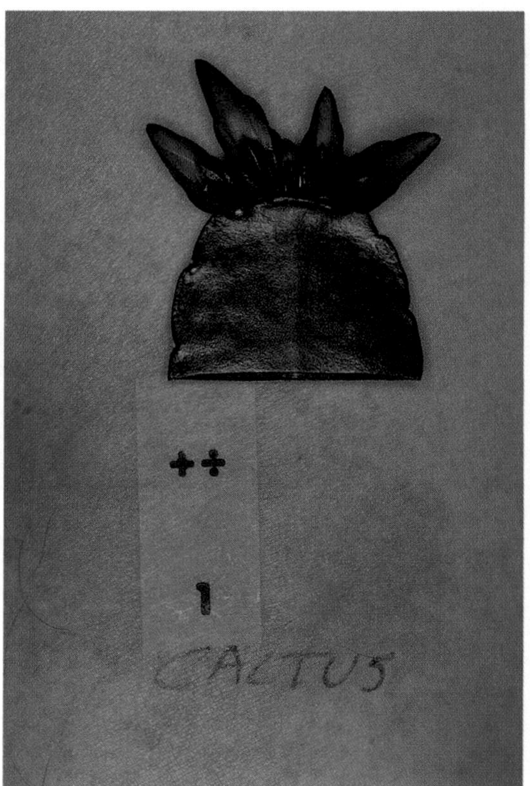

Figure 7.97 A 41-year-old man developed rhinitis, conjunctivitis and facial pruritus while working as a wholesaler of plants. A particular cactus was suspected, and a prick test to this plant, seen here, was positive. A patch test was negative. He was unable to completely avoid this cactus, and the symptoms persisted.

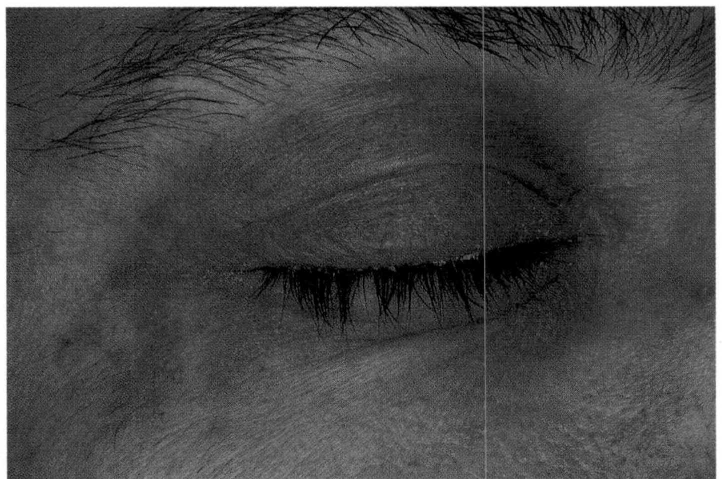
(a)

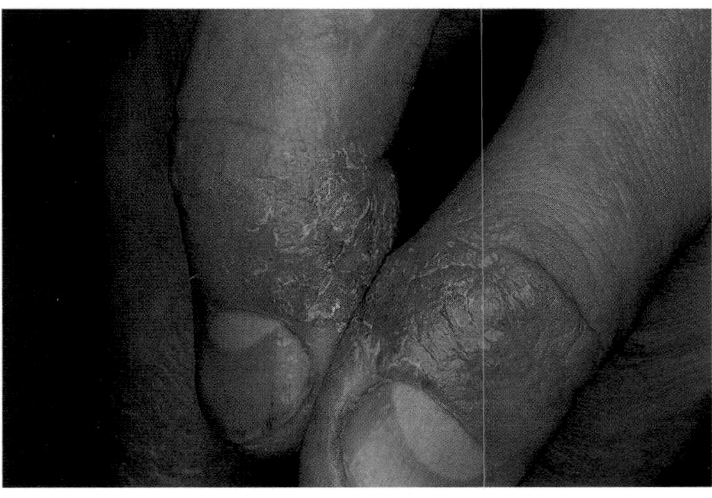
(b)

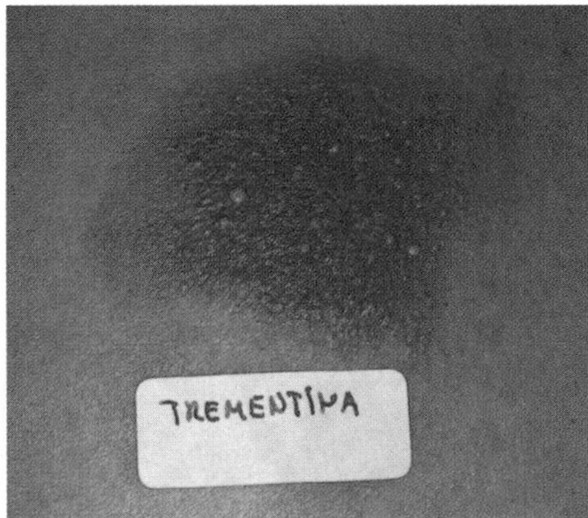

(c)

Figure 7.98 This carpenter developed dermatitis of the face (**a**) and hands (**b**) due to allergy to oil of turpentine; the patch test is seen in (**c**). This allergen is derived from pine by various methods of distillation, and can vary in allergenicity depending on the country of origin owing to variation in δ-3-carene content (Hjorth and Wilkinson, 1968).

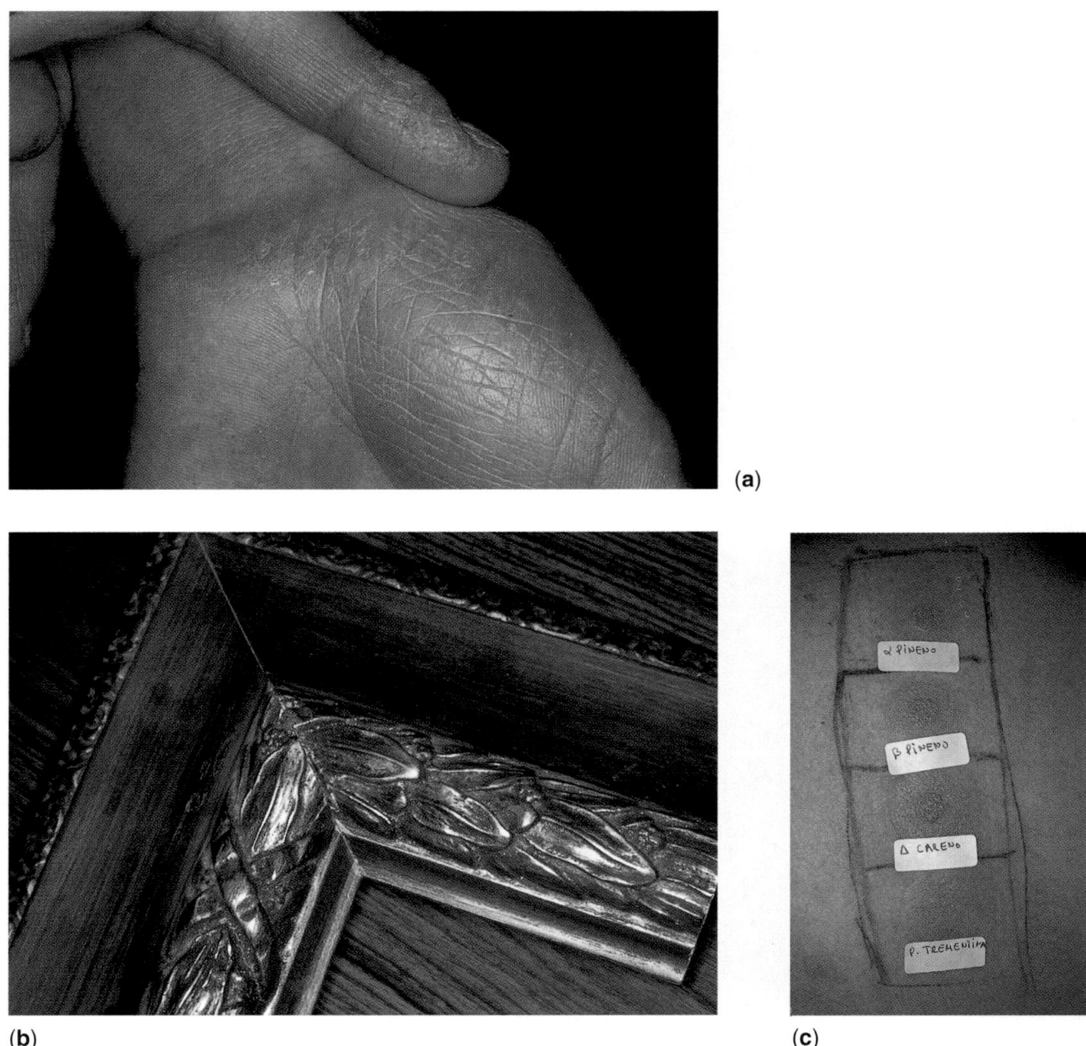

(**a**)

(**b**) (**c**)

Figure 7.99 The hand dermatitis seen in (**a**) was caused by handling picture frames, like the one seen in (**b**). The frames were treated with oil of turpentine, and the patient was allergic to several components of turpentine, as seen in (**c**): α-pinene, β-pinene and δ-3-carene.

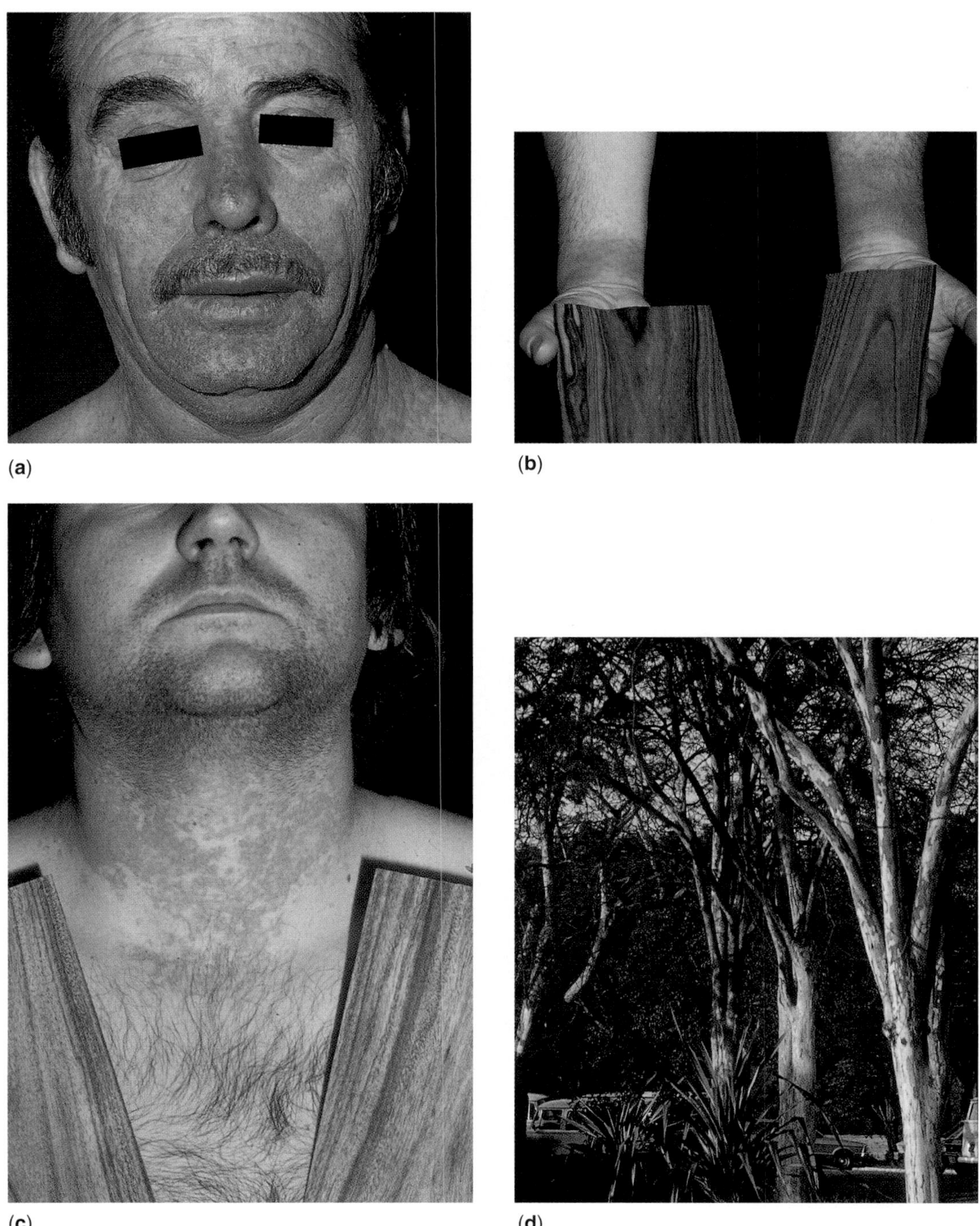

(a) (b) (c) (d)

Figure 7.100 (**a**) This man made cabinets for television sets from Brazilian ironwood, also known as 'pao ferro' (*Machaerium scleroxylum*) (Roed-Petersen et al, 1987). He developed rhinitis and conjunctivitis, as well as dermatitis. (**b**) The way in which the wood was handled. (**c**) A colleague had lesions more akin to erythema multiforme; (**d**) Brazilian ironwood (Conde-Salazar et al, 1980).

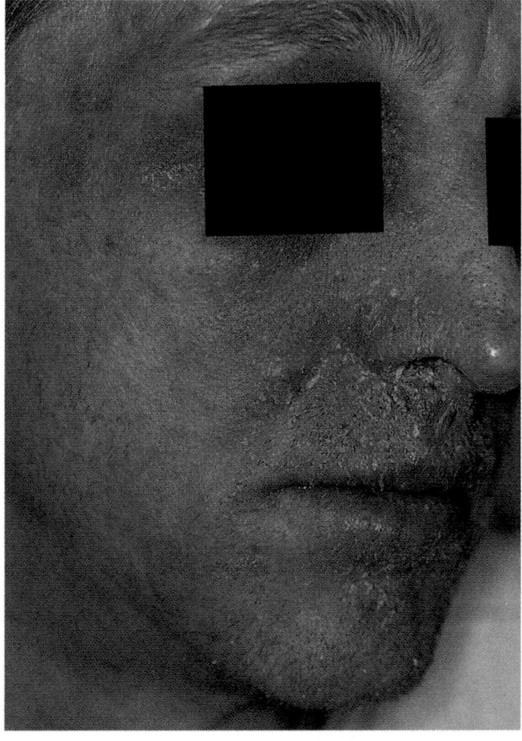

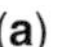

(a)

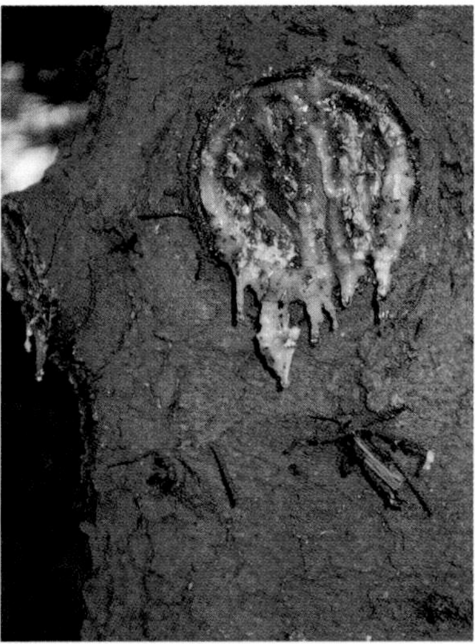

(b)

Figure 7.101 (**a**) This 39-year-old man developed dermatitis on his face after working in a factory where pine boxes were made. Patch testing showed that he was strongly allergic to colophony. The dermatitis faded only after he gave up his job. (**b**) Colophony, discharged from a pine tree after cutting off the branches.

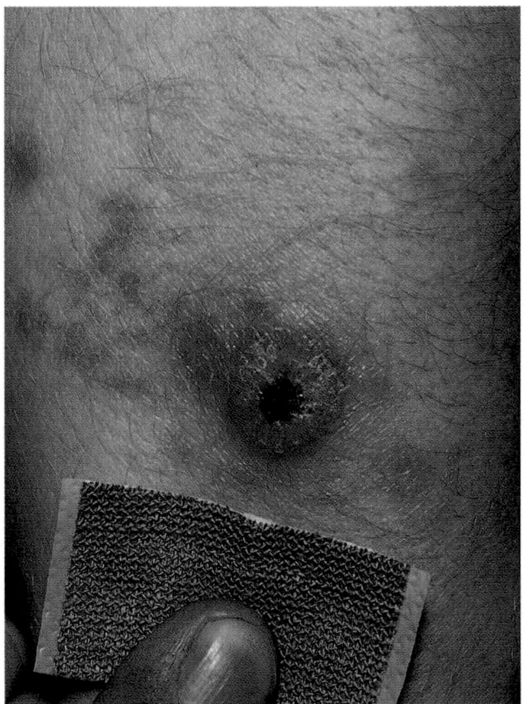

Figure 7.102 Colophony dermatitis can be suspected if a patient develops dermatitis under certain types of adhesive tape. The adhesive used in tapes containing colophony is very sticky.

Photography and Graphic Arts

There are many occupations in the category of photography and the graphic arts, and many different types of product are used. Some knowledge of working methods is required in order to identify sources of irritation or sensitization in these occupations. The most important occupations are printing and the reproduction of documents and photographs.

Printing processes involve the use of a variety of substances that are possible causes of contact dermatitis, for example:

- printing ink contains potential irritants;
- lithographic processes may expose workers to chromates;
- the photosensitive plates used in photolithography contain resins (epoxy, acrylics, etc.) that are powerful sensitizers;
- chemicals used to clean machinery may be irritants.

In addition there are various methods for reproducing original documents and drawings; those used most frequently are:

- photocopying (the electrostatic method; Rank-Xerox);
- the thermal method (Thermofax);
- the diazo method (Amonax, Dylene, Ozalid, ferrocyanide papers).

Each of these methods uses different chemical products capable of causing irritant or allergic contact dermatitis.

Working techniques in most commercial photographic processing laboratories are now completely automated, so that any contact with possible allergens (colour developers) is accidental or caused by cleaning equipment without suitable protection.

A variety of patterns of contact dermatitis can result from photographic chemicals, including common eczematous, lichenoid or airborne patterns. Colour developing chemicals, which are chemically related to paraphenylenediamine and are known by initials and numbers such as CD2, CD3, CD4 and CD6, have caused lichen planus-like reactions (Canizares, 1959). Cross-reactions between colour developers and paraphenylenediamine are not predictable, and may or may not occur (Rustemeyer and Frosch, 1995).

The common irritants and allergens are listed in the boxes on the following page.

Photography

Photography: Irritants	Photography: Allergens
Antioxidants	Amidol
Reducing agents	Chromates
	Colour developers (CD2, CD3, CD4, CD6)
	Formaldehyde solution
	Glutaraldehyde
	Hydroquinone
	Metol
	Paraphenylenediamine
	Pyrocatechol
	Pyrogallol
	Resorcinol
	Triazines

Graphic arts

Graphic arts: Irritants	Graphic arts: Allergens
Emulsions	Acrylates
Ink	Chloroacetamide
Machine-cleaning agents	Chromates
Organic compounds	Cobalt
Paper	Colophony
	Epoxy resins
	Formaldehyde solution
	Nickel
	Pigments
	Turpentine

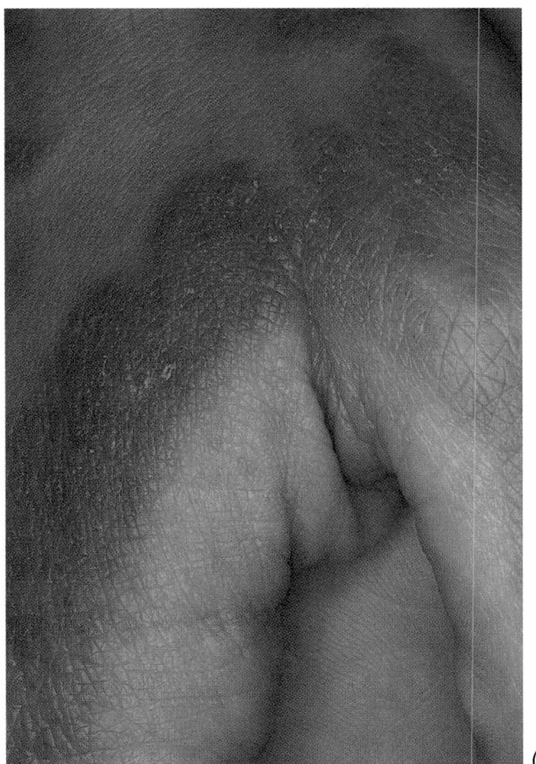

(**a**)

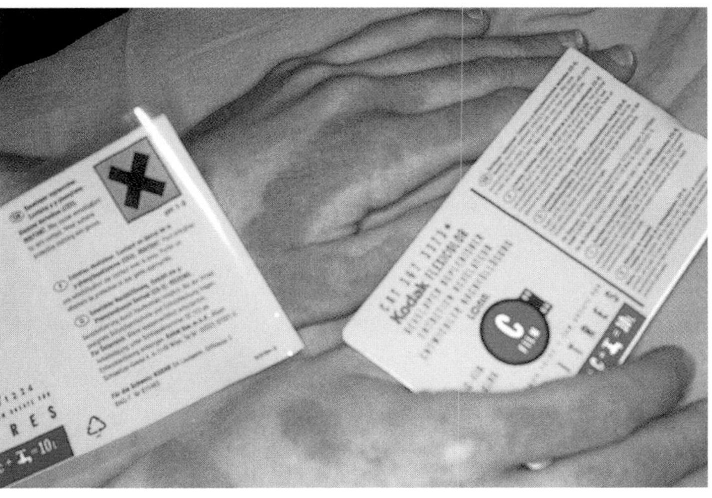

(**b**)

Figure 7.103 (**a**, **b**) Mild dermatitis of the hands is seen during the healing process in this photographer. Patch testing revealed sensitization to CD2, CD3, CD4 and metol. Metol is also known as *p*-methylaminophenol sulfate, and is used in black and white developing.

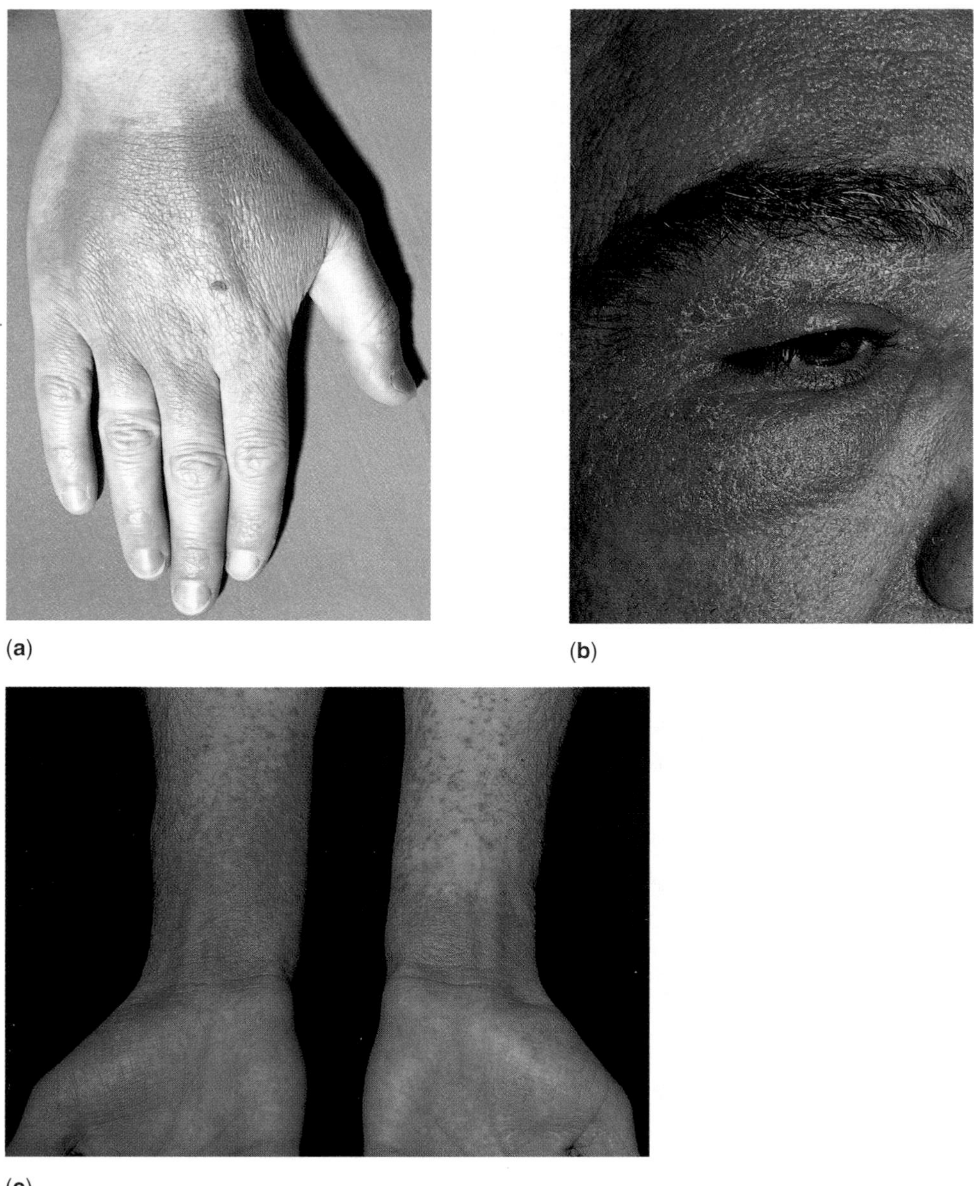

(a) (b)

(c)

Figure 7.104 Colour film developer, as noted in the introduction to this section, can cause a variety of morphological patterns of dermatitis. (**a**) Violaceous erythema more closely associated with lichenoid dermatitis. This is in contrast to the more traditional morphology of Figure 7.103, in which the allergens were the same, except for the addition of metol (Figure 7.103b). Here the violaceous change is not as apparent. CD2 and CD3 were also responsible for the facial dermatitis seen in (**b**). It was not clear whether airborne or ectopic contact was responsible for the facial localization. The wrist dermatitis in (**c**) again shows violaceous erythema (Conde-Salazar et al, 1982b).

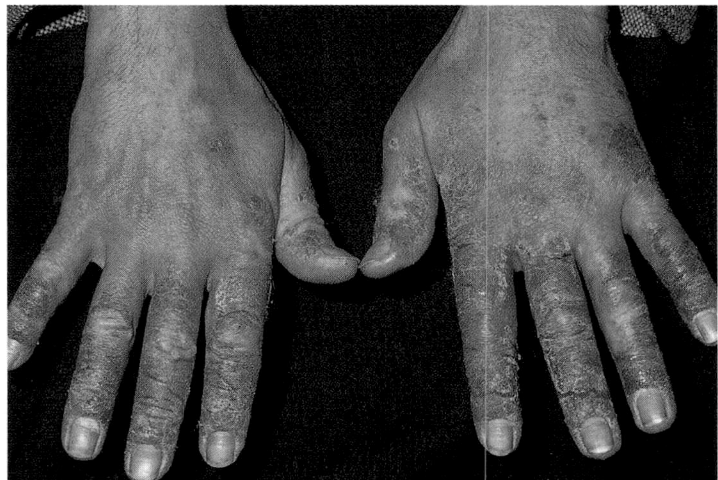

(a)

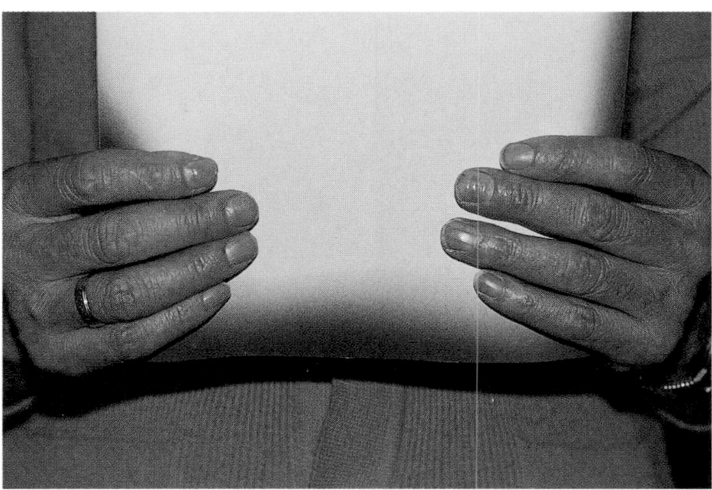

(b)

Figure 7.105 Allergic contact dermatitis was caused by diazonium compounds encountered when reproducing drawings. (**a**) The hand dermatitis. (**b**) The patient holding the diazoprints that contain the diazonium salts (Conde-Salazar et al, 1982a).

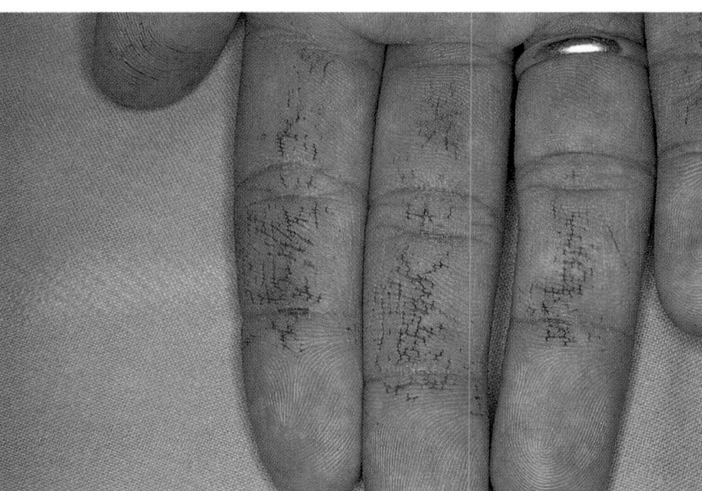

Figure 7.106 'Tattoo' lesions of the palmar aspects of the fingers in a graphic arts worker. Various inks and colours were responsible for this non-allergic skin change.

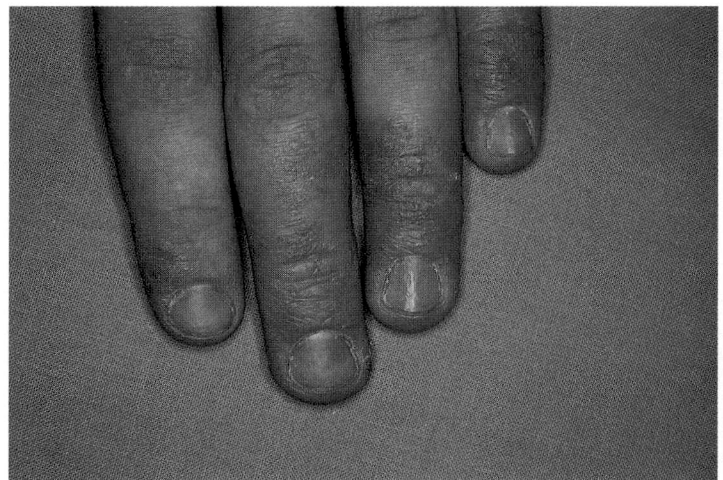
(**a**)

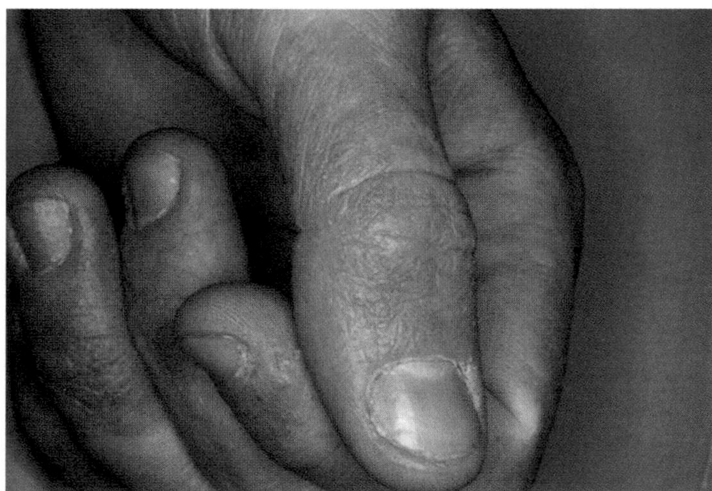
(**b**)

Figure 7.107 (**a, b**) This graphic arts worker was allergic to cobalt.

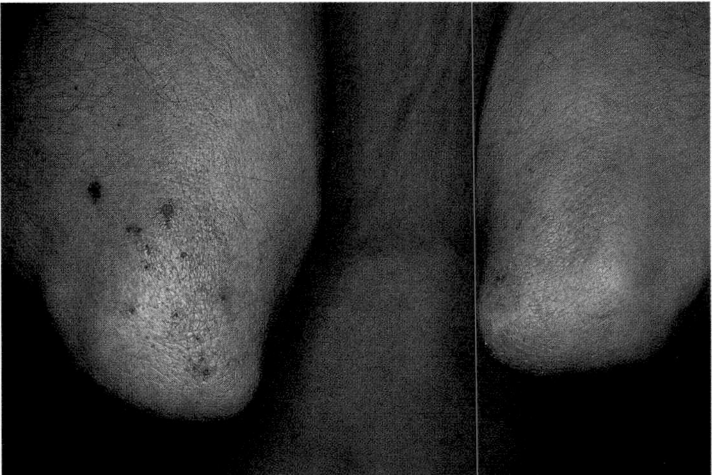

(a)

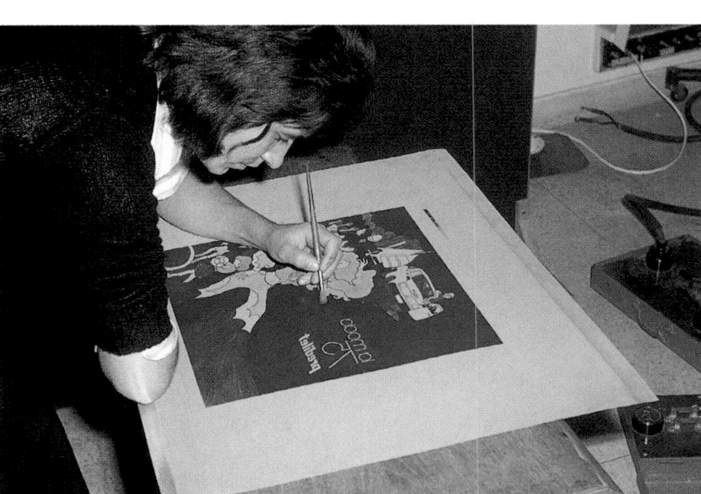

(b)

Figure 7.108 (**a**) Another example of a graphic arts worker who was allergic to cobalt. In this case the dermatitis was on the elbows. (**b**) The pattern of exposure.

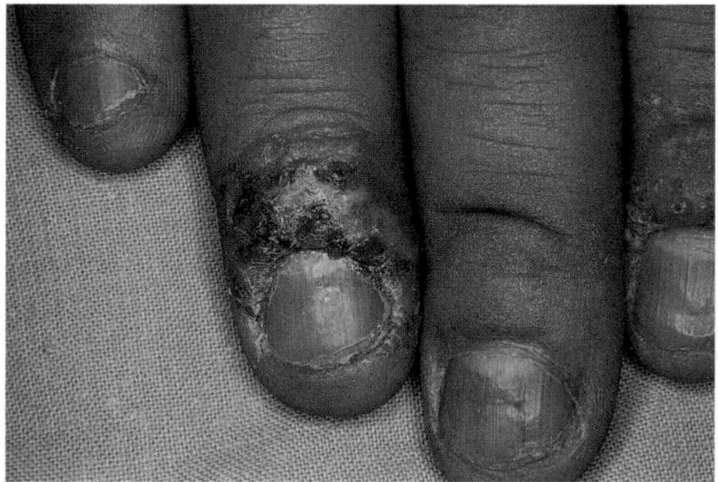
(**a**)

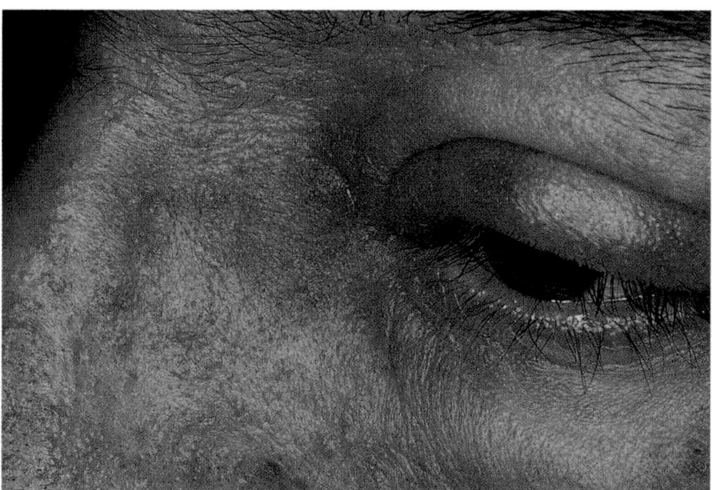
(**b**)

Figure 7.109 Lithography can expose workers to chromates. In (**a**) the fingers were affected, and in (**b**) an airborne exposure was believed to have caused the face and eyelid dermatitis. Both workers were patch-test positive for chromate.

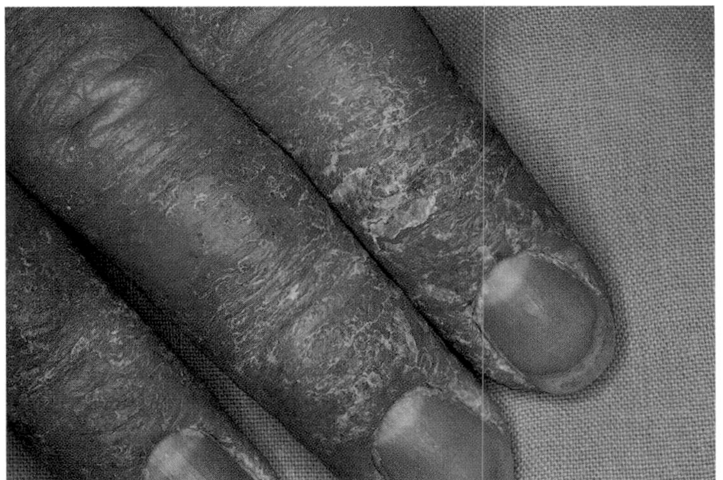
(a)

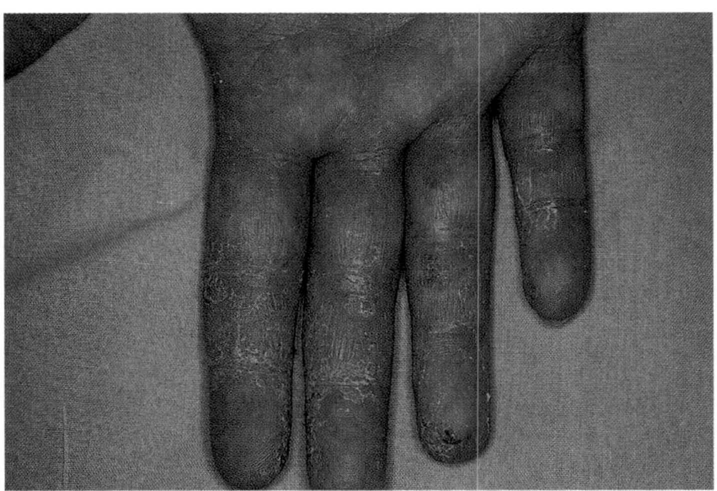
(b)

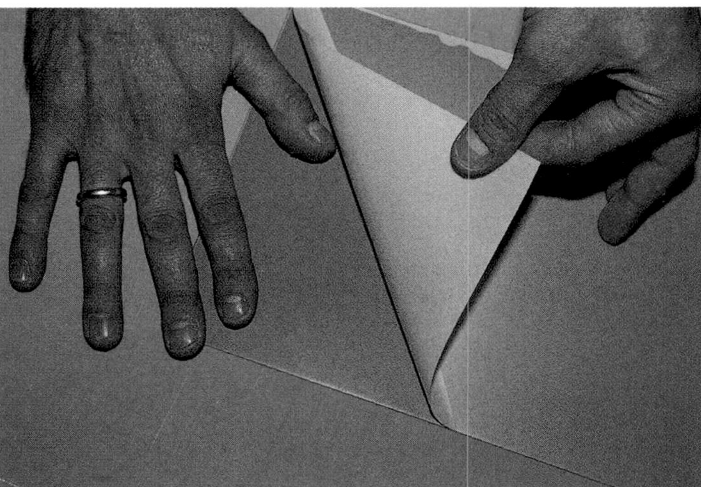
(c)

Figures 7.110 (**a, b**) Nyloprint was the source of this allergic contact dermatitis of the hands. This is an ultraviolet-cured acrylate system, and the route of exposure is demonstrated in (**c**), in which the patient is lifting a plastic layer that protects the prepolymer. Upon being irradiated with UV light, the prepolymer is transformed into a non-sensitizing polymer.

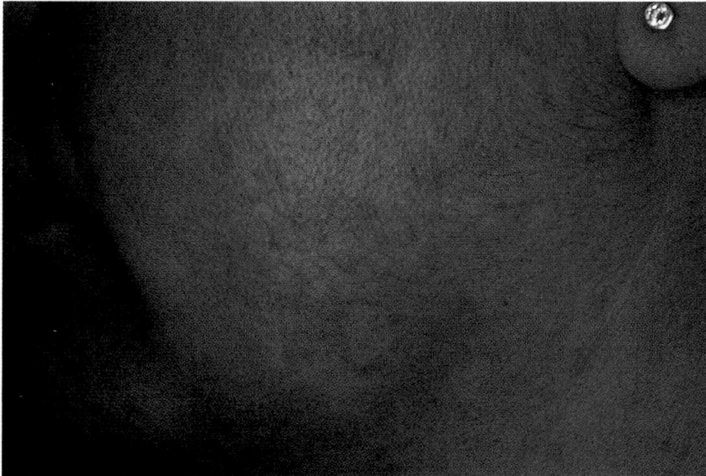

Figure 7.111 This facial allergic contact dermatitis was caused by airborne epoxy–acrylate present in an ultraviolet-cured coating used to print lottery tickets.

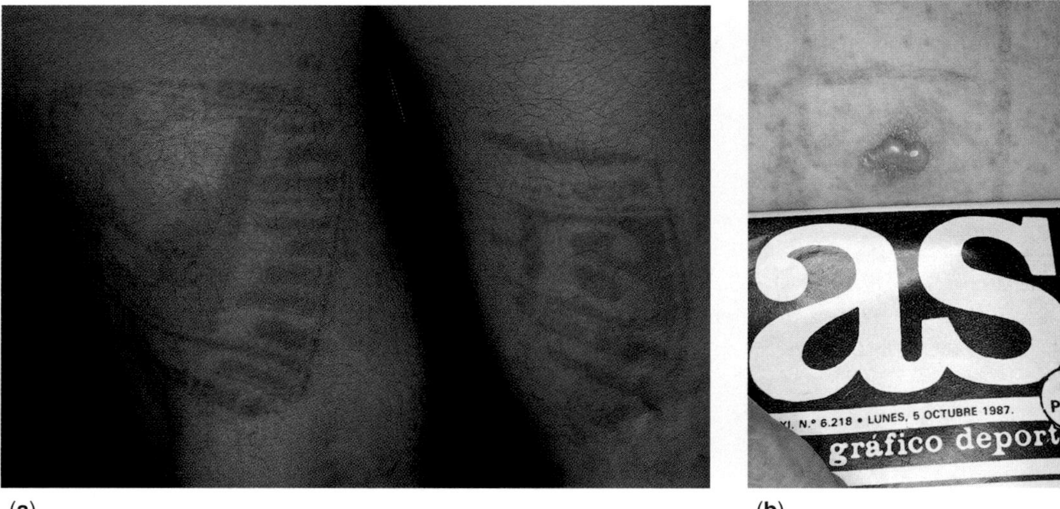

(**a**) (**b**)

Figure 7.112 (**a**) The dermatitis of this woman was caused by aminoazotoluene in newsprint. (**b**) The positive patch test to aminoazotoluene (Conde-Salazar et al, 1991b).

REFERENCES

Benezra C, Ducombs G, Sell A, Foussereau J (1985) *Plant Contact Dermatitis.* Burlington, ON: BC Decker.

Bruze M (1986) Detection of contact allergy to phenol formaldehyde resins. *Contact Dermatitis* **14**:127.

Camarasa JG, Conde-Salazar L (1987) Occupational dermatoses in sanitary workers. In: *Dermatology in Five Continents* (Orfanos CE, Sradler R, Gollnick H, eds). Berlin: Springer-Verlag: 1045–8.

Canizares O (1959) Lichen planus-like eruptions caused by a color-film developer. *Arch Dermatol* **80**:81–6.

Christensen LP, Kristiansen K (1995) Isolation and quantification of a new tuliposide (tuliposide D) by HPLC in *Alstroemeria. Contact Dermatitis* **33**:188–92.

Conde-Salazar L (1990) Rubber dermatitis: clinical forms. *Dermatol Clin* **8**:46–55.

Conde-Salazar L (1993) Dermatitis de contacto professional. *Rev Española de Alergia e Immunologica Clinica* **8**: 19–25.

Conde-Salazar L, Zambrano Zambrano A (1979) Ulceras por cromo. *Medicina y Seguridad del Trabajo* **108**:40–2.

Conde-Salazar L, Garcia A, Raffensperger F, Hausen B (1980) Contact allergy to the Brazilian rosewood substitute *Machaerium scleroxylon* Tul. (pao ferro). *Contact Dermatitis* **6**:246–50.

Conde-Salazar L, Romero L, Guimaraens D (1982a) Allergic contact dermatitis from diazo paper. *Contact Dermatitis* **8**:210–11.

Conde-Salazar L, Guimaraens D, Harto A, Romero L (1982b) Dermatitis de contacto por reealadores de color. *Actas Dermo-Sif* **73**:231–40.

Conde-Salazar L, Guimaraens D, Romero L, Harto A (1984) Sensibilidad de contacto a resina Para-terciario-butil-fenol formol. *Med Cutan Ibero Lat Am* **12**:449–56.

Conde-Salazar L, Romero L, Guimaraens D, Gonzalez MA (1988a) Dermatitis alergica de contacto por acrilatos en odontologo y protesico dental. *Actas Dermo-Sif* **79**:13–16.

Conde-Salazar L, Guimaraens D, Romero L (1988b) Occupational allergic contact dermatitis from anaerobic acrylic selants. *Contact Dermatitis* **18**:129–33.

Conde-Salazar L, Meza B, Guimaraens D, Cannavo A (1991a) Dermatosis profesionales por Bioban CS-1246 y Bioban p-1487 en metalurgicos. *Actas Dermo-Sif* **82**:675–9.

Conde-Salazar L, Gonzalez MA, Guimaraens D, Meza B (1991b) Allergic contact dermatitis from newspaper ink. *Am J Contact Derm* **2**:245–6.

Conde-Salazar L, Gorospe M, Guimaraens D (1993a) A new source of sensitivity to epoxy resin. *Contact Dermatitis* **28**:292.

Conde-Salazar L, Del Rio E, Guimaraens D, Gonzalez MA (1993b) Type IV allergy to rubber additives: a 10-year study of 686 cases. *J Am Acad Dermatol* **29**:176–80.

Conde-Salazar L, Cannavo Alonso A, Guimaraens D, Juanena D (1993c) Dermatosis profesionales en la industria metalurgica: revision de 269 casos. *Actas Dermo-Sif* **84**:339–45.

Conde-Salazar L, Gonzalez MA, Guimaraens D (1994) Sensitization to epoxy resin systems in special flooring workers. *Contact Dermatitis* **31**:157–60.

Conde-Salazar L, Guimaraens D, Villegas C et al (1995a) Occupational allergic contact dermatitis in construction workers. *Contact Dermatitis* **33**:226–30.

Conde-Salazar L, Baz M, Guimaraens D, Cannavo A (1995b) Contact dermatitis in hairdressers: patch test results in 379 hairdressers 1980–1993. *Am J Contact Derm* **6**:19–23.

Conde-Salazar L, Luelmo L, Guimaraens D et al (1997) Alergia al latex: estudio de 35 casos. *Med Cutan Iber Lat Am* 315–23.

Conde-Salazar L, Rojo S, Guimaraens D (1998) Occupational allergic contact dermatitis from cyanoacrylate. *Am J Contact Derm* **3**:188–9.

Dempsey KJ (1982) Hypersensitivity to Sta-Lok and Loctite anaerobic sealants. *J Am Acad Dermatol* **7**:779.

Fisher AA (1975) 'Hypoallergenic' surgical gloves and gloves for special situations. *Cutis* **15**:797.

Fisher AA (1982) Fiberglass vs mineral wool (rock wool) dermatitis. *Cutis* **29**:412.

Fisher AA, Dooms-Goossens A (1976) Persulfate hair bleach reactions. Cutaneous and respiratory manifestations. *Arch Dermatol* **112**:1407–9.

FDA (Food and Drug Administration) (1991). Allergic reactions to latex-containing medical devices. *FDA Med Bull.*

Hamman CP (1993) Natural rubber latex protein sensitivity in review. *Am J Contact Derm* **4**:4.

Hausen BM, Schulz KH (1978) Occupational allergic contact dermatitis due to leatherleaf fern *Arachnidodes adiantiformis* (Forst) Tindale. *Br J Dermatol* **98**:325–9

Hjorth N, Wilkinson DS (1968) Turpentine sensitivity. *Br J Dermatol* **80**:22.

Hogan DJ, Dannaker CJ, Maibach HI (1990) The prognosis of contact dermatitis. *J Am Acad Dermatol* **23**:300–7.

Holness DL, Nethercott JR (1995) Work outcome in workers with occupational skin disease. *Am J Ind Med* **27**:807–15.

Kanerva L, Joanki R, Estlander T (1992) Allergic contact dermatitis from non-diglycidyl ether of bisphenol A epoxy resins. *Contact Dermatitis* **24**:52.

Lamminpaa A, Estlander T, Jolanki R et al (1996) Occupational allergic contact dermatitis caused by decorative plants. *Contact Dermatitis* **34**:330–5.

Le Coz C, Goossens A (1998) Contact dermatitis from an immersion oil for microscopy. *N Engl J Med* **339**:406–7.

Lobel E (1995) Post-contact chronic eczema: pension or rehabilitation? *Australas J Dermatol* **36**:59–62.

Lushniak BD (1995) The epidemiology of occupational contact dermatitis. *Dermatol Clin* **23**:671–80.

Mathias CG (1988) Occupational dermatoses. *J Am Acad Dermatol* **19**:1107–14.

Meding B, Swanbeck G (1990) Occupational hand eczema in an industrial city. *Contact Dermatitis* **22**:13.

Mitchell JC, Rook A (1979) *Botanical Dermatology.* Vancouver, BC: Greenglass.

Murer AJ, Poulsen OM, Roed Petersen J, Tuchsen F (1995) Skin problems among Danish dental technicians. A cross-sectional study. *Contact Dermatitis* **33**:42–7.

Neldner KH (1972) Contact dermatitis from animal feed additives. *Arch Dermatol* **106**:722.

Nethercott JR, Holness DL (1991) Contact dermatitis associated with exposure to oils and coolants. In: *Exogenous Dermatosis: Environmental Dermatitis* (Menné T, Maibach HI, eds). Boca Raton, FL: CRC Press: 365–73.

Noojin RO (1954) Brief history of industrial dermatology. *Arch Dermatol* **70**:723–31.

Ortiz de Frutos J, Conde-Salazar L (1996) Dermatosis alergicas de contacto profesionales. Actualizacion 1995. *Dermatología 1994–1996*: 97–112.

Price SM, Popkin GL (1976) Barbers' interdigital hair sinus. *Arch Dermatol* **112**:523–4.

Rietschel RL (1984) Role of socks in shoe dermatitis. *Arch Dermatol* **120**:398.

Rietschel RL, Fowler JF Jr (1995) *Fisher's Contact Dermatitis.* Baltimore, MD: Williams and Wilkins.

Rietschel RL, Huggins R, Levy N et al (1984) In vivo and in vitro testing of gloves for protection against UV-curable acrylate resin systems. *Contact Dermatitis* **11**:279–82.

Roed-Petersen J, Menné T, Nielsen KM et al (1987) Is it possible to work with pao ferro (*Machaerium scleroxylum*, Tul.)? *Arch Dermatol Res* **279**:S108–10.

Rustemeyer T, Frosch PJ (1995) Allergic contact dermatitis from colour developers. *Contact Dermatitis* **32**:59–60.

Rycroft RG, Calnan CD (1976) Dermatitis industrials. *Br J Hosp Med (Ed Español)* **7**:1279–85.

Samitz MH, Epstein E (1962) Experimental cutaneous chromate ulcers in guinea pigs. *Arch Environ Health* **5**:463.

Schmidt H (1978) Contact urticaria. *Contact Dermatitis* **4**:230.

Storrs FJ (1988) Permanent wave contact dermatitis: contact allergy to glyceryl monothioglycolate. *J Am Acad Dermatol* **11**:74–85.

Susitaival P, Husman L, Hollmen A et al (1995) Hand eczema in Finnish farmers. *Contact Dermatitis* **32**:150–5.

Tacke J, Schmidt A, Fartasch M, Diepgen TL (1995) Occupational contact dermatitis in bakers, confectioners and cooks. A population-based study. *Contact Dermatitis* **33**:112–17.

Taylor JS (1982) The pilosebaceous unit. In: *Occupational and Industrial Dermatology* (Maibach HI, Gellin GA, eds). Chicago: Year Book Medical Publishers: 125–36.

Turk K, Rietschel RL (1993) Effect of processing cement to concrete on hexavalent chromium levels. *Contact Dermatitis* **28**:209–11.

Veien NK (1987) Occupational dermatoses in farmers. In: *Occupational and Industrial Dermatology*, 2nd edn (Maibach HI, ed). Chicago: Year Book Medical Publishers: 436–46.

Veien NK, Hattel T, Justesen O, Nørholm A (1980) Occupational contact dermatitis due to spiramycin and/or tylosin among farmers. *Contact Dermatitis* **6**:410.

8

Unique Cases

Contact dermatitis can present with unusual morphology or can be due to an unusual set of circumstances. These cases can be both instructive and of clinical interest. In some of the following examples, teaching points have broad applicability, while in others the point is a narrow one.

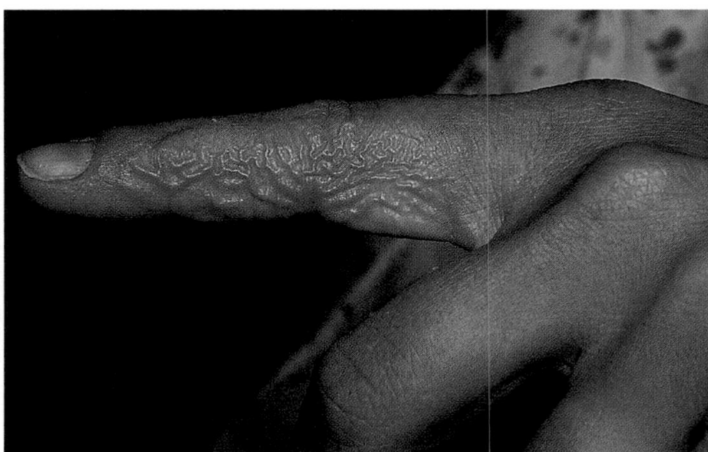

(a)

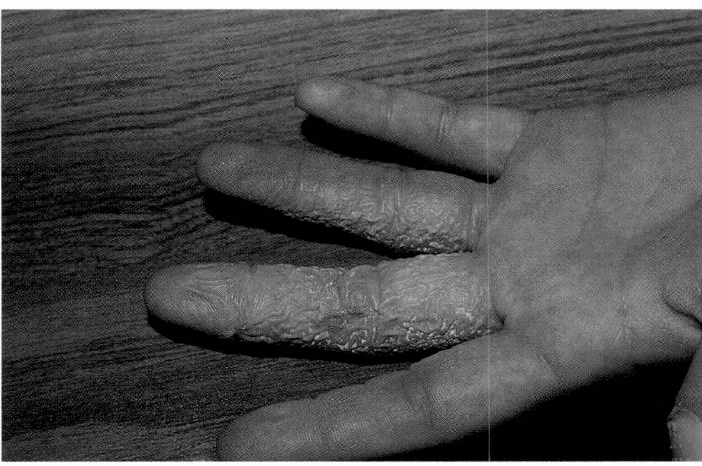

(b)

Figures 8.1 (**a**, **b**) The corrugation of the finger seen here occurred within hours of exposure to a solvent used to remove laundry labels glued into clothing. The solvent was 90% dimethylformamide and 10% glycol ethers. The changes lasted a week.

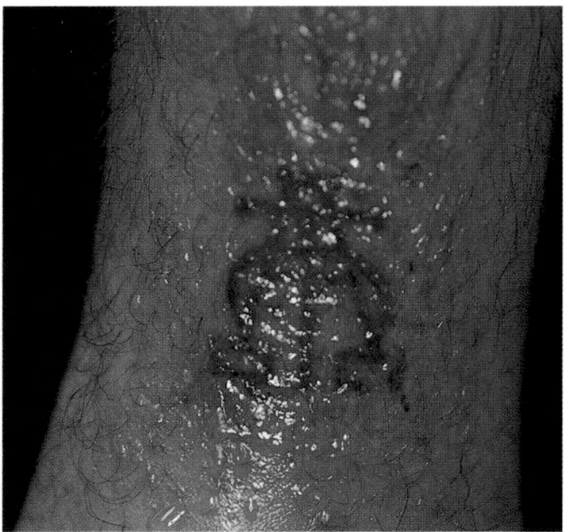

Figure 8.2 This young man was a college student who had his ankle tattooed. He developed dermatitis that was attributed to the presence of the tattoo by two physicians, who recommended removal of the tattoo. They failed to inquire about the use of topical medications, and he failed to mention that the tattoo parlour had instructed him to use a neomycin-containing topical antibiotic to prevent infection. He continued to use this preparation for a month, not realizing that he was allergic to the neomycin component of the medication. The tattoo was not the problem and did not need to be removed.

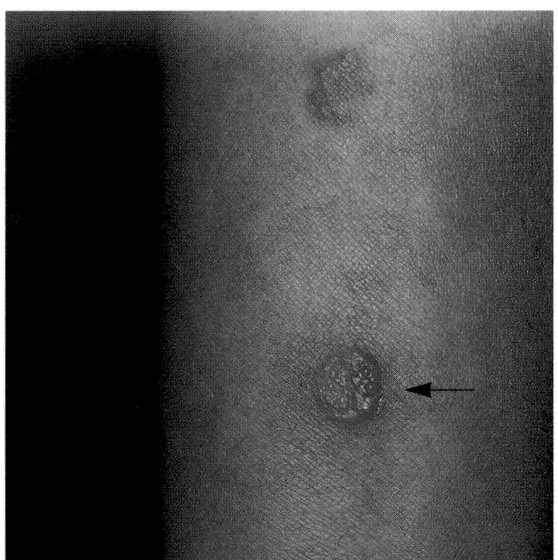

Figure 8.3 Although the quality of this picture is poor, the patch test reactions on this young woman's arm illustrate the specificity of the cutaneous immune system. She was a dermatology technician who was instructed to patch test several volunteers with maleic acid. She volunteered herself, and the patch test in the lower portion of this figure is a day 2 reaction (arrow): it is crisply circular. The reaction above this is not as crisp, and no patch test was applied to this site. She had forgotten that six years earlier, while working for another dermatology researcher, she had become sensitized to maleic acid and had been tested on the upper arm at that time as well. The less prominent reaction is recall of that antecedent reaction, and demonstrates the specificity of the skin's memory of prior events.

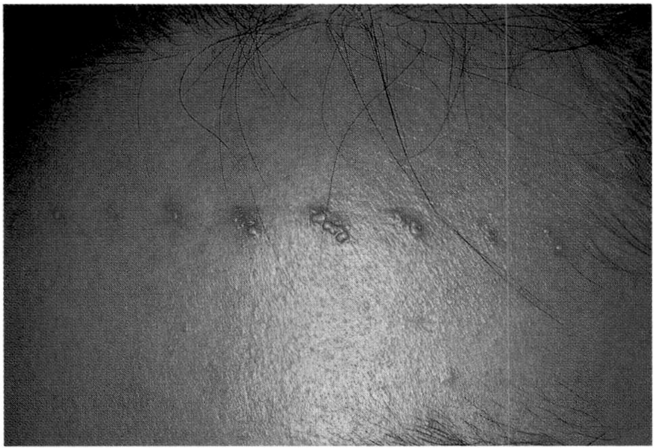

Figure 8.4 The pustules on the forehead of this young woman occurred within 24 hours of wearing a decorative metal headband as part of a costume. The metal decorations were diamond-shaped with somewhat sharp edges, accounting for the repeated pattern. Pustular reactions to occluded metals is not an allergic event, and is seen as a patch test artefact at times. This is more common among persons with atopic dermatitis, and can be induced by pricking the skin of an atopic person and then applying an occlusive patch test to a metal, such as nickel (Uehara et al, 1975).

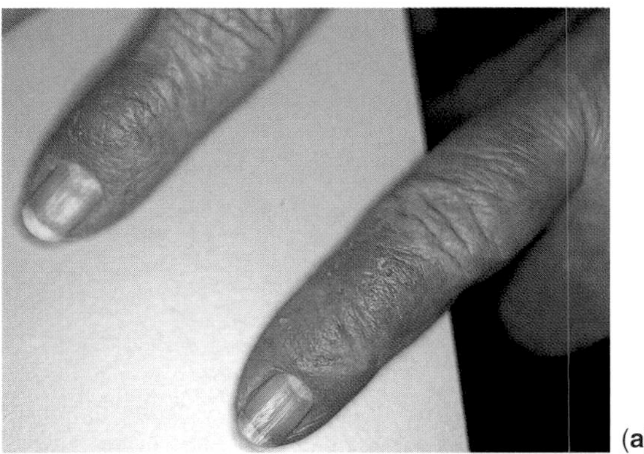

(**a**)

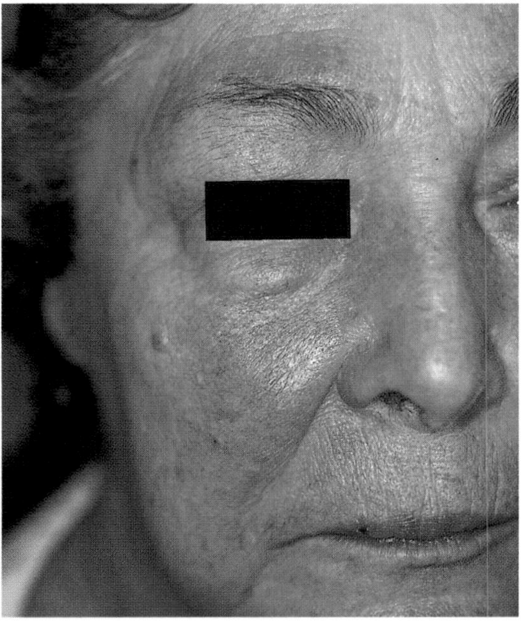

(**b**)

Figure 8.5 This woman had dermatitis of her fingers (**a**) and face (**b**) that persisted, despite treatment. Patch testing with the screening series of the North American Contact Dermatitis Group did not reveal the source of her eruption. Her problem began shortly after her husband suffered a stroke and she began to handle and administer his medications. Patch tests to his medications revealed a reaction to quinidine and his nitroglycerin patch. When she handled his medication with forceps and allowed him to apply his own nitroglycerin patch, her dermatitis cleared completely.

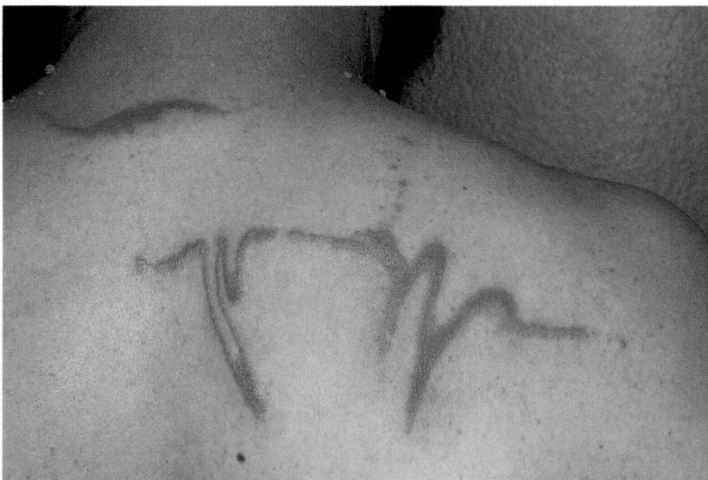

Figure 8.6 A peculiar skin reaction occurred after mediastinoscopy. The agent thought to be responsible was iodine, used as an antiseptic (Mochida et al, 1995).

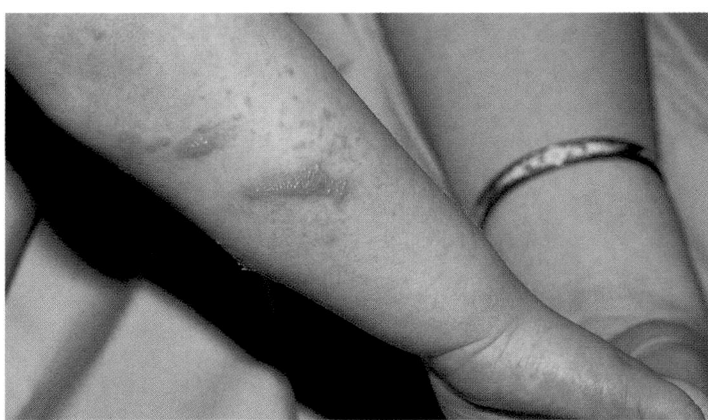

(a)

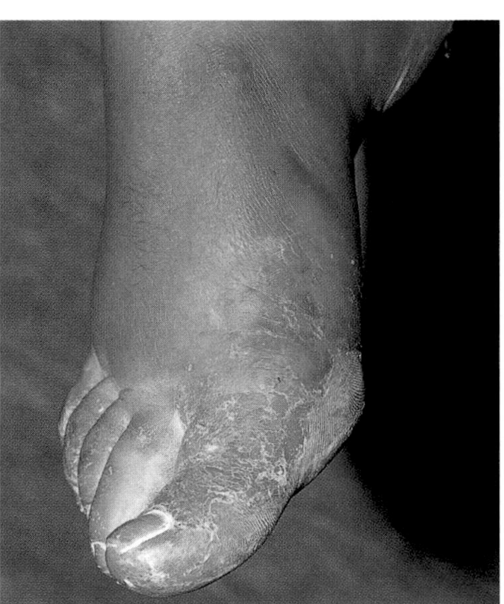

(b)

Figure 8.7 (**a**) Contact dermatitis to vegetation frequently causes linear streaks of dermatitis occurring in directions that do not conform to anatomical structures such as lymphatic channels. This dermatitis was due to contact with a plant. (**b**) Lymphangitis may be a complication of severe allergic contact dermatitis (here caused by shoe material).

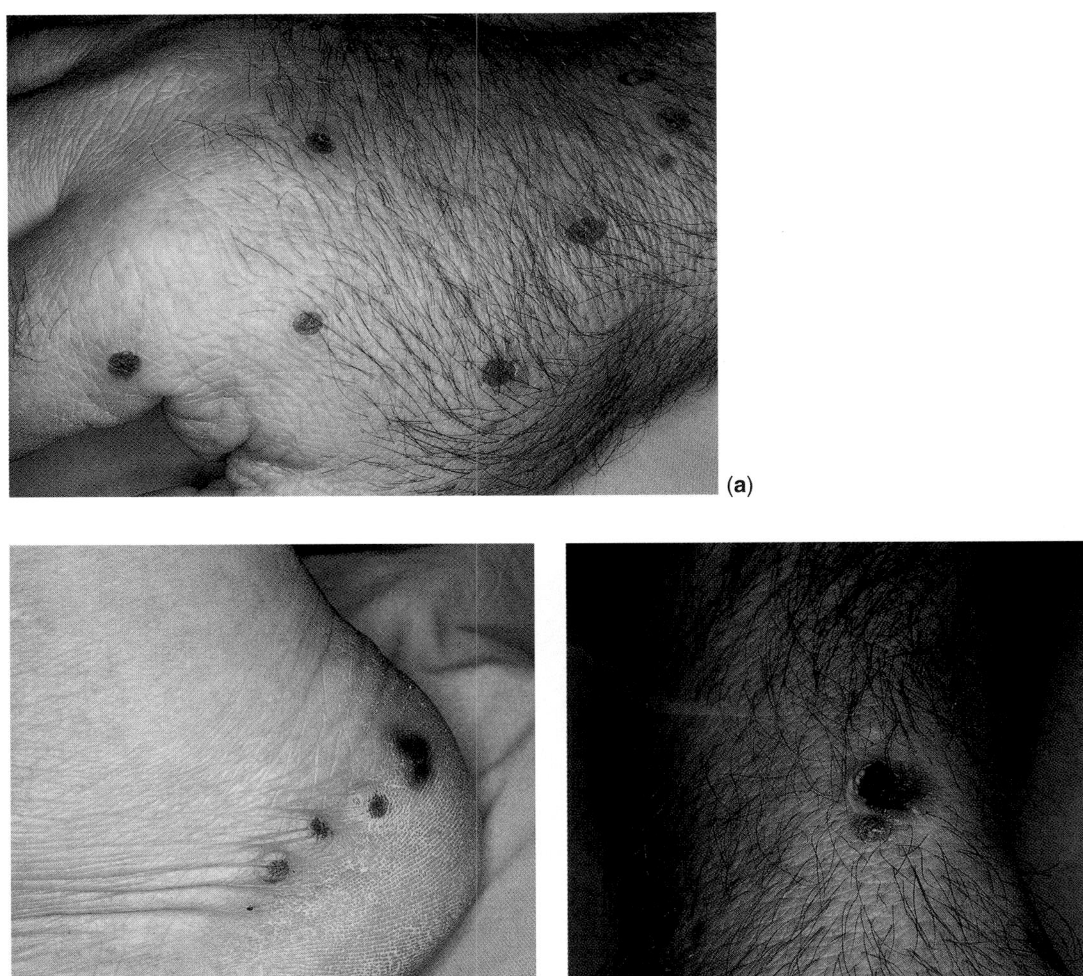

Figure 8.8 This patient had irritant lesions (burns) in various parts of the body, including the hands (a), feet (b) and abdomen. He consulted a dermatologist because he feared that some of the lesions were infected. At the time, he was treating joint pain with an unconventional treatment known as the Moxa technique. This consisted of applying powdered artemisia plant to specific points (determined by acupuncture) and then setting fire to it (c) (Conde-Salazar et al, 1991).

CONNUBIAL CONTACT DERMATITIS

Connubial contact dermatitis occurs when one spouse uses a substance to which he or she is not allergic, but to which the other spouse reacts following skin contact. When the partners are not married the correct term is consort dermatitis (Morren et al, 1992; Fisher, 1994).

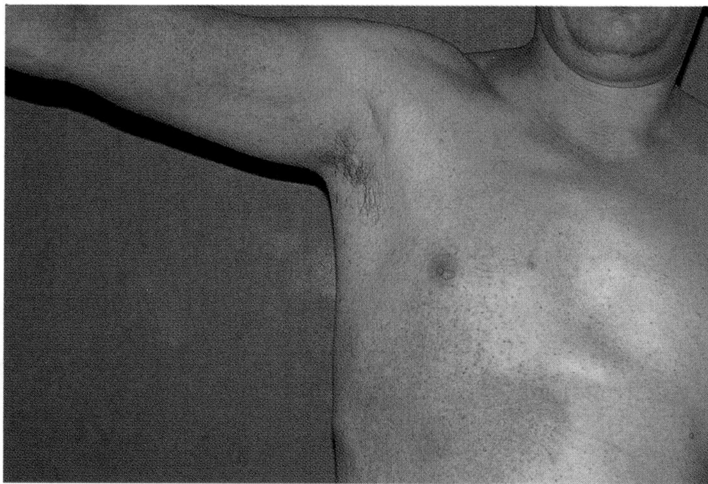

Figure 8.9 The dermatitis on the right trunk and arms was caused by exposure to etofenamate, a non-steroidal topical drug used by the patient's spouse on her left shoulder (Guerra et al, 1992).

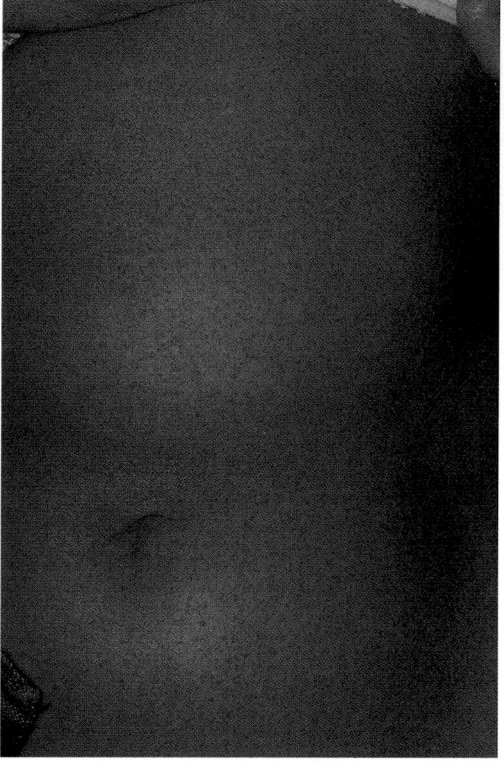

(**a**)

(**b**)

Figure 8.10 At times, the amount of material transferred from one partner to the other is such that only a folliculitis-like eruption will occur, as in this 24-year-old woman who did not use sunscreen, although her partner did. Her case was incorrectly diagnosed as recurrent and disseminate infundibulofolliculitis, until the connection with her partner's sunscreen use became apparent. (**a**, **b**) A positive patch test to individual sunscreen ingredients demonstrated that homosalate was the cause of this eruption. This substance was contained in the sunscreen in question (Rietschel and Lewis, 1978).

Figure 8.11 This young man had no dermatological problems until he married. His dermatitis was follicular and confined to the anterior trunk. He was asked to bring his wife's skin care products in for testing. He brought in a shopping bag full of skin-care products, and once these were in the dermatology clinic his eruption cleared. He had a folliculitis-like patch test reaction to glycerol and light mineral oil. A biopsy of the patch test reaction showed epidermal spongiosis and no evidence of folliculitis. The eruption cleared owing to his wife's avoidance of skin-care products containing glycerol and mineral oil.

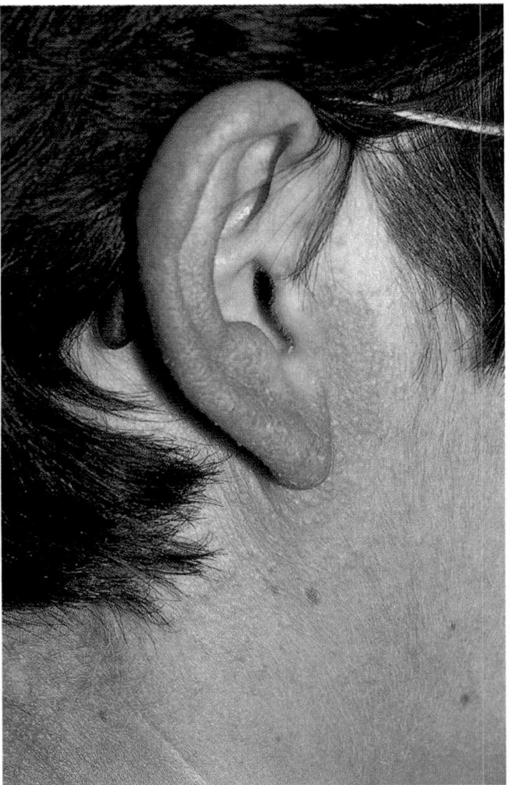

(**a**)

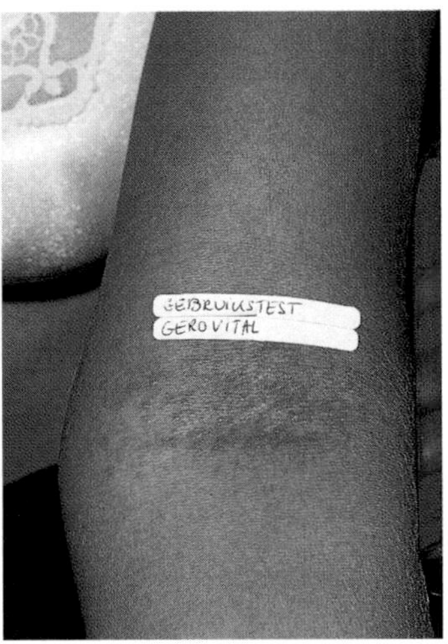

(**b**)

Figure 8.12 (**a**) This woman developed allergic contact dermatitis on the ears, as well as on the eyelids and neck, due to a pillow contaminated with a procaine-containing hair lotion used by her husband. (**b**) A positive repeated open application test (ROAT) in this procaine-sensitive woman.

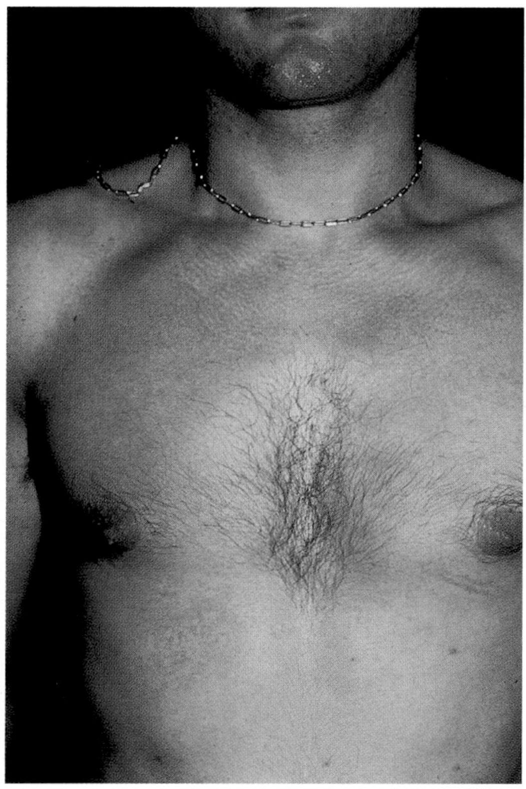

(a)

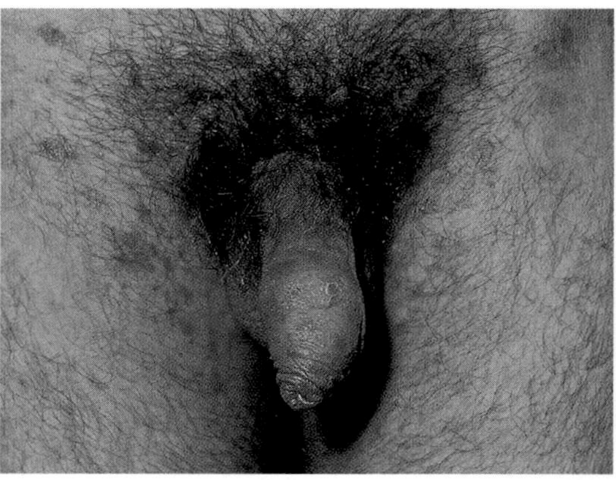

(b)

Figure 8.13 (**a**) Connubial dermatitis on the chest in a young man caused by the perfume used by his fiancée. (**b**) Lesions in the genital area in the same patient. (Courtesy of JM Mougeolle, Nancy, France.)

REFERENCES

Conde-Salazar L, Gonzalez MA, Guimaraens D, Fuente C (1991) Burns due to moxibustion. *Contact Dermatitis* **25**:332–3.

Fisher AA (1994) Management of 'consort dermatitis' due to combined allergy: seminal fluid and latex condoms. *Cutis* **54**:66–7.

Guerra L, Piraccini BM, Adami F et al (1992) Contact dermatitis due to etofenamate. *Contact Dermatitis* **26**:199.

Mochida K, Hisa T, Yasunaga C et al (1995) Skin ulceration due to povidone–iodine. *Contact Dermatitis* **33**:61–2.

Morren M-A, Rodrigues R, Dooms-Goossens A, Degreef H (1992) Connubial contact dermatitis: a review. *Eur J Dermatol* **2**:219–23.

Rietschel RL, Lewis CW (1978) Contact dermatitis to homomethyl salicylate. *Arch Dermatol* **114**:442–3.

Uehara M, Takahashi C, Ofugi S (1975) Pustular patch test reactions in atopic dermatitis. *Arch Dermatol* **111**:1154–7.

Appendix

European and US Standard Patch Test Series

European Standard Patch Test Series

Serial No.	*Substance*	*Concentration*[a]
1.	Potassium dichromate	0.5% pet
2.	Neomycin sulfate	20% pet
3.	Thiuram mix (tetramethylthiuram disulfide, tetraethylthiuram disulfide, tetramethylthiuram monosulfide, dipentamethylenethiuram disulfide, 0.25% each)	1% pet
4.	Paraphenylenediamine free base	1% pet
5.	Cobalt chloride, hexahydrate	1% pet
6.	Benzocaine	5% pet
7.	Formaldehyde	1% aq
8.	Colophony	20% pet
9.	Clioquinol	5% pet
10.	Balsam of Peru	25% pet
11.	*N*-isopropyl-*N*'-phenyl-*p*-phenylenediamine	0.1% pet
12.	Wool alcohols	30% pet
13.	Mercapto mix (mercaptobenzothiazole, *N*-cyclohexylbenzothiazyl sulfenamide, dibenzothiazyl disulfide, morpholinylmercaptobenzothiazole, 0.5% each)	2% pet
14.	Epoxy resin	1% pet
15.	Paraben mix (methyl *p*-hydroxybenzoate, ethyl *p*-hydroxybenzoate, propyl *p*-hydroxybenzoate, butyl *p*-hydroxybenzoate, 4% each)	16% pet
16.	*p-tert*-Butylphenol–formaldehyde resin	1% pet
17.	Fragrance mix (cinnamyl alcohol, cinnamaldehyde, eugenol, α-amylcinnamaldehyde, hydroxycitronellal, geraniol, isoeugenol, oak moss absolute, 1% each; sorbitan sesquioleate, 5%)	8% pet
18.	Quaternium-15 (Dowicil 200)	1% pet

[a] pet, petrolatum; aq, water.

19.	Nickel sulfate, hexahydrate	5% pet
20.	Methylchloroisothiazolinone–methylisothiazolinone	0.01% aq
21.	Mercaptobenzothiazole	2% pet
22.	Sesquiterpene lactone mix (alantolactone, dihydrocostus lactone, costunolide, 0.033% each)	0.1% pet
23.	Primin	0.01% pet

TRUE Test System

The 24 TRUE Test allergens are as follows:

PANEL 1

Serial No.	*Substance*	*Concentration*
1.	Nickel sulfate	200 μg/cm^2
2.	Wool alcohols	1000 μg/cm^2
3.	Neomycin sulfate	230 μg/cm^2
4.	Potassium dichromate	23 μg/cm^2
5.	Caine mix	630 μg/cm^2
6.	Fragrance mix	430 μg/cm^2
7.	Colophony	850 μg/cm^2
8.	Epoxy resin	50 μg/cm^2
9.	Quinoline mix	190 μg/cm^2
10.	Balsam of Peru	800 μg/cm^2
11.	Ethylenediamine dihydrochloride	50 μg/cm^2
12.	Cobalt chloride	20 μg/cm^2

PANEL 2

Serial No.	*Substance*	*Concentration*
13.	*p-tert*-Butylphenol–formaldehyde resin	40 μg/cm^2
14.	Paraben mix	1000 μg/cm^2
15.	Carba mix	250 μg/cm^2
16.	Black rubber mix (PPD mix)	75 μg/cm^2
17.	Methylchloroisothiazolinone–methylisothiazolinone	4 μg/cm^2
18.	Quaternium-15	100 μg/cm^2
19.	Mercaptobenzothiazole	75 μg/cm^2
20.	Paraphenylenediamine	90 μg/cm^2
21.	Formaldehyde	180 μg/cm^2
22.	Mercapto mix	75 μg/cm^2
23.	Thimerosal	8 μg/cm^2
24.	Thiuram mix	25 μg/cm^2

In North America, the above 24 allergens are thought to comprise a screening series that can be supplemented with additional allergens for a more comprehensive evaluation. The additional allergens that have been used by the North American Contact Dermatitis Group are as follows:

Serial No.	*Substance*	*Concentration*
25.	Diazolidinyl urea	1% pet
26.	DMDM hydantoin	1% pet
27.	Imidazolidinyl urea	2% pet
28.	Bacitracin	20% pet
29.	Mixed dialkyl thioureas	1% pet
30.	Methylchloroisothiazolinone–methylisothiazolinone	100 ppm aq
31.	Paraben mix	12% pet
32.	Methyldibromoglutaronitrile–phenoxyethanol	1% pet
33.	Fragrance mix	8% pet
34.	Glutaraldehyde	0.5% pet
35.	2-Bromo-2-nitropropane-1,3-diol	0.5% pet
36.	Sesquiterpene lactone mix	0.1% pet
37.	Thimerosal	0.1% pet
38.	Propylene glycol	30% aq
39.	Oxybenzone	3% pet
40.	Chloroxylenol (PCMX)	1% pet
41.	DMDM hydantoin	1% aq
42.	Diazolidinyl urea	1% aq
43.	Ethyleneurea melamine–formaldehyde	5% pet
44.	Methyldibromoglutaronitrile–phenoxyethanol	2.5% pet
45.	Butylhydroxyanisole	2% pet
46.	Glutaraldehyde	1% pet
47.	Sodium gold thiosulfate	0.5% pet
48.	Ethyl acrylate	0.1% pet
49.	Glyceryl thioglycolate	1% pet
50.	Toluenesulfonamide–formaldehyde resin	10% pet
51.	Methyl methacrylate	2% pet
52.	Cobalt chloride	1% pet
53.	Tixocortol-21-pivalate	1% pet
54.	Budesonide	0.1% pet
55.	Imidazolidinyl urea	2% aq

An alternative comprehensive evaluation would be to use the European Screening Series for the first 23 allergens, again supplemented by the above allergens 25–55.

Index

Abbreviations: CD, contact dermatitis

Aclomethasone dipropionate, 177
Acrylates, 179, 237–41, 249–51
  face, airborne source, 294
  hands/fingertips/nails, 91, 104, 249, 250, 251
    graphic arts workers, 293
    health care workers, 237–41
  medical devices, 183, 184
Acupuncture points, 303
Acupuncture staples, 68
Acute CD
  examples
    mild to moderate, 4
    moderate to severe, 5
    severe, 6
  histopathology, 14, 15
  management, 39–41
Adhesive tape, colophony, 284
Aftershave, 70
Agave americanus, 201
Agriculture, 217–22
  rubber
    components, 217, 259
    latex, 262
Airborne dermatitis, 143–9, *see also* Inhaled allergens
  Juniperus spp., 202
  occupational exposure, 276
    to chromates, 262, 292
    to epoxy resin, 242, 243
    in health care workers, 236
    in lithographers, 292
  topography, 49
Alkali burns, cement, 5, 224, 225, 226
Allergens, 135, *see also specific (types of) allergens*
  common, 1
    in agriculture, 217
    in construction industry, 224
    ears, 58
    extremities/genitalia, 72
    eyelids, 53
    face, 49
    feet, 107
    in graphic arts, 286
    hair-care products, 271, 272
    hands, 78
    in health care, 231
    in medical devices, 178
    metals and metalworking fluids, 263
    mouth/lips, 56
    nails, 103
    in photography, 286
    in plants, 196, 277
    in rubber, 252
    trunk, 60
  in delayed-type hypersensitivity, 14
  irritant reaction to non-standard allergens, 32
  medications as, 158
  photo-, *see* Photoallergic reactions
  route of reaching skin, 47
  substitution, 39
  systemic CD, 116
  tests, 21–38, 307–9
    with plant allergens, 196
  textiles/clothing/shoes, 208

Allergic CD, *see also* Photoallergic reactions
  acute
    mild to moderate, example, 4
    moderate to severe, example, 5
  chronic, example, 8
  common allergens, 1
  hands/fingers, 91, 101
  histopathology, 16
  irritant CD and, interweaving/co-existing, 1, 32
  management, 39
  mechanisms (immunology), 12, 13
  risk factors, 17
  subacute, examples, 7
  traditional concepts, 2–3
Alstroemeria, 91, 204, 205, 279
Aluminium hydroxide, 169
Aluminium subacetate, 40
Amalgam, 57, 195, 239
Amantadine, derivative, 56
Aminoazotoluene, 294
Aminophylline, ethylenediamine sensitivity and, 117
Ammonium compounds, quaternary, 191
Ammonium persulfate, 271
Amniotic fluid, bovine, 221, 222
Amputees, 179–80
α-Amylase, 155
Amyl salicylate, 171
Anaphylaxis (in IgE-mediated hypersensitivity/contact urticaria), 150
  ammonium persulfate, 271, 276
Angioedema, 159
Anthraquinone dye, 59
Antifungal agent, 220
Antimicrobials, photoallergy, 135, *see also specific drugs*
Antioxidants, rubber, 252
  feet, 109
  hands, 98
  paraphenylenediamine-derived, *see* Paraphenylenediamine-derived compounds
  trunk, 64
Antiperspirants, 69, 70
Antiviral drug, 56
  cream carrier, 77
Arms, sources of CD, 48, *see also* Extremities
  airborne, 202
  epoxy resins, 245
  thiurams, 261
  topical medications, 165, 166, 168, 169, 174
Artemisia plant, 303
Atopic dermatitis
  feet, 112
  hands in, 89, 97
    and concomitant locations, 88
    systemic CD affecting, 125
  as irritant CD risk factor, 14
Atranorin, 189
Axillary CD
  examples, 62, 69, 70
  sources, 48, 60
  systemic, 122
Azo dye, 111, 209

'Baboon syndrome' CD, 122, 176
Balsam
  Chinese, 167
  Peru, 96
    staining, 33
    systemic CD, 123
'Barber's hair sinus', 272
Barrier creams, 44
Bay leaf, 116
Beau's lines, 103, 104
Benzalkonium chloride, 159
Benzoin tincture, 178
Benzoyl peroxide and benzoic acid, 151, 159
Bioban CS-1246, 269
Biology, contact dermatitis, 12
Birch pollen, prick test, 36
BisGMA, 183
'Black heel', 131
Black light device, 28
Black rubber mix, 74, 180, 229, 252, 256, 257, 258
Bleach, 64
  hair, 5, 271, 276

Blisters, *see* Bullae
Bone cement, acrylate, 240
Bovine amniotic fluid, 221, 222
Brassiere materials, 60, 61
Brazilian ironwood, 283
Bricker bladder, 181
Budesonide, 176, 177
Building industry, 223–30
Bullae/blisters
  in acute dermatitis
    in allergic CD, 4
    in irritant CD, *6*
  feet, *6*
  hands/fingers, 4, *99*
  phytophotodermatitis, 137, 138, 139
  3–plus reaction in patch test, 31
Burow's solution, 40
Buttocks
  mechanical dermatitis, 131
  systemic reactions affecting, 122, 176
  topical medications affecting, 166, 176

Cactus, 201, 280
Camomile, 163
Carba mix, 61
δ-3–Carene, 281, 282
Cassia oil, 151
CD2/3/4/6 (colour developers), 285, 287, 288
Cellulose acetate, 59
Cement, 223, 224–8, *see also* Bone cement
  burns (alkali), 5, 224, 225, 226
Century plant, 201
Cephalosporins, 235
Cetrimide, 168
Chamber systems, 23, *see also* Scratch-chamber test
  example reactions, 25, 26, 27
Cheek CD, sources of, 48
Cheilitis, *see* Lips
Chin, sources of CD, 48
Chinese balsam, 167
Chinoform, 170
Chloracne, 270, 271
Chloramphenicol, 158
Chloroacetamide, 148
Chlorocresol, 32
Chloronaphthalenes, 271
Chromium/chromates
  airborne, 145
  back, 194
  extremities, 73
  feet, 109, 195, 212
  hands, 98, 124, 145, 193, 227, 228, 292
    non-eczematous CD, 126
    systemic CD, 124
  neck/face, 145, *266*, 292
  typical body distribution, 192
Chronic CD, 8
  histopathology, 14, 15
  management, 41–2
Cinnamon-containing substances, 151
Classification of dermatitis, 1
Clioquinol, 170
Clonidine, 185
Clothing/textiles, 60–5, 207–12, *see also* Footwear
  dyes, 29, 65, 75, 208, 209, 210
  purpuric patterns, 126
Coal tar, therapeutic use, 45
Coal-tar derivatives, 270
Cobalt, 227
  thigh, 73, 228
Cod, 38
Coins, 73, 263
Colophony (rosin), 7
  adhesive tape, 284
  Chinese balsam ointment, 167
  herbal product, 203
  pine boxes, 284
  wound dressing, 172
Colour developers, 285, 287, 288
Compositae, 196, 200
Condom, rubber urinal, 181
Connubial CD, 304–6
Consort CD, 304–6
Construction industry, 223–30
Contact urticaria, *see* Urticaria
Coolants, 267–9
Corrugations, finger, 299

Corticosteroids, topical
  adverse effects, 41, 42
    allergic CD, 112, 160, 175–7
  applications, 43
    acute CD, 40–1
    irritant CD, 45
    subacute/chronic CD, 41–2
  examples, 43
  relative potencies, 44
Cosmetics, 51, 185–91, *see also specific ingredients and types of cosmetics*
  subacute irritant CD, 7
Cost of occupational skin disease, 11
Cows
  amniotic fluid, 221, 222
  dander, 222
Creams
  barrier, 44
  hydroquinone-containing, 105
  steroid-containing, 41–2
  udder, 95
Creosote, 4
Crown bonding agents, 57
Cyanoacrylate, 251
Cyclist's bottom, 131
Cyclohexyl-phenyl paraphenylenediamine, 109

Dandelion, 200
Dander, cow, 222
Delayed-type hypersensitivity, allergens causing, 14
Dental materials, 57, 195
  health care workers, 237–41
Deodorants, 69, 189
Depigmentation, *see* Hypopigmentation/depigmentation
Dermatitis, classification, 1
Dermatographism, white, 88, 89
Dermatophytes (ringworm; tinea)
  feet, 97, 108
  hands, 86, 97, 132
Desquamation, 8
Detergent, washing, 62
  scented, 62
Developers
  black and white, 287
  colour, 285, 287, 288
Diallyl disulfide, 206, 279
Diazonium compounds, 289
N,N'-Dibenzylcarbamyl chloride, 64
Dibromodicyanobutane–phenoxyethanol, 71, 164, 186, 187
Dichromates, *see* Chromium/chromates
Diethylthiorurea, 210, 212
Digits of hand, *see* Fingertip/pulp reactions; Hand and finger dermatitis; Nails
Dimethylformamide, 6, 299
Dimethylglyoxime test, 194
Diphenyl-paraparaphenylenediamine, 256
Disinfectant, 233
Disperse blue-106, 209
Disperse orange, 65, 75
  patch test, 29, 65, 75
Disperse yellow, 65, 75
  patch test, 29, 65, 75
Dorsal dermatitis
  feet, footwear and, 107, 108, 109, 110, 112, 195
  hands, 93, 94, 95, 96
    palmar dermatitis with, 102
Dough, 152
Drug reactions, *see* Medications and drugs
Drug therapy
  acute CD, 40–1
  irritant CD, 45
  phototherapy plus, 45–6
  subacute/chronic CD, 41–2
Dyes
  footwear, 211
  hair, 50, 51, 190, 273–5
  patch test, 29, 65, 75
  spectacle frame, 59
  stocking, *see* Stocking dye
  textiles, 29, 65, 75, 208, 209, 210
Dyshidrosis, lamellar, 87

Ears, 58–9
  airborne CD behind, 146, 149, 202
  common sources of CD, 48, 58
    metals, 58, 192
    topical medications, 160, 161, 166

Ectopic dermatitis
face/eyelids
acrylic nails, 250
nailpolish, 52, 55
plant allergens, 197, 198
neck, from nailpolish, 52, 55
Edema, *see* Oedema
Elastic components, 64
Elbow
nickel, *see* Nickel
systemic CD, 123
flexures, 119
Electrical nerve stimulation
peroneal, 182
transcutaneous, 183
Electronic printed circuit boards, 246
Electroplating and chromates, 266
Environmental risk factors
allergic CD, 17
contact urticaria/protein CD, 17
irritant CD, 15
Epidemiology, 11
occupational CD, 215–16
Epoxy resin, 59, 242–6
in medical devices, 183, 184
occupational exposure, 148, 241, 250
airborne, 242, 243, 294
Erysipelas, 173
Erythema
acute CD, 4
reflex, 28
violaceous, 288
Erythema multiforme, 126
Ethylenediamine sensitivity, 145
aminophylline and, 117
Etisazole, 220
Etofenamate, 304
Eucerin, 164
European Standard Patch Test Series, 307–8
Euxyl K100 (methylchloroisothiazolinone–methylisothiazolinone), 71, 164, 186, 187, 230
Euxyl K400, 187
Extremities, 72–8, *see also specific parts*
common sources of CD, 48
amputee prostheses, 179–80
dyes, 75, 209
fragrances, 7, 74
topical medications, 166
Exudation in acute allergic CD, 4
Eyebrows, sources of CD, 48
Eyelash curlers, rubber component, 54
Eyelids, 52, 52–5
airborne allergens, 236, 276
chromates, 266, 292
airborne irritants, 147
common sources of CD, 48, 53
factitious dermatitis, 133, 134
lower, 48
protein CD, 154
systemic CD, 122
topical medications affecting, 158–60
upper, 48
dermatitis syndrome (UEDS), 52, 53

Face, 49–57, *see also specific parts*
airborne CD, 146, 147, 148, 202, 236, 266, 276, 292, 294
common sources of CD, 48, 49
cosmetics as, *see* Cosmetics
rubber chemicals, 256
systemic CD, 116, 117
topical medications
CD caused by, 161–4
CD treatment with, 41
Factitious dermatitis, 133, 134
Farming, *see* Agriculture
Fasteners, metal, 67
Foot, *see* Feet
Fibre insulating material, 229
'Fiddlers neck', 129
Finger dermatitis, *see* Hand and finger dermatitis *and entries below*
Finger rings, 91, 92
Fingernails, *see* Nails; Nailpolish
Fingertip/pulp reactions
allergic, 91, 101
in health care workers, 235, 237–41
plants, 91, 206, 278, 279
resins, 246, 248, 249, 251
other, 101
Fingerwebs, 93, 96

Finn chamber, example reactions, 25, 26, 27
'Fixed' dermatitis, 102
Flexural dermatitis, 119
Floor wax stripper, 8
Florists, 205, 278, 280
Folliculitis, 270
  connubial CD, 304, 305
Food allergens, common, 36
Feet, 107–12
  non-eczematous CD, 126, 128, 131
  sources of CD, 48, 107
    chemicals, 108, 109, 110, 111, 195, 251
    topical medications, 171–4, 175
Footwear/shoes
  alternatives, 107
  reactions in makers of, 248
  reactions to, 107, 108, 109, 110
    allergic CD complicating treatment, 175
    chromates in leather, 109, 195
Forearms, *see* Arms
Forehead CD, sources of, 48
Formaldehyde, 172, 207, *see also p-tert*-butylphenol-formaldehyde resin; Tosylamide–formaldehyde
  in coolants, 269
  in health care, 234
Fragrances, *see* Perfumes/scents/fragrances
Frictional, CD, 127, 129, 131, *see also* Mechanical dermatitis
Furocoumarins, *see* Psoralens

Garlic, 91, 206, 279
Genetic risk factors for allergic CD, 17
Genitalia, 77
  common sources of CD, 48, 72
    medical devices, 181
    topical medications, 170
  connubial CD, 306
  systemic CD, 122
Geraniol, 74
Giant hogweed, 138–9
Gloves
  protective, 43, 154, 239
  reactions to, 234
    leather gloves, 98
    nickel button on steel mesh gloves, 264
    rubber gloves, *see* Rubber gloves
Glucocorticoids, *see* Corticosteroids
Glycerol, 305
Glyceryl (mono)thioglycolate, 191, 271
Glycol ethers, 299
Goggles, swim, 55
Graphic arts, 285, 289–94
Grass pollen, prick test, 36
Green pepper, 37
Grenz ray treatment, 45
Guttate psoriasis, 81

Hair, embedded fragments, 272
Hair-care products, 190–1, 271–6
  bleach, 5, 271, 276
  dye, 50, 51, 190, 273–5
  lotions, 50, 161, 191, 305
    perming, 191, 271
Halogenated compounds, 270, 271
Hand and finger dermatitis, 78–106, *see also* Fingertip/pulp reactions; Fingerwebs; Nails
  common sources, 48, 78
    acrylates, *see* Acrylates
    agricultural workers, 218, 219, 220, 221, 222
    construction workers, 227, 228, 229, 230
    epoxy resins, 241, 244, 245, 246
    hair-care products, 272–6
    health care workers, 232, 233, 234, 235, 237, 239, 240, 241
    nickel, *see* Nickel
    plants/woods, 91, 141, 203, 204, 205, 206, 278, 279, 281, 282
    p-tert-butylphenol-formaldehyde resin, 247, 248
    rubber chemicals, 94, 98, 153, 229, 231, 253–5, 257–60
    topical medications, 167, 168
  concomitant other locations, 88–90
  dermatophytes, 86, 97, 132
  diagnostic algorithm, 78–9

epidemiology, 11
non-eczematous CD, 126, 127, 128, 130, 132
non-eczematous dermatoses (non-CD) in, exclusion, 80–7
patterns/morphology, *79*, 91–102
prognosis in occupational causes, 11
steroid therapy, 41, 43
systemic, 115, 116, *119*, 120, 121, 123, 124, 125
unique reactions, *299*
Haptens, 12
sensitization, *see* Sensitization
Health care, 230–41
Heel, friction purpura, 131
Heracleum mantegazzianum (giant hogweed), 138–*9*
Herring, 154
Hexafluorosilicate, 10
Hexamidine, 161
Hip prosthesis, bone cement, 240
Histamine control (prick test), *36*
Histopathology, 14
Hogweed, giant, 138–*9*
Homosalate, 304
Hyacinths, 278
Hydrocortisone allergy, 112, *160*
Hydroquinone, 105
Hyperkeratotic dermatitis, *see* Keratotic/hyperkeratotic dermatitis
Hyperpigmentation, *9*
in chronic irritant CD, 8
floor wax stripper, 8
nickel, *9*, 58, 104, 234
in phototoxic reactions, 127, 141
thiuram, 104
Hypersensitivity
delayed-type, allergens causing, 14
immediate-type, *see* Immediate-type hypersensitivity
Hypopigmentation/depigmentation, post-inflammatory
agents causing
metals, *67*
in patch test, 34
p-tert-butylphenol-formaldehyde resin, 110
feet, 110
waist, *67*

Immediate-type hypersensitivity, *see also* Anaphylaxis
in contact urticaria/protein contact CD, 14, 150
in patch tests, 35
Immunoglobulin E-mediated hypersensitivity, *see* Immediate-type hypersensitivity
Immunology
contact dermatitis, 12
contact urticaria, *see* Urticaria
photoallergic reactions, 12, 134
Incidence, occupational CD, 215–16
Individual factors
allergic CD, 17
contact urticaria/protein CD, 17
irritant CD, 14
Infected hand dermatitis, secondarily, 84
Inhaled allergens
common, *36*
prick tests, 35
Inks
reactions to, *289*
use in patch test, 28
Insulin pumps, 184
Interdigital dermatitis, *93*
Iodine, 302
Iridium-192 dermatitis, 106
Irritant CD
acute, examples
mild to moderate, 4
moderate to severe, 5
severe, *6*
allergic CD and, interweaving/co-existing, 1, 32
biology, 12
chronic, examples, 8
common irritants, 1
agriculture, 217
construction industry, 224
in graphic arts, 286
hair-care products, 272
health care, 231
metal lubricants, 263

Irritant CD – *continued*
photographic chemicals, 286
plant and wood-related occupations, 277
diagnostic criteria, 3
hands, 91
management, 43–5
pustular reactions, 10, 34, 301
risk factors, 14–16
subacute, example, 7
traditional concepts, 2
Isoeugenol, 69
N-Isopropyl-*N'*-phenyl-*p*-phenylenediamine (IPPD), 252, 256
feet, 109
hands, 98, 259

Jogger's nipple, 130
Jugular region, photodermatitis, 136
Juniperus spp., 202
Juvenile plantar dermatitis, 128

Kathon CG (methylchloroisothiazolinone-methylisothiazolinone), 71, 164, 186, 187, 230
Kayak rower's keratotic papules, 130
Keloid at patch test site, 34
Keratolysis exfoliativa, 86
Keratotic/hyperkeratotic dermatitis, 8, 100, 128
chromates, 227, 228
kayak rower's, 130
palmar psoriasis vs, 82, 100
plants causing, 204, 206
resins, 248, 249
rubber components, 253, 259
Knuckles, 93

Lamellar dyshidrosis, 87
Langerhans cells, 12
Lanolin, 51, 73
Latex, 252
rubber gloves, 236, 262
Laurel oil, 116
Leather
chromates in, 98, 109, 195, 212
p-tert-butylphenol-formaldehyde resin in, *see p-tert*-butylphenol-formaldehyde resin
Leatherleaf fern, 280
Lettuce, 200
Lichen, 203
Lichen planus, 85
amalgam reaction vs, 195
Lichenification
in atopic dermatitis, 89
in chronic irritant CD, 8
Limbs, *see* Extremities
Lime, 127, 141
d-Limonene, 170
Lincomycin, 166
Lips (cheilitis), 56–7
common sources of CD, 48, 56
lettuce, 200
Lithography, 292
Location of lesions, *see* Site
Lubricants, metal, 262, 267–70
Lymphangitis, 302

Machaerium scleroxylum, 277, 283
Machine cooling lubricants, 267–9
Maleated soya bean oil, 189
Maleic acid sensitization, 300
Management, 39–46
Mascara, 53
Mechanical dermatitis, 130–1, *see also* Frictional CD
buttocks, 131
feet, 112
hands/fingers/wrists
occupational causes, 82, 101, 218, 229, 230
sport-related, 130
nails, 103
neck, 128
trunk, 9, 130
Medical devices, 177–85, 301
Medications and drugs (humans), 157–77
photosensitizing, 143
topical, 73, 157–77
connubial CD, 304
in first aid boxes (construction site), 223

unique cases, 300, 301
Medications and drugs (veterinary), 217, 219, 220
Mephenesin, 171
Mercapto mix, 307
Mercaptobenzothiazole, *61*, *64*, *78*, 180
footwear, 108, 212
patch test, 31, *64*
Mercury, 57, 195, *239*
Metal(s), *66–8*, 192–5, 262–71, *see also specific metals and metal salts*
ears, 58, 192
extremities, 73, *76*, *77*, 123
in amputee prostheses, 180
graphic arts worker, 291
eyelids, 54
hands/fingers, *92*, *96*, 102, 104, 119, 120, 121, 192, 193
graphic arts worker, 290
health care workers, 234, 235
neck, *66*, *129*
shoulder, *68*
systemic CD, 118, 119, 120, 121, 123
trunk, *9*, *66–8*, 118, 119
wristwatch strap, 193
Metalworking fluids, 262, 267–70
common irritants/allergens, 263
8–Methoxypsoralen + UV, 45–6
Methyl methacrylate, 104, 239, 249
p-Methylaminophenol sulphate, 287
Methylchloroisothiazolinone–methylisothiazolinone, 71, 164, 186, 187, 230
Methyldibromoglutaronitrile–phenoxyethanol, 71, 164, 186, 187
α-Methylene γ-butyrolactone, 204
Metol, 287
Micropore tape, 25
Milking equipment
cleaning fluid, *219*
rubber components, *259*
Mineral oil, 305
Minoxidil, 158
Moisturizers
arm reactions, 72
facial reactions, 51
in irritant CD management, 44
Mouth, 56–7
dental materials, 57, 195
Moxa technique, 303
Musk, *69*, 142, *189*

Nails (i.e. fingernails), 103
artificial acrylic, 250
sources of CD, 48
Nailpolish, 186
facial/eyelid dermatitis, 52, 55
neck dermatitis, 71
Naphthol AS, *63*
Neck
common sources of CD, 48
example reactions, 4, *66*, *70*, 71
non-eczematous CD, 128, *129*
photodermatoses, *136*
topical medications affecting, 160
Neomycin, *59*, *160*, 165, 300
primary sensitization, 34
Neoprene rubber, 212
Nerve stimulation, electrical, *see* Electrical nerve stimulation
Newsprint, 294
Nickel, 192, 193–4, 263–5
dimethylglyoxime test, 194
ears, 58, 192
elbows, 123
graphic arts worker, 291
extremities, 73, *76*, *77*
in amputee prostheses, 180
eyelids, 54
face (spectacle frame), 194
hands/fingers, *92*, *96*, 102, 104, 119, 120, 121, 193, 263, 267
graphic arts worker, 290
hairdressing implements, 275
health care workers, 234, 235
neck, *66*, *129*
shoulder, *68*
systemic CD, 118, 119, 120, 121, 123
trunk, *9*, *67*, 119
typical body distribution, 192
urticarial contact reaction, 118
wristwatch strap, 193
Nipple, jogger's, 130
Nitroglycerin, 185, 301
Non-eczematous CD, 125–34

Non-eczematous dermatoses (non-CD), exclusion in hand dermatitis, 80–7
North American CD Group, additional patch test allergens, 309
Nose, sources of CD, 48
Nostrils, sources of CD, 48
Nummular dermatitis, 88, 90
Nyloprint, 293

Oak moss, 189
Occupational CD, 215–97, *see also specific allergens and irritants*
  factitious, 133, 134
  hands, *see* Hand and finger dermatitis
  prevention, 18
  topography and sensitization source, correlation between, 49
Occupational skin disease, cost, 11
Oedema, angioneurotic, 159
Oil, 94, 132
  heavy, 270
  maleated soya bean, 189
  mineral, 305
Oil-based lubricants, 270
Oil of turpentine, 281, 282, *see also* Colophony
Ointments, steroid-containing, 41–2
Oleoresins, *see* Colophony; Turpentine
1–plus reaction, 30
Onion, 91
Oral cavity, *see* Mouth
Orthodontic braces, 178
Orthopaedic surgeons, 240, 241

Paint
  preservative in, 230
  sprayed, 148
Paint primer, 126
Palmar dermatitis, 97–102
  dorsal and, 102
  systemic, 120, 121
  in weightlifters, 130
Palmar peeling, 86
Palmar psoriasis, 81
  hyperkeratotic dermatitis vs., 82, 100
Palmo-plantar pustulosis, 84
'Pao ferro', 277, 283
Papules
  feet, 112
  fingers, 86
Papulovesicular CD, topical medications, 161, 162, 168
Parabens, 125, 164, 182
  patch test mix, 307
p-methylaminophenol sulphate, 287
Paraphenylenediamine
  in coolant, 269
  hair dye, 50, 51, 190, 273–5
  staining, 33
Paraphenylenediamine-derived compounds (incl. rubber antioxidants), 252, 256
  eyelids, 54
  feet, 109
  hands, 98, 259
Paraphenylenediamine mix (black rubber mix), 74, 180, 229, 252, 256, 257, 258
p-tert-butylphenol-formaldehyde resin, 148, 179, 180
  in leather belt, 211
  leather handbag maker's hands, 247
  in shoes, 110, 211
  shoemaker's hands, 248
Parsley, 140
Parsnip, 140
Patch test, 21–34
  examples, 29–34
    aminoazotoluene, 294
    artefacts, 32, 301
    chromium/chromates, 194, 227
    cobalt, 227
    colophony, 203
    crown-bonding agent, 57
    dyes, 29, 65, 75
    etisazole, 221
    garlic/diallyl disulphide, 206
    geraniol, 74
    Juniperus spp., 202
    Kathon CG, 71
    medications, 161, 162, 165, 169, 171, 177
    Naphthol AS, 63

rubber chemicals, 31, *64*, 74, 252, 256, 261
tosylamide-formaldehyde resin, 52, 71
turpentine components, 281, 282
Standard Patch Test Series
European, 307–8
US, 308–9
systems, 23
TRUE, *see* TRUE test system
technique, 21–3
tixocortol pivalate, 160
Penicillins, semi-synthetic, 235
Pepper, green, 37
Perfumes/scents/fragrances, 185, 186, 188–9
axilla, *69*, 70
connubial CD, 306
extremities, 7, 74
face/neck, 4, 70
hands, *96*
patch test mix, 307
photoallergy, 135, 142, 189
Permanganate bath, 40
Peroneal nerve electrical stimulator, 182
Personal hygiene products, *69–71*
Peru balsam, *see* Balsam
Peruvian lily (*Alstroemeria*), 91, 204, 205, 279
Pesticides, 217, 218, 271
Petrolatum-based allergens, Finn chambers, 27
Pharmaceuticals, *see* Drug therapy; Medications and drugs
Phenol, 6
Phenylbutazone, 167
Phenyl-cyclohexyl paraphenylenediamine, 256
Philodendrons, 201
Photoallergic reactions, 134–43
allergens, 135
fragrance, 135, 142, 189
immunology, 12, 134
Photochemotherapy, 45–6
Photography, 285, 287–8
Phototoxic reactions, 134–43
hyperpigmentation, 127, 141
Phytophotodermatitis, *see* Plants
Pigmentary abnormalities, *see* Hyperpigmentation; Hypopigmentation
Pine, 281, 284, *see also* Colophony; Turpentine
α-Pinene, 282
β-Pinene, 282
Pityriasis amiantacea (tinea aminatacea)-like dermatitis, 50, 191
Pityrosporum ovale, 35, 37
Placebo-controlled oral challenge in systemic CD, 118
Plant(s), 136–41, 196–207, 277–85, *see also* Woods
common allergens, 196, 277
hand/finger(tip) reactions, 91, 141, 203, 204, 205, 206, 278, *279*, 281, 282
photoreactions to (phytophotodermatitis), 135
airborne, 144
examples, 127, 136–41, 144
unique cases, 302, 303
Plantar dermatitis (sole), 112, *see also* Palmo-plantar pustulosis
footwear and, 107
juvenile, 128
Plastic allergen, swim goggles, 55
Plastic spectacle frame dye, 59
Plastizote, 107
Poison ivy, 5, 39, 199
Poison oak, 199
Pollen, prick test, 36
Pompholyx, 99
Potassium dichromate, *see* Chromium/chromates
Potassium permanganate bath, 40
Potatoes, 152
Prednicarbate, 177
Pre-malignant lesion, periungual, 106
Preservatives
cosmetics, 185–6, 186–7
body lotion, 71, 72
hair lotion, 161
medical devices, 182
paint, 230
pharmaceuticals, 164
systemic CD, 125

Prevalence, 11
Prevention of CD, primary and secondary, 18
Prick test, 35–8
  examples, 36–8
    ammonium persulfate, 276
    cactus, 280
    potato, 152
    rubber, 153
  technique, 35
Primer, 126
Primin, 196, 197
Primula, 197, 198, 199, 278
Printed circuit boards, electronic, 246
Printing processes, 285
Procaine, 305
Prognosis
  hand dermatitis, 11
  occupational CD, 11, 216
Prostheses
  amputee, 179–80
  dental, 237–41
  hip, bone cement, 240
Protein CD, 14, 35
  contact urticaria resulting in, 35, 150
  examples, 154, 155
    agriculture, 221, 222
  risk factors, 17
Pruritic dermatitis
  arms, 169
  hands, 99
    construction worker, 229
    dairy farmer, 222
    with nickel, 264, 265
  legs, 63, 78
    with medical devices, 180, 182
  trunk, 61, 63, 169
Psoralens (furocoumarins)
  phototoxic reactions, 127, 135, 141
  UV plus (PUVA therapy), 45–6
Psoriasis, hands, 80–3
  hyperkeratotic palmar dermatitis vs., 82, 100
  irritant CD superimposed on, 95
Pulp of finger, *see* Fingertip/pulp reactions
Purpuric patterns, causes
  clothing, 126
  friction, 131
  sulfanilamide cream, 174
Pustular dermatitic reactions, 10, 34, 301
Pustular psoriasis, 83
Pustulosis, palmo-plantar, 84
PUVA, 45–6

Quaternary ammonium compounds, 191
Quinidine, 301
Quinones in exotic woods, 205

Radiodermatitis, nail region, 105, 106
Reflex erythema, 28
Resins, 242–51, *see also specific types*
Resorcinol monobenzoate, 59
Respiratory allergens, prick tests, 49
Ring dermatitis, 91, 92
Ringworm, *see* Dermatophytes
Risk factors
  allergic CD, 17
  contact urticaria/protein CD, 17
  irritant CD, 14–16
Rivets, metal, 67
Rockwool fibres, 54
Rosewood, 197
Rosin, *see* Colophony
Rowers, mechanical CD
  hand, 130, 131
  rump, 131
Rubber (mainly rubber additives)
  in agriculture, *see* Agriculture
  extremities, 74, 180, 252–62
  eyelids, 54
  face, 256
  feet, 108, 109, 212
  forearms, 261
  hands, 94, 98, 153, 229, 231, 253–5, 257–60
  in medical devices, 180, 181
  patch test, 31, 64, 74, 252, 256, 261
  trunk, 60, 64
  typical distribution, 253
Rubber gloves
  protective, 154, 239
  reactions, 94, 153, 229, 231, 260, 261
    latex, 236, 262

Scaling, 8
Scalp
  hair-care products affecting, 50, 51, 190, 191
  medications applied to
    CD caused by, 158
    CD treatment with, 41
  sources of CD, 48
Scanpor tape, 27
Scents, *see* Perfumes/scents/fragrances
Scratch-chamber test, 35
  positive examples, 37, 38, 152, 155, 221
Sealants, 249
Seborrhoeic dermatitis, 88
Sensitization, *see also* Hypersensitivity
  to haptens, 12, 13
    primary (in patch test), 33, 34, 277
  site of lesions and source of, correlation between, 47–9
Sequelae of CD, 9
Sesquiterpene lactones, 116, 200, 280
Setting lotion, 50, 191
Shampoo, 273
  scented
    face/neck, 4
    hands, 96
Sheath, rubber urinal, 181
Shoes, *see* Footwear
Silica particles, 225
Sinus, 'barber's hair', 272
Site of lesions, 47–114
  airborne dermatitis, 143
  hand dermatitis and concomitant dermatitis in other regions, 88–90
  metal dermatitis, 192, 193
  photoallergic and phototoxic reactions, 135
  sensitization source and, correlation between, 47–9
  systemic CD, 115
  textile dermatitis, 207
  with topical medications, 157
Skin tests, *see* Patch test; Prick test
Soap, hands, 92, 96
Sodium hydroxide, 219
Sole, *see* Plantar dermatitis
Solvents, 299
Sorbic acid, 151
Soya bean oil, maleated, 189
Spanish moss, 203
Spectacle frame
  dye, 59
  nickel, 194
Sport-related mechanical CD, 130–1
Spouse, skin contact, 304–6
Staining of skin with test substances, 33
Stasis dermatitis, reactions to topical medications, 173, 174
Steroids, *see* Corticosteroids
Stethoscope, nickel, 235
Stocking dyes, 75, 111
  patch test, 29, 75
Stomatitis, 56–7
Straw, 218
Strimmer's dermatitis, 141
Subacute CD
  examples, 7
  management, 41–2
Subungual pre-malignant lesion, 106
Sulfanilamide, 162, 168, 174
Sulfuric acid vapour, 149
Sunlight, *see also* Photoallergic reactions; Phototoxic reactions; Ultraviolet light
Sunscreens, 304
  photoallergy, 135, 142
Surfing shoe, 212
Sweating, palmar dermatitis, 97
Swim goggles, 55
Systemic CD, 115–25
  with steroids, 176

T cells, 12, 13
Tea tree oil, 170
TEA-oleylpolypeptide, 161
TENS, 183
p-tert-butylphenol–formaldehyde resin, *see under* Para-
Tetramethylthiuram disulfide, 255
Textiles, *see* Clothing
Theophylline, ethylenediamine sensitivity and, 117
Therapy, 39–46
Thimerosal, 77, 117
Thiourea, 210, 212

Thiuram/thiuram derivatives
  hands and forearms, 234, 254, 255, 261
  lips, 54
  nails, 104
  patch test, 31
  patch test mix, 307
3–plus reaction, 30
  bullous, 31
Tinea, *see* Dermatophytes
Tinea amiantacea-like dermatitis, 50, 191
Tixocortol pivalate, 112, 160
Tobacco powder, factitious dermatitis, 134
Toluene sulphonamide–formaldehyde resin, *see* Tosylamide–formaldehyde resin
Topical medications, 73, 157–77
Torso, *see* Trunk
Tosylamide–formaldehyde (toluene sulphonamide–formaldehyde) resin, 52, 55
  patch test, 52, 71
Toxicodendron radicans (poison ivy), 5, 39, 199
Transcutaneous electrical nerve stimulation, 183
Transdermal patches, 185, 301
Treatment, 39–46
Triamcinolone acetonide, 175
3,4,6–Trichloropyridazine, 33
Trichophyton rubrum, 86, 132
Tricresyl acetate, 59
Triglycidylisocyanurate, 146–7
Triphenyl phosphate, 59
Tromantadine, 56
TRUE test system, 23, 308
  positive reaction example, 25
Trunk/torso, 60–71
  phytophotodermatatis, 136
  sources of CD, 48, 60
    clothing/textiles, 60–5, 210, 211
    topical medications, 166, 167, 169
Tulip, 278
  tulip bulbs, 91, 278
Tulipalin A, 204
Tuliposide, 279
Turpentine, 281, 282, *see also* Colophony
2–plus reaction, 30
Tylosin, 219

Udder cream, 95
Ultraviolet light
  in photoallergic reactions, 134, 140, 142
  psoralen plus (therapeutic use), 45–6
United States Standard Patch Test Series, 308–9
Unna boot, 182
Urinal condom, rubber, 181
Urushiols, 196
Urticaria, contact, 14, 150–5
  agriculture, 221, 222
  anaphylaxis risk, *see* Anaphylaxis
  immunological, 14
    latex, 236, 252, 262
    other causes, 150
  nickel, 118
  non-immunological, 14, 151
    causes, 14, 150
  risk factors, 17
US Standard Patch Test Series, 308–9
Usnic acid, 203
UV, *see* Ultraviolet light

Vaccines, aluminium hydroxide in, 169
Van der Bend chamber, example reaction, 25
Vasculitic allergic CD, sulfanilamide, 174
Vegetation, *see* Plants; Woods
Vehicle ingredients (cosmetics), 189
Vesicles, *see also* Papulovesicular CD
  forearms, 96
  hands/fingers, 4, 96, 99, 119
    in protein CD, 154
    in systemic CD, 120, 121, 124
  in mild to moderate acute allergic CD, 4
  in moderate to severe acute allergic CD, 5
  poison ivy, 5, 199
Veterinary medications, 217, 220, 221
Veterinary practitioner, 221, 222
Vioform, 170
Violaceous erythema, 288

Violin, neck reactions, 129
Virginiamycin, 163
Vitamin E, 126

Washing detergent, *see* Detergent
Watch-strap metal, 193
Weed strimmer's dermatitis, 141
Weightlifter's palmar dermatitis, 130
Welding flux, 111
Wetsuit, 210, 212
Wheat, 152
White dermatographism, 88, 89
Woods, 223, 281–4
  exotic/tropical, 205, 223
Wool socks, 126
Wristwatch strap, nickel, 193

Zippers, 66